THE POLITICS OF HOSPITAL PROVISION IN EARLY TWENTIETH-CENTURY BRITAIN

STUDIES FOR THE SOCIETY FOR THE SOCIAL HISTORY OF MEDICINE

Series Editors: David Cantor
Keir Waddington

TITLES IN THIS SERIES

FORTHCOMING TITLES

THE POLITICS OF HOSPITAL PROVISION IN EARLY TWENTIETH-CENTURY BRITAIN

BY

Barry M. Doyle

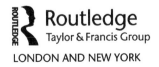

Routledge
Taylor & Francis Group

LONDON AND NEW YORK

First published 2014 by Pickering & Chatto (Publishers) Limited

Published 2016 by Routledge
2 Park Square, Milton Park, Abingdon, Oxfordshire OX14 4RN
711 Third Avenue, New York, NY 10017, USA

First issued in paperback 2015

Routledge is an imprint of the Taylor & Francis Group, an informa business

BRITISH LIBRARY CATALOGUING IN PUBLICATION DATA

Doyle, Barry M. author.
The politics of hospital provision in early twentieth-century Britain. – (Studies
for the Society for the Social History of Medicine)
1. Hospitals – Great Britain – History – 20th century. 2. Hospital care – Political aspects – Great Britain – History – 20th century. 3. Medical policy – Great
Britain – History – 20th century.
I. Title II. Series
362.1'1'0941'09041-dc23

ISBN-13: 978-1-138-66299-5 (pbk)
ISBN-13: 978-1-8489-3433-7 (hbk)

Typeset by Pickering & Chatto (Publishers) Limited

CONTENTS

For Ros, Fergus and Nuala and to the memory of my
Mother and Father, Ramona and Michael.

ACKNOWLEDGEMENTS

This book has its genesis in research I undertook at Teesside University into the politics and finances of the hospitals of Middlesbrough. The success of that work owed much to the support of Professor A. J. Pollard and Dr Richard Lewis, who encouraged me and helped secure funding from South Tees Hospital Trust and the AHRC along with a grant from the Wellcome Trust. When I was looking to extend the research on Middlesbrough I became increasingly interested in the part local party politics might have played in determining the type of hospital service provided. Leeds and Sheffield quickly emerged as the most likely comparators as the first had a peculiarly contested municipal record while the latter was the first major city to return and maintain a Labour administration. The next stage of this project benefitted from a small grant from the Wellcome Trust WT079543, which permitted a three-way comparison of Middlesbrough, Leeds and Sheffield. I was assisted in this part of the project by Robina Weeds and Dr Charlie McGuire at Teesside and Dr Alan Guakroger and Dr Paul Atkinson at the University of Huddersfield. Together they provided me with excellent support, helped to amass a significant body of material and provided me with insight and ideas. Thank you all very much.

I am extremely grateful to the Wellcome Trust who made the writing of this book possible by awarding me a one year Wellcome Trust Research Fellowship WT094109MA. This gave me the academic year 2011–2 free from my role as head of History, English, Languages and Media at the University of Huddersfield and I would like to thank the university for allowing me the opportunity to apply for the leave and Professor Mike Russ, Dean of the School of Music, Humanities and Media, for his support. Also thanks to Professor Paul Ward for covering as head of department and Dr Janette Martin for taking on the role of lecturer to assist Paul. Completing the book was made possible by a sabbatical from the history subject area at Huddersfield and I would like to thank all my colleagues for covering for me, especially to Dr Pat Cullum and Dr Sarah Bastow, the subject leaders who supported the initial application and managed the period of leave.

Writing the book was made easier knowing I had a contract. Professor Keir Waddington, series editor for the Social History of Medicine series, has been incredibly supportive from the beginning to the end of the project. He was understanding, but firm, with deadlines and prompt and helpful with comments. I would also like to thank the two referees whose advice and incisive criticism made this a significantly better book. In addition to Keir and the referees, Paul Atkinson, Paul Ward, Professor Keith Laybourn and Dr Rosemary Wall read parts of the manuscript and provided very helpful advice. Thanks to each of you for your time and support. Numerous colleagues commented on conference and seminar papers which fed into the book, but I would particularly like to thank Professor John Stewart, who encouraged the original idea, and my long suffering friends Graham Ford, Anthony McElligott and David Nash.

Dr Alysa Levene, John Stewart, Professor Martin Powell and Dr Becky Taylor gave me access to their spread sheets of interwar municipal health spending which proved very useful. My research assistants and I received assistance from the staff at the West Yorkshire Archives, Leeds, the Brotherton Library, Leeds, Leeds City Library Local Studies Department, Sheffield City Archives, Sheffield University Archives, the National Archives and Oxford Brookes University Library. Part of Chapter 5 was originally published in a slightly different form as 'Eggs, Rags and Whist Drives: Popular Munificence and the Development of Provincial Medical Voluntarism between the Wars', *Historical Research*, 86:234 (2013), pp. 712–40. I am grateful to Dr Nick Hayes and the editors of *Historical Research* for permission to reproduce the material here.

Finally I would like to thank my family. I had no idea how much of an effort would be required by Ros, Fergus and Nuala when I took on this project. They have given constant, unstinting and loving support and I can't thank them enough. It really would not have been possible without you.

LIST OF TABLES

INTRODUCTION

At the beginning of December 1946 the Sheffield Hospital Contributors' Association met for its one hundredth quarterly meeting. The association invited a number of local dignitaries to the meeting and also the Minster of Health, Aneurin Bevan, MP. Mr Bevan was, unfortunately, unable to attend but wrote urging the contributors to welcome, not fear, the new service. For:

> what is it we are taking away from the Hospitals? – not their independence, not their special characters and their treasured local associations, but only their anxieties – above all, their anxieties about money, and the difficulties that will disappear when each Hospital no longer stands alone. And at last we are to have a Hospital service in the true sense; from our present chaos of 3,000 Hospitals – some of them superlatively good, some by no means faultless, and almost none organically linked with their neighbours – we intend to create a single great service ... they will still be, not 'State' Hospitals, but your Hospitals – it will be your service and for you, with our help, to make of it what you can and will.[1]

In these few lines Bevan encapsulated many of the perceived characteristics of the pre-National Health Service (NHS) hospital system – financial anxiety, individualism and a chaotic lack of organization. Yet he also had to recognize some of its strengths – independence, voluntary effort and a sense of commitment and ownership. Most significant, however, was the importance of place, the rooting of the hospital system in the locality which was embodied in organizations like the Sheffield Hospital Contributors' Association. This book considers how hospital systems developed in a local context in the thirty years before the NHS and explores how the social, economic and political structures and cultures of specific places shaped the development of institutional treatment, especially Bevan's points of anxiety – finance and co-operation.

Viewing the development of hospital systems from the locality is essential to understanding hospitals before Bevan, for even among health historians much of the debate surrounding the strength of pre-NHS hospital provision has been based on national aggregate data, evidence drawn from London, and a patchy understanding of the wider experience of urban hospital systems in this period.[2] Moreover, although there have been some important regional studies,[3] there have been few attempts to compare how hospital services developed in provincial cities or on a regional basis and in particular there has been little discussion of how these were shaped by local economic, social and political cultures.[4] Moreover, the politics of hospital provision remains largely unexplored.[5] For while there has been considerable discussion of debates at a national level involving parties, civil servants and various peak organizations,[6] studies of the factors shaping local decision-making remain rare. This is especially the case in relation to the involvement in, and attitudes of, local Labour parties and labour movements to hospital provision[7] which is often read off from national evidence and studies of bodies like the Socialist Medical Association.[8]

This book addresses these lacunae through an exploration of hospital politics in two Yorkshire cities – Leeds and Sheffield – in the first half of the twentieth century, with a particular focus upon the interwar years when public attitudes to hospitals shifted sharply from distrustful dependence to hopeful expectation of access and cure. This era was marked by the transition in voluntary hospital funding with its associated impact on access and management;[9] by the growth of municipal services, especially in the aftermath of the break-up of the poor law;[10] and by an eagerly anticipated – though not always realized – development of co-ordination and co-operation across the sectors.[11] Moreover, it saw the decline of many of the traditional diseases and threats of urban life and the emergence of new health challenges associated with affluence – including road accidents, cancer and the desire for institutional childbirth – creating a demand for specialist services influenced by local needs and crossing the existing rigid boundaries between voluntary and public hospitals.[12] In exploring the development of local hospital systems, it focuses on the experience of joint working in Leeds and Sheffield demonstrating that developments in this sphere were not linear. Underpinning the study is a recognition of the importance of the economic and social environment of the two cities and how this affected both demand for services and the ability of the locality to provide an adequate, integrated service.[13] Particular attention is paid to the role of class and gender in shaping service provision. Overall, the book argues that social and economic diversity, which influenced both the need for and the ability to provide adequate hospital services, is fundamental to understanding the diversity of provision across the nation in this period.

As this brief overview suggests, over the past twenty years historians have gone some way towards revising our understanding of hospital provision, management and politics in the half century before the inauguration of the NHS. Yet important and influential negative views remain evident. Writing in its official history, Charles Webster drew on Bevan's ideas to suggest that the NHS was 'designed to bring order' to a piecemeal collection of institutions 'deficient in system and planning' for which 'urgently required modernization and improvement was held back by such limitations as anachronism, administrative complexity, duplication, parochialism, inertia and stagnation'.[14] Webster's work has been highly influential in shaping perceptions of interwar health care and the view that hospital access was governed by the elite; that voluntary hospitals were teetering on the verge of bankruptcy; that municipal and poor law hospitals were stigmatizing and inferior; and that the two systems were in constant conflict to the detriment of an effective service for the population. This remains the widely accepted view in general textbooks and popular culture.[15]

However, recent national studies of voluntary hospitals by Gorsky, Mohan and Powell and of municipal provision by Levene, Powell, Stewart and Taylor have challenged some of these assumptions through excellent macro-level statistical analyses and some illuminating case studies of a range of less familiar locations, such as Barnsley and Newport.[16] This work has demonstrated the patchy nature of provision before the Second World War though the source base has provided a rather pessimistic and external reading of the local experience. In many cases the Ministry of Health and other surveyors, such as Political and Economic Planning (PEP) tended to focus on the weaknesses in the system whilst playing down the massive improvements in service over the twenty-five years following the First World War.[17] Pickstone has drawn attention to this tendency for contemporaries and historians to counterpose the general pattern of existing hospital services 'to some ideal distribution of facilities; the difference is said to demonstrate the necessity of reform'.[18] Cherry is more optimistic about the progress of hospital provision and challenges the traditional narratives, with their focus on the big London hospitals and crisis moments like 1922 and 1938.[19] Together this work shows that both voluntary and municipal sectors adapted their funding base and responded to growing demand by expanding beds, buildings and specialisms and in some cases began to work with each other and the central state.[20] However, in general it lacks the richness of the local study and remains sceptical about the ability of either the voluntary or the municipal sector to deal with the challenges of increasing medical sophistication and rising costs. Moreover, it tends to show expansion of provision, rather than explain how it happened or why it might happen differently in different places.

To see how systems operated on the ground we need to turn to the relatively small number of fine local studies which do exist, including Pickstone's pioneering examination of the north-west of England, Rivett's survey of London, Mohan's work on the north-east, and various town studies by Gorsky, Cherry, Reinarz and Hayes.[21] While Pickstone and Mohan do explore the development of both the municipal and the voluntary hospital sector, their material on specific towns is in most cases exemplary rather than detailed, with the former providing good evidence for Manchester and Preston but less on the other towns of Lancashire, while Mohan tends to steer clear of the big cities and focus on the smaller towns. Levene et al. do touch on aspects of the activities of the voluntary sector, as does Welshman, but this is not their key concern, while Reinarz makes no references to local authority provision so that, to date, only Gorsky has attempted a study of both sectors in one town.[22] These, and other specialist works focusing on the general history of hospitals, the growth of provision from place to place and the emergence of specialist services, have provided some insight into how the stock of hospitals expanded and how the work of the institutions became more complex, scientific and expensive.[23] Some have measured the provision of local services against a univeralist norm, but as John Pickstone observes, it was not that places failed to 'conform to some national plan' but rather that localities produced a 'variety of systems, formal and informal' in turn shaped by their political ecology.[24] As Levene et al. have shown for the municipal sector, local needs and resources as well as political cultures could demand that some areas of provision were privileged and others more or less neglected. Although historians of the public sector have observed this decision-making process it has played little or no part in our understanding of the distribution of voluntary general and specialist institutions. Indeed these continue to be viewed in a highly individualistic manner, with an emphasis on the interests of donors or doctors while other structural or political factors are downplayed.[25]

Yet the central contention of this book is that the form of hospital services provided, the way they were paid for and the nature of the politics and governance of that provision were all shaped by local economic and social factors and their impact on class and gender structures and relations. To this end the opening chapter reviews the economic, social and political development of Leeds and Sheffield in the later nineteenth and early twentieth century, paying particular attention to how these shaped, and were shaped by, class and gender relations. In particular, attention is focused on the contrast between the masculine, proletarian society created by Sheffield's heavy industrial economy, with its physical risks and limited employment roles for women, and the more middle-class and 'female' environment deriving from the diverse service and light manufacturing base in Leeds which provided opportunities for women in textiles, clothing and commerce. Together these factors shaped union power, voluntary organizations and local politics producing divergent forms of party competition for municipal control. Both anti-socialist and Labour strategies are addressed with particular attention paid to the way in which economic and social structures influenced the composition, ideology and focus of left and right, shaping the policy priorities and development of services demonstrated by municipal and voluntary providers.

Thus how hospitals came into being, survived and developed is the subject of Chapter 2. Paying particular attention to the growth of sites, buildings and bed numbers in the voluntary, poor law and municipal sectors, it explores the acute and general medical services along with municipal provision for infectious diseases, pulmonary and non-pulmonary tuberculosis. Mental health inpatient services are not included in the study as neither Leeds nor Sheffield county borough had direct responsibility for mental health patients. These were accommodated in asylums managed for the cities and the West Riding County Council by a county board with five institutions across West Yorkshire.[26] It explores the factors influencing the expansion of the hospital estate, including finance, ideology and need and examines the largely overlooked growth of ancillary services, technological developments and administrative facilities between the wars which proved as necessary as extra beds in the campaign to satisfy the demand for mass health care.[27] Chapter 3 assesses the substantial increase in patient numbers which transformed the hospital from a site for the sick poor to a centre for popular health care. The question of who attended hospital has been rather overlooked in the recent debates over finance and specialization with considerable uncertainty remaining around issues of class, age and especially gender. Therefore, this chapter reviews the number and types of patients admitted and where they were admitted to – including inpatient, outpatient and casualty services – examining the role of the almoner, another neglected topic, in gatekeeping access and considering the extent to which patient demographics were shaped by local socio-economic structures.

Building on these findings, Chapter 4 considers the extent to which specialist departments emerged, from traditional specialisms like ear, nose and throat (ENT) and skin complaints to more unusual departments like mental health outpatients. Furthermore, drawing on the ideas of Cooter and Sturdy, it examines the extent to which institutions invested in the organization and management of patients, especially through larger, more complex outpatient departments. These findings are brought together in an investigation of two specific areas where service provision was influenced by local needs and cultures – orthopaedics and the management and healing of accidental bone damage; and the challenge of the growing demand for institutional childbirth. Although the development of these services was part of national trends in the 1930s, they had very different outcomes in Leeds and Sheffield with the prevalence of workplace accidents promoting the creation of specialist orthopaedic services supported by industry and the labour movement in Sheffield, while the extensive maternity provision in Leeds suggests a link with both the more significant role of women in the economy and service provision.

Thus existing local and regional studies provide an essential long-term view of provision in the provinces but they give only a limited picture of how local hospital systems developed and none really address the issue of the politics of local hospital provision. Therefore, the second half of the book focuses on the hospital politics of the two cities, addressing finance, policy and co-operation. Recent research by Cherry, Gorsky and Mohan, Gosling, Reinarz, Daunton,

Hayes and Doyle has pointed to the importance of new forms of funding for both state and voluntary provision in the first half of the century.[28] Building on mutualist models from the late nineteenth century the interwar period saw the flowering of contributory schemes of varying types from works collections and Saturday Funds to full-scale citywide organizations with hundreds of thousands of members.[29] Debate has surrounded whether or not these schemes were sustainable, whether they would have allowed the voluntary sector to continue to expand, whether they were mutualist or 'merely' insurance schemes, and whether they represented a democratic alternative to both elitist voluntarism and state control. Current historiography favours the belief that they were part of a transition from voluntary to state with, as Daunton argues, the population increasingly choosing the certainty and simplicity of the state.[30]

Similarly, as Powell and others have shown, changes in the funding of and to the local state, especially appropriation and the growth of specific central funding for non-acute illness and disease, allowed for the expansion and increased professionalization of the state sector.[31] Municipal provision also moved towards delivering universal services especially for those not always covered by the voluntary sector, such as women and children, the elderly and the terminally ill.[32] However, the extent to which the municipal sector was improving, whether it was or even could compete with the voluntary sector, and the extent to which it was contributing to the development of urban and even regional systems remains uncertain. Recent work has also highlighted the strength of elements of voluntarism throughout the interwar period, especially community based fundraising, endowments, appeals and legacies. These served to strengthen a sense of ownership and democratized investment in, as well as use of, hospitals as community resources.[33]

In light of these historiographical developments, Chapter 5 explores the major forms of hospital finance, paying particular attention to the development of workers' contributions, the changing shape of voluntary income and donations and the growing role of the state both locally and nationally. In particular, it investigates the impact of the differing types of workers' funds – the Leeds Workpeople's Hospital Fund (LWHF) and Sheffield's Penny in the Pound scheme – on the management and administration of the voluntary hospitals and on issues such as access to treatment. It also provides an analysis of the shape of municipal hospital spending and assesses the growing role of patient payments in the ability of both the voluntary and state sectors to meet increased demand. Yet despite an enduring interest in hospital finance, few local studies have addressed the part played by ideology and party in the shaping of services, with a tendency to focus on structural issues rather than party as a determinant of policy choice.[34] Hospital politics have been explored by Stewart in his studies of the Socialist Medical Association and by Willis's work on Sheffield and Bradford whilst Taylor, Stewart and Powell's macro study has touched on the inspectors' views of the influence of local politics in the early 1930s.[35] But in general this is a topic which is largely ignored and is in need of further investigation, not least because the outcomes are indeed complex and the impact of party and ideology is highly variable, strongly influenced by local economic and social factors.

Chapter 6 highlights the role of party, the labour movement and the traditional elite – as well as the medical profession and academics – in the nature and extent of hospital provision and explores the management of poor law and municipal hospital services, both at the political level of council committees and their membership and within the services, considering the role of the medical officers of health, medical superintendents and consultants from both sectors. It shows that local political cultures and the ideologies they created strongly influenced services. In particular it examines the way the labour movement debated the appropriate role of the state and the voluntary providers, questioning the degree to which labour opposed the voluntary approach and traditional elites limited the development of the state sector. The distinctive hospital politics of Leeds and Sheffield are highlighted and the underlying reasons for these differing approaches is assessed with particular emphasis on the form of the local labour movement, the importance and nature of mutualist structures and the size and strength of the traditional elite.

The central element of the critique of interwar hospitals was their failure to co-operate in the development of a rational system – although there is a tendency to assert rather than prove that relations between and within the sectors remained poor throughout the period. Manchester, Birmingham, Oxford, Bristol and Liverpool are usually highlighted as areas with good levels of co-operation, but these are frequently presented as exceptions.[36] Certainly there is much evidence of limited development such as Mohan's study of Durham and Northumberland which offers a very pessimistic view based on the survey reports of 1930–4, as does Levene et al.'s examination of West Hartlepool, but a number of other towns show gradual collaboration, including Barnsley, Middlesbrough and Aberdeen, where the Medical Officer of Health (MOH) was instrumental in negotiating integration; Newcastle, where collaboration was clearly quite advanced; and Leicester, where joint working was also progressing.[37] Moreover, Gorsky has shown the importance of medical schools in both Aberdeen and Bristol in bringing the disparate elements together, as has Pickstone in his study of Manchester. On the other hand, less has been written about individuals involved in the hospital management or doctors, including consultants and medical superintendents.[38]

Drawing together these elements, the final chapter examines the extent to which these cities were able to develop a hospital system in the fifty years prior to the establishment of the NHS. It considers the growth of integrated working within the voluntary sector and the local state's efforts to join up the elements of council and poor law provision after 1929. It then explores the ways in which state and voluntary hospitals competed and co-operated, looking especially at the role of the workers' funds and medical schools in promoting joint working and the sharing of resources. Moreover, as much co-operation took place at an operational level it will investigate the role of medical, administrative and social and political actors in facilitating or blocking integration. Finally, the chapter assesses the growing pressure for a regional approach to hospital services and the role this played in promoting or limiting joint working.

Overall, this revisionist literature has provided a new framework for assessing the hospital sector in the first half of the twentieth century which acknowledges growth in capacity, capability and specialization, increased financial resources and the suggestion of a nascent cross-sector system at least in some urban areas. However, conclusions on each of these areas remain tentative whilst the place of politics, especially the role of traditional elites and the labour movement, remain under-researched. In order to address some of these issues this study will deploy a comparative case study approach to explore how hospital systems developed and whether they developed to meet the needs of their localities. By comparing two similarly sized industrial cities, it will examine how systems grew from local demand, local resources and how they met – or did not meet – the challenges they faced. To achieve this it will make use of Pickstone's concept of 'political ecology' which encompasses the 'complex interrelations between the hospitals and the communities they were built to serve'. In particular, it will follow the way he 'tried to show how the formal and informal structures of hospitals and similar institutions were related to the economic, social and political structures of the cities or towns or villages which created them'. In his survey of hospital provision in the Manchester region Pickstone noted that 'towns which to a dis-tant observer might seem similar, in fact showed remarkably different patterns of medical services – differences which can be explained by, or at least linked to, these different political structures'.[39] This holistic urban history approach has not been widely adopted by hospital historians in the ensuing twenty-five years. It does inform Welshman's work on Leicester, but was not deployed by Mohan or Gorsky, or Cherry for his East Anglian study.[40] This study employs it to com-pare two Yorkshire cities to investigate a wider range of stakeholders and policy formers and attempt a broader analysis of the economic, social and cultural backgrounds than Pickstone was able to achieve in a regional study.

To this end the book utilizes case studies of Leeds and Sheffield, cities which were chosen because, while physically close and on the surface quite similar, being industrial cities in northern England with populations of around half a million, they actually differ quite significantly in their economic and social make-up, their regional role and their local politics. For these reasons they offer fertile ground to explore five key issues: what hospital services were available in the cities and how did these grow and change over the period of study; in what ways did local cultures impact upon the approach to specific medical concerns of the interwar period such as maternity and orthopaedic services; how were these services funded both by the local and central state and by the voluntary sector; what were the key political factors determining the operation of hospital services, especially the role of the labour movement, the traditional elite, medical professionals and institutions like medical schools and the city health department; and to what extent had a unified hospital system emerged by the 1940s.

In addressing these issues particular attention has been paid to the economic, social and political development of the towns.[41] Little research has been undertaken on their medical services. Sheffield has received attention from Tim Willis and Steve Cherry[42] as well as from a number of traditional medical historians.[43] Leeds is less well served, relying heavily on the largely antiquarian work of Stephen Anning.[44] Given their centrality and their significant place in the regional hierarchy of the NHS, the neglect of their hospital systems seems strange and in need of revision. The choice of Leeds and Sheffield as case studies is based largely on their political make-up, their economic structure, regional position and the fact that they had important medical infrastructure, including large general hospitals, extensive municipal services and medical schools. Politically Leeds proved to be one of the most polarized and complex cities of the interwar period with control of the council see-sawing between Labour and a dominant Conservative party, while Sheffield was the first major provincial city to fall to Labour (in 1926) and the party dominated for the rest of the interwar period.[45] How these political landscapes and the social and economic structures which created them affected hospital policy, practice and provision is a key focus of this book.

Overall the book contends that the heavy industrial nature of the economy of Sheffield, with its relatively small middle class and heavily unionized male workforce, created both different medical needs and labour movements to those in Leeds, with its more diverse economy, large female workforce and old middle class. This diversity was underpinned by different forms of hospital funding – contributory schemes or mutualist collection funds – and political responses to the local working arrangements. However, it shows that co-operation and co-ordination were neither linear and consistent, nor always at their most fruitful, in organized committees. In particular it challenges the accepted view of Sheffield as possessing a highly sophisticated integrated service while revealing productive relations between voluntary and municipal sectors behind the political posturing in Leeds. Thus, while these towns were moving at different speeds towards a hospital system, each moved a long way towards unified working over twenty-five years, underlining Pickstone's view that close attention to the local reveals how 'these different arrangements illustrate the range of potential systems of which the NHS was but one'.[46]

1 LEEDS AND SHEFFIELD: ECONOMIC, SOCIAL AND POLITICAL CHANGE

General histories of hospital services in the first half of the twentieth century often highlight the variability in provision between towns, pointing to the serendipitous and illogical foundations of voluntary hospitals and the restrictions imposed by finance and political preference on local authorities.[1] Yet this, as Pickstone has noted,[2] under-estimates the fact that local need shaped by economic, social and political structures was often the vital component in determining hospital services in the fifty years before the NHS. Admittedly, a number of studies have demonstrated the importance of local financial resources and political cultures on the form services took but these rarely consider how socio-economic structures may have created specific needs resulting in unique patterns of provision. Thus, to understand fully the influences on hospital services, finance and management regimes in Leeds and Sheffield, it is necessary to explore their changing urban ecology.[3] In particular, we need to explore how the fate of both the individual hospitals and the broader citywide provision were determined by longer-term developments in economic specialization, class structure, the role of gender in the workforce and the scale and nature of trade unionism along with shorter-term factors such as the impact of unemployment and the outcome of municipal elections. This chapter will show that the relative strength of the middle class in Leeds and the working class in Sheffield along with the markedly different role of gender in the two labour markets played a central part in shaping the form, function and finance of their hospital services.

Leeds and Sheffield are industrial cities in the West Riding of the county of Yorkshire, with Leeds situated on the River Aire, at the heart of the county, while Sheffield is in the far south adjoining Derbyshire and Nottinghamshire. Leeds was well placed to act as a focal point for the adjacent woollen towns, had strong east–west transport links by water, rail and road and was favourably positioned for expansion. Sheffield, however, is tucked in a bowl of hills, with poor communications in any direction (except by water) and with few close neighbours except the town of Rotherham. Despite these different geographical features, both cities played a major part in England's economic development and were significant population centres by the late eighteenth century. As Table 1.1 shows, during the nineteenth century they rose to prominence, and by the turn of the twentieth century ranked as the fourth and fifth provincial cities in England. A marked spurt in the second quarter of the nineteenth century saw Leeds' population more than treble between 1801 and 1851, but growth then slowed with a quarter of a million inhabitants added in the second half of the century, giving an overall eightfold rise for the century. The experience in Sheffield was similar, with almost 200 per cent growth in the later nineteenth century while a combination of in-migration and a healthy birth rate saw it pass Leeds by the First World War. The interwar period saw only marginal expansion in either city, most of it as a result of boundary changes.[4]

Table 1.1: Population growth, Leeds and Sheffield, 1801–1931

	Leeds	Sheffield
1801	52,276	45,755
1851	172,270	135,310
1901	428,968	380,793
1911	445,550	454,632
1921	458,232	490,639
1931	482,809	511,757

Source: Morgan, 'Demographic Change', p. 48; Crook, 'Population', pp. 482–3.

Initial growth occurred in the urban core and the immediate fringes as courts and yards were filled in and vast estates of back-to-back houses were constructed. In the second half of the nineteenth century population growth shifted to the suburbs creating distinctive and lasting social segregation in both cities. In the Leeds parish of Headingley-cum-Burley the number of inhabitants increased sevenfold in the second half of the century, creating a dense middle-class enclave. South of the river, working-class Hunslet and Holbeck were joined by Armley and Bramley while Potternewton in the north-east, the focus of the developing tailoring trades and of Jewish immigration, saw the number of inhabitants increase eightfold between 1881 and 1914. Conversely, from 1891 the population of the city centre and some of the inner suburbs south of the river began to decline. Thus, the third quarter of the century was characterized by the development of heavy industry south of the river, the late Victorian and Edwardian period saw the emergence of the north-east as a centre of light manufacturing matched by the growth of middle-class Headingley.[5] In Sheffield, however, topography constrained urban development. The traditional industries of crucible steel and cutlery (the light trades) were concentrated in the city centre and inner suburbs hemmed in by hills. The area to the west and south-west became the focus for middle-class suburbs while only the Don valley to the north-east proved favourable to the large-scale development of the heavy trades of specialist steels and armaments. This led to the rapid expansion of housing in the Brightside Bierlow and Attercliffe registration district where the population rose from 38,000 to 125,000 between 1861 and 1901.[6] Only after 1900 did the city begin to fill in to the south-east and north-west with both private speculators and the local authority contributing equally to a 50 per cent increase in the number of homes in the city.[7]

As with most rapidly developing industrial cities of the nineteenth century, house building was characterized by a period of in-filling in the city centre, then by the development of working class suburbs of cheap, often back-to-back, housing. As a legacy of this, interwar Leeds still had 13,000 back-to-back properties and there was a greater proportion of the population living in just three rooms than the average for county boroughs.[8] The situation was similar in Sheffield, where poor housing and rapid population growth were exacerbated by the hilly terrain. Such conditions were conducive to the spread of infectious diseases, especially tuberculosis (TB), and were amplified by inadequate sanitation. In Sheffield, the dominant form of excrement removal was the privy and the ash-pit while in Leeds these were supplemented by the trough water closet, which proved unsuitable for domestic use. These systems attracted flies and probably accounted for much of the infantile diarrhoea endemic in both cities until the full adoption of water closets in the 1930s. The mixing of residential and industrial properties, especially in the city centres and inner suburbs, exposed much of the population to very high levels of air pollution described, in the case of Sheffield, by the Ministry of Health inspector Donelan as 'a vast expanse of murky haze overlying the city like a pall'.[9] Although industrial change eased the situation for northern Leeds, south of the river in Holbeck and Hunslet, air pollution was a significant problem which concerned the Medical Officer of Health (MOH) throughout his thirty years in office. A range of witting and unwitting developments reduced the health risks of the urban environment; in addition to water closets, slum clearance, bigger houses and more conscious urban zoning, the replacement of the horse by the motor car helped to reduce the fly population, diminishing the transmission of enteritis.[10] But these changes could also bring new problems. The motor car produced shocking levels of road accident victims, while relocation to new suburban housing brought significant increases in costs leading to short-term reductions in living standards as well as separating populations from many of the health-care services which remained in the city centres.

Sheffield: Economic Developments

Sheffield had a narrow economic base with a social structure more like a single industry town than a complex central place. The professional, commercial and transport sectors of the population were small while the metalworking staple industries dominated the working population.[11] These staple industries were formed around five interlocking sectors – crucible and specialist steel production; cutlery and edged implements; armaments and heavy steel; toolmaking; and engineering. Initial industrial strength was based on crucible steel and cutlery, small-scale handcraft processes in which human skill and strength predominated. Crucible steel was a high-value product manufactured in relatively small quantities, often to order. Cutlery was even more small scale and flexible, run by 'little mesters', the vast majority of whom employed fewer than fifty workers and many less than five. By the later nineteenth century much of the industry relied on outworkers and had acquired the characteristics of a sweated trade, employing mainly older males, younger females and youths.[12] Moreover, although public demand for cutlery and the other domestic output of the Sheffield light trades was growing between the wars, expansion was in cheap, mass-produced goods rather than the high-value specialist products of the city.[13]

Sheffield's third area of production was specialist steels, especially alloy steels for the tool industry, and stainless steel. Despite retaining a world leading position in this sector between the wars it was a relatively small part of the economy in employment terms, insufficient to compensate for the jobs lost in cutlery and armaments. Companies like Vickers and John Brown emerged as the nation's leading armour and munitions producers, and employment numbers in the heavy trades passed those in the traditional sector, reaching 70,000 by the end of the Great War. Such numbers were unsustainable, falling to just 47,000 by 1931.[14] Unemployment in this sector was particularly severe as this was relatively unskilled work and those laid off had few alternatives to the dole. However, from 1935 tariffs, rationalization and rearmament helped the industry to emerge from depression[15] while recovery was accelerated by the Second World War which gave a huge boost to the local economy.[16] The experience of the heavy trades was mirrored in engineering. Although some parts, like high-speed tools, held up, those supplying the mining industry, transport and heavy engineering suffered badly. Thus, the high levels of interconnectedness within the local economy which linked light and heavy trades with steelmaking and engineering created a vicious downward cycle resulting in fifteen years of depression in the local economy and a significant impact on hospital services in the city.[17]

Thus, from 1920 the structural unemployment that would dog the city first became apparent with a sharp rise to 49,500 unemployed in 1921 (32.5 per cent of registered workers), further problems during the strike year of 1926[18] and becoming most severe during the great depression when it peaked at 60,000 unemployed in 1932 (over one-third of the registered workers). Even in more prosperous times there was a hard core of around 25,000 (15 per cent) constantly out of work. Specific trades were hit particularly hard. At the bottom of the slump, more than half of ironworkers and steelworkers were unemployed, along with 42 per cent in cutlery and around one-third in engineering. Yet for those in work, conditions were generally good and wages could be high in engineering and the heavy trades.[19] Beyond the metal trades, although mining was also badly hit there is evidence to suggest a growth in non-manual labour with the number of men employed in commerce and finance increasing by more than 50 per cent. As in the First World War – although in a slightly more managed and directed way – the Second World War brought full employment back to the city, providing an element of stability and prosperity which had been missing for almost twenty years.

These economic conditions had significant health effects. Work in steel, armaments and mining was characterized by accidents and injuries along with specific conditions such as 'grinder's lung' and rheumatism.[20] As a result, health services in the city targeted the treatment of such conditions, especially fractures, adult orthopaedics and physiotherapy, for long-term damage.[21] The city also experienced damaging levels of air pollution; around 380 tons of soot a year fell on Sheffield city centre in the early 1930s and probably more in periods of full industrial production. Such levels were known to have an impact on respiratory diseases, and this is evident in the 1920s, though the situation was less severe than that recorded in Middlesbrough.[22] More ambiguous were the health effects of long-term unemployment and poverty. Tania McIntosh has shown that some workers in the city experienced long-term worklessness lasting up to three years, but historians remain divided on the effect of such conditions on morbidity and mortality. Pessimists like Webster, Mitchell and Laybourn have argued strongly for adverse health outcomes while more optimistic analyses have been provided by Winter and McIntosh.[23] These factors will be explored further below.

Class, Gender and the Labour Market

Sheffield had an unusual social structure for a city of its size. There were few commercial or administrative functions[24] while the business class was also atypical. The persistence of little mesters in the light trades meant most firms were small[25] and even in iron and steel the majority of all firms were of limited size: just twenty firms employing more than two hundred workers and only a dozen more than a thousand.[26] As such there were few great fortunes made in the city and only a small group of comfortably off businessmen who were brought together in the Master Cutler's Company.[27] Rather, Sheffield should be characterized as a proletarian city. It was also a very masculine place, as steelmaking and heavy engineering was physically demanding work that encouraged a culture of manliness while providing few opportunities for women's work. Early marriage and relatively large families were the norm until the First World War while McIntosh estimates that only 10 per cent of married women worked outside the home.[28] Admittedly, opportunities for female employment did increase between the wars, particularly in shops, offices and distribution, where the numbers employed grew by 25 per cent, but this did little to change the overall gender divisions within the labour market.[29]

Yet despite the predominance of male metalworkers the labour movement was not homogenous or particularly united. The unions in the light trades retained close links to the Liberal party[30] but the emergence of socialist organizations in the heavy trades created divisions which led to the formation of two umbrella organizations: the Sheffield Federated Trades Council (SFTC), based largely on the light trades and sceptical about the new Labour Representation Committee (LRC), and the Sheffield Trades and Labour Council (STLC), a socialist body which drew its membership from the heavy trades and dominated the LRC.[31] However, the war and the major strides made by labour generally saw the two organizations unite in 1920 and for much of the interwar period the Trades Council was in the hands of moderates promoting broadly labourist policies. The STLC's broad basis meant it was accepted as the voice of labour in developing corporatist responses to the crises experienced by the city – including that affecting the hospitals. Indeed, the dominance of a small group of steel magnates in philanthropy and metalworking unions in the labour movement meant that hospitals concentrated on the health concerns of the adult male workforce first and foremost while their prominent position in hospital governance left few spaces for women to play an active role. This intersection became most obvious in the response to the post-war financial crisis at the voluntary hospitals which saw the foundation of the Penny in the Pound workers' contributory scheme. This highly successful initiative, which was raising £250,000 by the later 1930s, brought together unions and employers to ensure free hospital treatment for male workers and their families and pioneered a corporatist approach to hospital finance which was eventually employed for capital as well as treatment costs.[32]

Health

Given the high and persistent levels of unemployment and poverty in interwar Sheffield, one might expect to see poor health indicators, yet this was not entirely the case. Despite a historiographical tendency to emphasize a close link between the depression and poor health in 'the north' – for example by Webster and Mitchell – Sheffield does not support such an interpretation.[33] From 1921 the Sheffield crude death rate began to track the national rate, sitting a little below it for most of the 1920s and drifting a little above it from the mid-1930s. The rate did spike due to outbreaks of smallpox and influenza in the 1920s and it also crept up between 1930 and 1933 but this was in line with the national trend.[34] Yet overall rates were stable across the period and not notably affected by the prevailing economic conditions. This is borne out by infant and maternal mortality patterns. In the former case the rate fell slowly during the 1920s, but the decline was marked in the 1930s and fell to below the national average. Indeed the biggest drop was recorded in the depression years of 1929–34, the infant mortality rate (IMR) first falling below the national average in 1933. McIntosh points to the successful clearance of all of the city's privies and ash pits which reduced the number of flies, as well as to factors such as slum clearance and rehousing on the new estates, and improved general nutrition for most. Furthermore, the MOH claimed some credit when he suggested falls in mortality and morbidity were 'a direct result of their labours in the gradual removing of insanitary conditions and the improvement of the environment'.[35] It is likely that municipal maternity and child welfare provision also contributed to the decline, especially the work of the large team of health visitors.[36] Even in that most stubborn of interwar death rates – maternal mortality – significant strides were made. The rate of four and five per thousand was a little above the national average for most of the 1920s, with particular problems at the Jessop Hospital for Women, where puerperal sepsis reached near epidemic proportions in 1926.[37] Yet by 1939 Sheffield rates were below the national average of 2.97 and though this owed something to sulphonamides, rates had been falling since the early part of the decade due to a sepsis isolation unit at the Jessop, the professionalization of domiciliary midwifery and overall improvements in domestic conditions. By the mid-1930s the MOH was of the opinion that most cases of maternal mortality were the results of attempted abortions rather than poor conditions or inadequate medical interventions.[38] Yet unlike the situation in Leeds or in some other large cities like Manchester, the council delivered most maternity and child welfare services, eschewing the mixed economy approach.[39] The Edwardian period had seen the foundation of a voluntary Motherhood League concerned mainly with the dissemination of information to mothers but this was wound up in 1919 and its functions taken over by the Health Department.[40]

Table 1.2: Annual crude birth and death rates and infant mortality (deaths per thousand births) in Leeds, Sheffield and England and Wales, 1920–39

	Birth rate			Death rate			Infant mortality		
	Sheffield	Leeds	E & W	Sheffield	Leeds	E & W	Sheffield	Leeds	E & W
1920–4	21.8	20.6	21.4	12.1	13.8	12.2	93	101.2	76.8
1925–9	16.6	16.4	17.2	12.0	13.6	12.2	83.2	88.2	70.8
1930–4	14.6	14.7	15.3	11.5	13.1	12.0	65.4	76.8	62.8
1935–9	15.3	14.8	14.9	12.0	13.3	12.0	52.8	63.4	55.4

Source: MOH Leeds, *Annual Reports*, 1920–39; MOH Sheffield, *Annual Reports*, 1920–39.

Furthermore, by the end of the 1930s, the city could boast some of the lowest attack and death rates in the country for the old killer diseases. In line with other large cities, it was free of smallpox for most of the interwar period – experiencing just one major outbreak in 1926–7 – and had also triumphed over typhoid. By

1938 Sheffield had the lowest rates of the northern industrial cities for the four main infectious diseases affecting children – measles, scarlet fever, diphtheria and whooping cough – with measles and whooping cough declining as killers at around the national rate in part due to a policy of hospitalizing the more serious cases. However, scarlet fever and diphtheria, which reduced in frequency and virulence during the first half of the 1920s, were epidemic between 1927 and 1937. Outbreaks of scarlet fever were recorded between 1927 and 1930 and again from 1934 to 1936, though in the latter case deaths were low. The diphtheria epidemic of 1934–7 was serious, however, with all cases hospitalized and deaths peaking at 70 from around 2,000 affected people in 1935. Yet both diseases were under control by the outbreak of the Second World War, with rates at or below the national average.

These falls in the classic infectious diseases mirrored a national trend, but more impressive, given the notable levels of air pollution in the city, was the triumph over the killer respiratory diseases of influenza, bronchitis and pneumonia. Other steel towns like Middlesbrough and its north-eastern neighbours recorded exceptional levels of mortality from these diseases in the early twentieth century.[41] Figures had been high in Sheffield, with over 2,000 deaths per annum from non-tubercular respiratory diseases before 1914, while the city seems to have suffered more heavily than Leeds during the influenza pandemic of 1918–19. However, both the incidence of and mortality from these diseases fell notably, especially from the later 1920s, with deaths from bronchitis dropping from 700 in 1919 to 131 in 1939, those from pneumonia halving in the same period and influenza fatalities declining to a rate significantly below the national average. Although smog could still be a cause of ill health – the MOH noting that an increase in mortality in 1926 was 'very largely attributable to atmospheric conditions which were marked almost throughout the year by excessive humidity and an abnormally small amount of sunshine'[42] – the general improvement probably owed much to the control of atmospheric pollution. In particular, the city was amongst the first to act on the Public Health (Smoke Abatement) Act of 1926 when the Sheffield and Rotherham Joint Smoke Abatement Committee was formed in April 1927. This body claimed good relations with the business community and sought their support to ensure the 'protection of the public from the noxious effects of industrial smoke' for without their 'cordial co-operation all legislation and all the efforts of Local Authorities are stultified'.[43]

This success with general respiratory diseases was matched by an effective pulmonary TB strategy which recorded a sustained fall in mortality from as early as 1919. However, although Sheffield had generally low levels of respiratory TB, this did not apply to workers in the cutlery industry, especially the grinders. Even in the early 1910s, over half the deaths among those described as grinders were caused by pulmonary TB, compared to one-eighth for the general adult population. The proportion remained high until the 1930s and, while only 2 per cent of the population, grinders still accounted for 8 per cent of TB deaths in the 1930s. Overall Sheffield had one of the lowest respiratory TB death rates of the big cities, matching that for England and Wales from around 1925 – yet it continued to have one of the highest notification and treatment rates for the disease, mainly amongst schoolchildren.[44]

In addition to 'grinders' lung', heavy industry and mining posed significant threats to the bodies of the workers. Accidents, especially broken bones, crushing and foreign bodies in the eye were common,[45] the Royal Infirmary noting:

> Although the greater frequency of accidents must be regretted, the Board hold the view that the increase shown in the above figures is due, in the main, to the larger number of works accidents which have occurred following upon the trade revival which the city has enjoyed during 1936.[46]

Accidents prompted a significant interest amongst the medical profession and charitable institutions in developing orthopaedic services and the care and rehabilitation of injuries while the prevalence of rheumatism amongst steelworkers led to the development of some specialist services. Conversely, the relatively limited role for women in the workforce meant their health needs were overlooked with maternity provision, both voluntary and municipal, particularly poor for much of the early twentieth century.[47] This weakness notwithstanding, Sheffield was clearly benefitting from the general improvements in health apparent nationwide. A different 'cause of death' profile was emerging that saw infectious diseases replaced by coronary and circulatory diseases while the number of deaths from cancer almost doubled. Moreover, there was a marked change in age at death with less than 10 per cent of deaths under the age of five years and over 40 per cent aged sixty-five and over, leading the MOH to comment in 1928 that 'we have now a population of considerably greater average age than we had in the past'.[48]

The ability to deal with this changing health environment was aided by the development in both Sheffield and Leeds of university medical schools. The Sheffield school – launched in the 1820s – was closely involved in the formation of the University of Sheffield and when that institution received its charter in 1905 the medical school was accommodated in buildings at Western Bank close to three of the four voluntary hospitals. The clinical and university teaching were united in a single faculty before the First World War, creating the influential Staff Club, while the work of Sturdy has shown that the school and the university derived much of its income and status from serving the community, especially in the case of the pathology and bacteriology departments. This underpinned the development of a strong research culture amongst the physicians which saw important breakthroughs in the understanding and utilization of nutrition, insulin and penicillin.[49] The medical faculty was important in urging the creation of a new funding regime for the voluntary hospitals after the First World War based on a centralized workers' fund, while their role in promoting the merger of the city's two voluntary general hospitals in 1939 and the building of a new super-hospital adjacent to the medical school proved significant.[50] However, they were less engaged with the municipal hospitals and did little to involve the municipal doctors in teaching beyond the minimal role of public health specialists. The 1945 surveyors found relations between the university and the public hospitals to be poor, the report commenting on the lack of teaching even in maternity wards.[51]

Politics and Political Cultures

Until 1948, local authorities remained the primary vehicle for the initiation and delivery of public services, with political and financial responsibility increasingly consolidated in the hands of the large, single-purpose county boroughs with party politics dominating their annual round of elections.[52] Although historians remain divided on the extent to which party and ideology shaped service delivery it is clear politicians responding to local conditions, needs and ideals determined the form and scale of provision.[53] Sheffield was made a county borough (along with Leeds) in 1888, giving it control over a very wide range of services including general public health and infectious disease control. The late Victorian authority municipalized water, electricity and trams while in the early twentieth century it was one of the first to undertake housing projects under the 1890 Housing of the Working Classes Act. Relief was administered by two Poor Law Unions, Sheffield and Ecclesall, each of which had a workhouse with separate infirmary accommodation at Fir Vale (Sheffield Union) on the northern edge of the city and at Nether Edge (Ecclesall) to the south-west. The unions were merged in 1925[54] while the responsibilities of the poor law were taken over by the council in 1929, including the hospital provision which was 'appropriated'.[55]

Municipal affairs in Sheffield saw the Conservatives dominate the council in the late nineteenth century and the Liberals in charge for much of the Edwardian era. The Conservatives attracted support from a broad range of electors and were the favoured party of the metal trades' employers by the Edwardian period.[56] There was a strong Lib/Lab tradition in the city focused on the independent cutlery workers which weakened the socialists and prevented a Labour breakthrough before the First World War. Indeed both the socialists and the Lib/Lab contingent had been marginalized on the council in part due to a covert anti-socialist alliance between the Liberals and Conservatives which minimized three-way contests.[57] Given the Labour party's poor performance and the movement's organizational and ideological divisions in the Edwardian era, its rapid rise to council dominance by 1926 is surprising. This owed something to leaders like steelworker Moses Humberstone (from the SFTC) and E. G. Rowlinson, the railwayman who led the Labour group, emphasizing practical issues over ideology aiming at efficient municipal socialism with an emphasis on health, housing and education. With a tripling of Labour seats on the council from 13 to 38 between 1919 and 1926, the party gained an outright majority which they held with just one year's break until the Second World War.

Labour success in 1926 owed something to fallout from the General Strike and coal strike, the improvements in Labour fortunes seen nationally and a number of local factors. Central among these was the perceived financial mismanagement by the Citizens' Alliance (CA), which had been formed by the Liberal and Conservative parties prior to the 1921 council elections.[58] Socialists pointed to the use of utility profits and borrowing to reduce rates while CA abolition of tenant compounding saw rate arrears rise. They were also accused of poor service delivery, including inadequate school accommodation on the new council estates and a limited housing policy which saw around 5,000 houses built (though this was at or above the national average for council completions).[59] Once in control, Labour remained the dominant party until 1932 when, in keeping with most Labour councils in Yorkshire, it was ejected.[60] However, this was short-lived and Labour returned to office the following year. The Progressives (as the Citizens' Alliance was now known) were unable to consolidate their weak grip on the inner-city wards while the memory of Macdonald's government began to recede and the means test was now the responsibility of a Progressive administration.[61]

Labour in Power

Sheffield Labour's first term of office was characterized by moderate reforms designed to make council services more efficient and democratic. This included financial reforms to provide a stable base for their service provision; the institution of a Direct Labour Organisation (DLO) which would be used for all council building; and an enlightened policy on poor relief and the subsequent transitional payments. On the other hand, their house-building programme was cautious, completions only passing the CA administration in 1932, while in some areas of health policy, like slum clearance and maternity and child welfare, the record was limited. It was only with appropriation of the hospitals that a more radical policy was adopted and even here the early development of the service was complementary to the work of the voluntary sector.[62]

Following their return to power in 1933, Labour became more ambitious, extending the role and power of the local authority. They instituted a rigorous slum clearance policy, constructing some 13,000 new homes in the later 1930s at completion rates considerably above the national average.[63] Expansion was also

seen in parks and gardens, in streets and sewers and in attempts at town planning. Social services were overhauled, moving away from the poor law principles
to the care of the elderly, sick and infirm. Moreover, health policy was radicalized
as plans were laid for major expansions of both traditional services like TB and
modern general hospital provision.[64] In most of this work the council backed
off from too close a relationship with the voluntary sector and the trend was
away from a mixed economy and towards full local state services. Thus, although
some joint health services remained, such as the Tuberculosis Dispensary and
the venereal disease clinics in the voluntary hospitals, in areas like maternity and
child welfare, no role was found for the charitable sector, with services focused
on the council-run central clinic. Here Labour was building on a traditional
arms-length approach to the voluntary sector shaped by both politicians and the
Health Department. However, in hospital services this policy was less apparent,
at least until the later 1930s, and how the public/voluntary mix developed over
this period will be a central concern of this book.

Leeds: Economic Developments

In marked contrast to Sheffield, the economic structure of Leeds was complex
and diverse – at one time the city being known as the place that made everything.
A manufacturing, commercial and transport centre, it dominated the West Riding textile district. Unlike the constricted physical location of Sheffield, Leeds
benefitted from a wide range of geographical advantages. It was

> [c]lose to valuable beds of limestone, an open valley, a navigable river, canals ... com-
> municating with the Mersey at Liverpool, the Ouse at Goole and ... the Humber ...
> and railways branching off in every direction ... These advantages give every possible
> facility for bringing raw materials, sending away manufactured goods, and for the
> access of men of business.[65]

To these natural benefits historians have added an adaptable business class and
an ability to attract migrant labour. Moreover, unlike Sheffield, which sat on the
boundary between three counties with competing interests and cultures, Leeds
was the dominant city and administrative capital of the West Riding. As a result,
many county-wide organizations were established in the city, including the voluntary hospitals, while the borough council developed good relationships with
most of the neighbouring authorities.

Leeds played a leading role in the development of the West Riding textile
industry, pioneering large-scale factory organization and acquiring a commercial
centre of markets, exchanges and banks.[66] From the mid-nineteenth century the
economy began to diversify in a virtuous cycle of interlinking developments led
by the growth of a wide-ranging engineering sector. Mainly concentrated along
the River Aire to the west of the city there were more than fifty branches of

engineering undertaken in the city employing 33,000 men in 1911 – one in five of the male workforce.[67] Its diversity and flexibility made it less susceptible to a general depression, though it was evidencing vulnerability by the Edwardian period with its continued dependence on iron rather than steel and on machines and mechanical engineering over tools or electrical products.[68] The late nineteenth century also saw the rapid growth of men's ready-to-wear clothing, based on the application of locally developed technology, particularly John Barran's bandsaw, which was capable of cutting up to one hundred pieces of cloth at once.[69] This, and the sewing machine, facilitated the mass production of suits, increasingly marketed by the producers in their own retail outlets. Pioneered by Hepworth, these shops introduced the bespoke ready-to-wear suit perfected by Montague Burton in the interwar period.[70] The majority of employees in this sector were women – 24,500 by 1921 rising to 31,000 ten years later – with many of the 12,000 men recent Jewish immigrants. By 1921 clothing was the largest employer of labour in the city, absorbing workers from the declining textile and footwear sectors and attracting women into the city for work.[71] There is even some suggestion it constrained the development of female non-manual labour between the wars in areas such as commerce.[72]

Leeds benefitted from the general growth of a consumer economy as local producers moved from the production of semi-finished goods – such as leather or cloth – to suits, coats and hats and footwear.[73] The city became a major centre of brewing with Tetley's in particular emerging as a regional force,[74] there were an increasing numbers of food producers supplied by the city's extensive market provision while Joseph Watson, Baron Manton, created a nationally prominent soap works.[75] Yet much as with the engineering sector, few of these businesses – with the exception of ready-made clothing – were tapping into the emerging sectors of the economy.[76] But together the larger concerns in the industrial sector underpinned middle-class development as well as creating some significant fortunes for men like Manton, Tetley, Burton and Brotherton that would feed into a sustained interwar charitable sector.

The manufacturing middle class were bolstered by a strong commercial sector including the private bank of Beckett's, the popular Yorkshire Penny Bank, a stock exchange and retail centre enhanced by the erection of elegant arcades.[77] These – along with the professionals maintained by a university town and centre of county justice – accounted for 11 per cent of the workforce in 1911. Moreover, the city retained a large rentier middle-class based on the wealth generated over one 150 years in industry and commerce.[78] This large middle class created opportunities for domestic servants – mostly young women – who fed into the clothing industry while the diversity of the economy was evidenced by the significant numbers of men employed in transport and the utilities who accounted for around 9 per cent of male employment in work that was often well paid, highly unionized and likely to be in the employ of the local authority.[79]

As Leeds was not as exposed as Sheffield to the interconnectedness of the heavy industrial sector, its experience of interwar unemployment was not as severe. The immediate post-war recession saw the numbers out of work rise to over 25,000 but, despite some disruption caused by the long-running coal dispute, the later 1920s were a period of relative stability with unemployment rates around the average for county boroughs and only marginally above the national figure (Table 1.3). The depression was slightly delayed in Leeds but by early 1931 unemployment was almost double that of January 1929 and remained high until 1933. In the aftermath of the depression, jobless figures fell at around the national average to sit at approximately 10 per cent by 1937. However, the effects of unemployment were not felt evenly across the city economy. The impact was greatest in declining sectors, such as textiles, footwear, chemicals, mining and engineering, the latter losing 10,000 employees between 1921 and 1931.[80] Conversely, the ready-made clothing sector continued to grow, reaching 43,000 workers in 1931, over one-third of the national total and one-third of all insured workers in the city. Moreover, 75 per cent of these employees were women and girls, a significant number of them married.[81] Overall, therefore, the more traditional elements of the Leeds economy suffered, including relatively high and persistent unemployment amongst adult males but opportunities grew in clothing as the city became more specialized from the nineteenth century.

Table 1.3: Unemployment in Leeds and average for counties and county boroughs, 1927–33

	No.	%	All counties	All county boroughs	National
1927	20,068	12.3	8	12.8	9.7
1928	16,498	10.1	8.8	10	10.8
1929	21,588	12.8	11.2	13.6	10.4
1930	22,462	13.4	11.1	14	16.1
1931	38,844	22.3	18.5	24.3	21.3
1932	35,108	19.6	20.9	23.4	22.1
1933	38,928	21.7	22.8	24.2	19.9

Source: TNA/MH66/711 Leeds Survey Report Appendix A.

Class, Gender, Ethnicity and the Labour Market

If Sheffield could be defined as a masculine city, then the predominance of women in the workforce made Leeds, to some extent, a women's city. Although not as dominant as in neighbouring Bradford, female labour force participation became more important between the wars as the ready-made clothing industry took off.[82] Thus, while the number of male workers in the city scarcely grew between 1921 and 1931, the number of women increased by one-sixth to a participation rate of 44 per cent, with women accounting for 36.5 per cent of the city's employees.[83] Although employees in the outwork and workshop sector remained poorly paid, those in factories like Burtons could expect regular wages and satisfactory modern conditions, including work canteens, pension schemes and occupational health facilities. Yet despite the female dominance within the industry there were still strong gender hierarchies, which meant that most women workers earned around 40 per cent of the salaries of equivalent males, with the male-dominated unions doing little to support female employees.[84]

Indeed unions in the clothing industry were relatively weak, as were unions generally in Leeds. The highly specialized nature of engineering meant that though some of the producers of heavy goods, like Kitsons,[85] did have large workforces of skilled men, most of the specialist areas were small-scale concerns, leading one historian to conclude:

> One of the city's largest industries, ready-made clothing, remained effectively unorganised, its workers in four main unions divided by sex, by race and by skill, and a weak trade union presence characterised most other industries.[86]

As this implies, the Leeds working class was subject to ethnic divisions absent from Sheffield. Although there was a sizable community of Irish descent in the city, some of whom played a part in the socialist movement, in general they retained a separatist approach to politics and failed to gain a foothold in any of the major industries of the city.[87] However, east European Jews, numbering about 15,000 by the First World War, stamped an important imprint on the social and economic structure of Leeds. Jewish immigrants settled mainly in the north-east of the city, the majority working in the clothing and tailoring industry by the 1890s.[88] In general, the Jewish trades retained some of the characteristics of the traditional tailoring industry, employing mainly men in workshops and outwork where wages and conditions were below those in the emerging ready-to-wear factories.[89] These weaknesses in labour organization had two outcomes: the development of mutualist organizations to protect workers from the vagaries of life, including an extensive co-operative movement, numerous friendly societies and the Leeds Workpeople's Hospital Fund; and the development of a strong socialist movement which dominated the trades' council and the Labour Party.[90] Together these trends shaped the development of hospital provision by marginalizing male, labourist approaches to service delivery in favour of independent mutualism on the one hand and ideological socialism on the other.

Of equal importance was the presence of a wider middle class in Leeds than in Sheffield.[91] The diverse nature of the Leeds economy and the tendency for the city's bourgeoisie to remain resident within its extensive boundaries ensured a large activist middle class, especially amongst its women. The prominent role played by the middle class in the city's Victorian voluntary organizations has been recorded by Morris and Gunn but their suggestions of bourgeois withdrawal from public engagement in the later nineteenth century is asserted rather than proved.[92] Rather, Leeds continued to present the air of a city with a deep and wide civic culture underpinned by a strong but integrated suburban identity.

Health

Although Leeds was more prosperous and middle class than Sheffield, surprisingly its health indicators were less impressive (Table 1.2). Thus while the death rate fell from a considerable high in 1919 it remained one or two points above the national average throughout the interwar period, rising sharply during the flu epidemic of 1929 and remaining high throughout the 1930s.[93] A final wave of infectious epidemics affected the city in 1929 with peaks in scarlet fever, measles and whooping cough cases and mortality. However, scarlet fever in particular, but also measles and whooping cough, became increasingly benign with case fatalities of less than one in a hundred during the 1930s. Diphtheria remained more serious until the mass inoculation campaign launched in 1935 which saw up to 30,000 children treated a year, slowly bringing incidence and fatality rates down to historic lows.

The poor general mortality figures owed much to a stubbornly high infant mortality rate – despite heavy intervention through infant and child welfare clinics. Influenced by the city's low birth rate, Dr Johnson Jervis – the MOH who assumed office in 1917 and remained in the post until 1946 – placed infant protection at the centre of his policy, promising in 1918 'to redouble our efforts to conserve our diminished resources in child life' and that:

> no expense should be spared in improving the housing and the sanitation of the community, in providing a pure milk supply, in stamping out venereal disease, in organizing safe conditions for maternity and disseminating a knowledge of mothercraft among present and future mothers.[94]

Although the city's IMR remained 16 points above the figure for Sheffield, Jervis could take comfort from that fact that his city saw a greater than average decline from 119 deaths per 1,000 births in 1919 to 57 per 1,000 in 1938, compared to a national fall from 84 to 50.

Much of the decline was due to a significant fall in deaths from diarrhoea and enteritis which by 1939 were around half the level of 1920, while neo-natal mortality rates had been cut by around one-third. But compared to other indicators infant deaths proved much more difficult to reduce, with marked fluctuations up until the mid-1930s and the commencement of a major slum clearance campaign. This was probably due to unresolved sanitary problems, including the presence of 8,000 ash pits in the city 'which because of their size and the volume of refuse they could accommodate ... were not only a nuisance in the sanitary sense but an attraction for flies, rats and other vermin',[95] while it was not until after 1927 that the city secured the power to deal with the nearly 10,000 trough closets in existence. In a similar vein Leeds's major health success was its taming of maternal mortality. Like Sheffield it had seen high figures in the 1920s, but mortality rates began to fall from the early 1930s to a rate well below the national average by 1939.[96] In 1946 the MOH regarded this as a 'notable achievement which amply justifies the time, labour and money expended' and he identified four key factors '(i) the greater skill and competence of doctor and midwife, (ii) the use of special drugs which aid the parturient woman to resist infection, (iii) the improved nutrition of the mother and (iv) the better facilities for her confinement'.[97] Amongst the latter was the growth of institutional birth, along with an extensive network of antenatal clinics.

The city was also successful in tackling respiratory diseases (bronchitis, pneumonia and influenza). These peaked in 1918 during the influenza pandemic, were still high in 1919 with over 2,000 deaths, but dropped to pre-epidemic levels of around 1,350 deaths in the early 1920s. The 1929 influenza epidemic pushed deaths back over 2,000; however, from this point rapid progress was made as annual mortality settled at around 700 for most of the 1930s and early 1940s – equivalent to a halving of the death rate in less than twenty years. Similar success was seen with TB, the number of fatalities from all forms declining from 719 in 1919 to 397 in 1939 and just 288 in 1946 as the fatality rate fell by two-thirds between 1919 and 1946. As a result of these changes the MOH was able to record in his final report that:

> The main causes of death in 1916 in order of numerical importance were heart disease, tuberculosis, bronchitis, pneumonia and cancer. In 1946 they were the same except that bronchitis was replaced by cerebral haemorrhage and there was a change in the order, cancer moving up to second place and pulmonary tuberculosis dropping to fifth place.[98]

Thus by the end of our period Leeds was demonstrating a 'modern' mortality pattern with the persistence of pneumonia reflecting the increasing age profile of the population. In 1918 over a quarter of all deaths were amongst those aged under one year while almost the same proportion were over the age of 65. Thirty years later, infant deaths had fallen to just 7 per cent of the total while those aged over sixty-five accounted for more than half of all mortality (57 per cent). This had a major impact on life expectancy and particularly on the mean age at death, which rose from 41 years in 1916 to 64 years by 1946.

A key feature of these changes was the increasing prominence of cancer deaths – as it was nationally – which rose from 500 at a rate of 1.17 in 1918 to

960 or 1.99 per thousand in 1946. These figures were notably higher than either Sheffield or the figures for England and Wales, leading the MOH to state that:

> It is sometimes said that the increase is apparent and not real and that it is due to improved diagnosis and the greater age to which the population is living. But whether apparent or real makes little odds to the general position which is worsening year by year and which in time ... will become so serious as to threaten the whole structure of the nation's health and security.[99]

Finding ways to deal with the disease preoccupied the medical profession, both voluntary and public, with both cities developing as regional treatment centres under the auspices of the British Empire Cancer Campaign and the Cancer Act.[100]

As the case of cancer shows, health metrics in Leeds were not particularly related to specific local factors. Unlike Sheffield, there were no occupational diseases, nor were housing conditions significantly different, with back-to-back housing widespread in both cities.[101] Indeed, the Ministry of Health inspector felt housing in the city was generally good while the MOH admitted that the newer back-to-back house 'makes a reasonably good dwelling' though he continued that 'there is nothing to commend the oldest type which is thoroughly bad in every respect and should be swept away'.[102] The depression may have had an effect on overall health, Maternity and Child Welfare clinics reporting evidence of ill health among mothers by 1933.[103] Yet, in comparison to Sheffield, health provision for women seems to have been good, with rather more general and specialist beds in the city for women than men.[104] This was underpinned by an active policy by the Health Department to support mothers and tackle infant and maternal mortality. Yet housing and slum clearance policies were more contested in Leeds than in socialist Sheffield and it was only in the later 1930s that significant inroads were made into demolishing the worst areas – 11,000 slums had been demolished by 1939 – while the municipal housing schemes 'made a notable contribution to the health of the city and have greatly improved its amenities'.[105] Furthermore, in both cities smoke abatement was a priority with the Leeds MOH making it a primary concern, ably assisted by the research of the chemist, Professor Cohen. Jervis commented in 1946 that thirty years earlier

> Leeds lived and moved and had its being (and some would add prospered) in a constant cloud of smoke and dirt ... But at what cost to its amenities and especially to the health of its people? The answer is to be found in the health statistics and particularly in the stunted growth and physical appearance of the children. The fogs of those early years of the century were things that had to be experienced to be believed for they were complete black-outs lasting sometimes for days and causing widespread misery, inconvenience and damage to life and property.

In claiming credit for the reduction in air pollution he pointed to stricter control of industrial smoke, tighter regulation of and improvement in boiler plant, the promotion of smokeless fuels like gas and electricity especially in homes and co-operation from the Gas and Electricity Departments, employers and the general public, concluding:

> it can justifiably be claimed that (i) fogs are less frequent and when they do occur, less dense and less irritating, (ii) that respiratory diseases have decreased, (iii) that rickets in children – a disease intimately associated with lack of sunshine – have practically disappeared and (iv) that the stature and appearance of the children have improved.[106]

Yet while emissions were markedly reduced and air quality improved, this may have owed as much to economic changes such as smoke-free clothing manufacture as to the work of the sanitary department.[107]

The changing health landscape of the city was delivered through partnerships between a range of voluntary agencies and a rapidly developing medical school. In contrast to the situation in Sheffield, Johnson Jervis supported and even promoted partnership, working with the voluntary sector in areas such as VD treatment, TB and maternity and child welfare. In common with many big cities venereal disease treatment was contracted out to the main voluntary hospital where it was managed by the MOH while attempts were made to join this up with treatment given in the poor law infirmaries and the mothers' homes.[108] In 1921 the council took over all of the institutional TB services including outpatients from the Leeds General Infirmary (LGI), sanatorium treatment and inpatient care although voluntary elements were retained as the Health Department continued to work with the Care Committee which looked after the 'social side of the Tuberculosis scheme'.[109] More significant joint working was seen in the area of maternity and child welfare where municipal services were delivered in tandem with an extensive voluntary operation run by the Leeds Babies' Welcome Association. Founded in 1908 by Ina Kitson Clark, the Welcomes provided the infrastructure on which the municipal system was based. In 1917 the municipality took over responsibility for the large number of maternity centres the Welcomes ran in working class areas of the city. As in other cities such as Bristol, Manchester and Liverpool, a division of labour was established whereby the council provided the medical services – doctors, health visitors, access to consultants – and the Welcomes maintained the premises, mobilized the volunteers to run the centres, undertook social and educational work for the Health Department and provided some access to clothing and other help to the poor mothers.[110] When Dame Janet Campbell[111] visited Leeds for the Ministry of Health in 1933 her opinion of the centres was positive and she noted that 'co-operation between the Voluntary Association and the Public Health Department is good' although she did suggest that the association 'would be none the worse for a stirring up occasionally, and might do more in the direction of model clothing, good posters and organised teaching'.[112] Similarly, Johnson Jervis was convinced that relationships with the Association 'have been of the happiest' and that 'under the combined aegis of the two bodies the work has prospered'.[113]

But the most important external player was the medical school, which acquired a permanent building next to the General Infirmary in 1894 and from 1904 formed part of the independent University of Leeds. This move reinforced the links between the teaching and clinical staff who shared an increasing number of personnel in a large and powerful medical faculty. Oversight of the university and clinical teachers remained separate until 1910 when, according to Anning, the desire to unite the teaching was driven (as at Sheffield) by the 'reasonable probability that a grant might be obtained for the School from the Board of Education provided that the clinical work at the Infirmary could be brought within the scope of their regulations for the clinical institution'.[114] As a result a board of the Faculty of Medicine was created to unite the Infirmary staff and in addition to the appointment of two salaried tutors the amalgamation also confirmed the right of female medical students to practise in the Infirmary.

As in Manchester, Bristol and Birmingham, the presence of a medical school acted as a neutral space where conflicts between the various groups involved in the delivery of hospital care could be negotiated and often resolved.[115] Thus, in Leeds, as in Sheffield, the faculty of the medical school played an important role in promoting innovation and hospital co-operation. In the early 1920s, led by Sir Berkeley Moynihan, the faculty pushed (unsuccessfully) for a new financial arrangement to be developed by the voluntary hospitals and promoted closer working arrangements with the municipal and even the poor law sectors. They made appointments from the municipal staff, including a chair for the MOH and a lectureship for the TB officer, and in the early 1930s promoted the merging of the faculties of the three main voluntary hospitals. By the later 1930s they were backing joint appointments with the municipal sector for new specialities so that by 1945 the close collaboration between the university, the municipal and the voluntary hospitals was favourably noted.[116]

Politics and Political Culture

The county borough of Leeds was active in municipal enterprise and had acquired control of gas, water, electricity and trams by 1900, seeking to improve services and set fairer tariffs as well as directing profits to a variety of projects including relief of the rates.[117] It extended its boundaries on a number of occasions, amassing a considerable acreage which would assist the council when it came to house building and redevelopment in the twentieth century. The poor law was administered by four boards until 1926 – Leeds and three others covering relatively small and poor areas. While Leeds had a very extensive workhouse complex[118] those in the suburban unions were of varying size and quality although this period saw improvements at each of the institutions.[119]

Party contests dominated local politics before the First World War. Victorian Leeds had been overwhelmingly Liberal but in the 1890s the council fell to the Conservatives[120] and although the Liberals returned briefly to power the rising strength of Labour was the key characteristic of the Edwardian period. The party experienced rapid success up to 1906 and though the anti-socialists fought back, in the three years after 1910 Labour made a sustained breakthrough, increasing their representation to sixteen council members.[121] The strength of Labour's political challenge has been attributed largely to the organizational weakness of the trade union movement in the city, which made an industrial strategy less likely to succeed. Although there were some notable industrial disputes,[122] local labour was more heavily influenced by socialists in the Independent Labour Party (ILP) and the British Socialist Party than by the big unions as had been the case in Sheffield.[123]

Significant Labour gains after the First World War initially prompted close co-operation between the older parties (though never a formal alliance). However, following the General Strike the Conservatives convinced five Liberals to defect before the November 1926 elections in which Labour made huge gains.[124] The Labour breakthrough, defections and the loss of aldermanic seats almost wiped out the Liberals and from this point onwards politics in Leeds was a two-party affair.[125] This did not particularly benefit the Labour party who struggled to gain and keep control of the council. Indeed they only managed two brief periods in charge – 1928–30 and 1933–5 – the Tories dominating municipal politics, especially the many new suburban wards created in 1930.[126]

What, then, was the effect on services of this highly contested period of local politics? The Leeds Labour Party developed a left-wing position between the wars matched by an aggressive anti-socialism on the part of the Conservatives. Yet, as in many big cities, Conservative policy was not narrowly non-interventionist.[127] In the 1920s the city built around 5,000 council houses in keeping with the pattern nationally. Moreover, the Conservative administration of the later 1930s were happy to continue with the policies initiated by the Labour administration of 1933–5,[128] especially their controversial slum clearance and housing programmes. Thus, in the three years before the outbreak of the Second World War the council built around 7,500 new homes and rehoused 10,000 households[129] on a combination of suburban estates and city centre redevelopments like Quarry Hill, conveniently located for much of the ready-made clothing industry.[130] There was also a notable change in the Tories' health policy during the 1930s. When the party took power in 1930 they reversed Labour's policy of appropriating the poor law hospitals to the Health Committee.[131] Unsurprisingly Labour made appropriation a priority in their second period of office, fighting the 1935 local elections in part on their record on health.[132] Yet the triumphant Conservatives honoured Labour's commitments to improving the fabric and role of the hospitals in the later 1930s and acted aggressively to expand the powers of the municipal service through the Joint Hospitals Council established in 1936.[133]

Conclusion

Leeds and Sheffield offer contrasting images of the early industrial city managing the difficult economic conditions of the interwar years. Although both had populations of around half a million and had played a leading part in the industrial revolution, by the First World War they had developed very different demographic, economic and social profiles which produced divergent political paths. Key elements stand out from this survey. Sheffield had a narrow economic base, dependent largely on elements of metalworking which produced a very masculine employment structure, strong trade unions and a limited role for women in economy, society and politics. Moreover, although a substantial place, it had little regional influence, its location on the border of three administrative counties and its lack of major civic, administrative or legal functions leaving it politically and socially isolated. Leeds, on the other hand, had a diverse economic base with a wide range of industries as well as a strong commercial sector. The main industry was dominated by women workers of all ages while the middle class was large and still closely involved in civic culture. Furthermore, its regional role was significant. It was centrally placed to build networks across Yorkshire, had major legal functions and was the focus of commerce, finance and exchange. It remained the social centre of the county, many of its voluntary associations, including its hospitals, linking city and county. Both cities developed strong Labour parties, but while the party in Sheffield was dominated by labourist aims, the one in Leeds was more ideologically driven.

Together these factors had a major impact on the emergence and form of hospital provision. As major centres they had to develop extensive general services for large populations and in this the hospitals they supported were broadly similar to those in other places like Newcastle or Bristol – though with fewer specialist institutions than the very large cities of Manchester and Birmingham.[134] But the way specialities developed was clearly influenced by economic and social factors. In particular, provision for women was strong in Leeds and relatively weak in Sheffield where, conversely, facilities for industrial accidents and for the treatment of fractures, damaged muscles and other orthopaedic conditions were extensive. Similarly, class structures and politics influenced the ways in which voluntary hospitals were financed and co-operation between the public and voluntary sectors developed. In Sheffield, a narrow middle class and prolonged economic crisis meant large-scale voluntary effort was quickly superseded by a corporatist approach to ordinary and extraordinary income generation, while Leeds remained able to mobilize large public appeals to supplement a diverse range of ordinary income sources. Ideology did constrain – on the surface – co-ordination of services between voluntary and public but the effects of this could be mitigated by individual clinical relationships and the influence of the medical schools. Finally, the generally positive trends in most disease profiles between the wars raised important issues for health-care providers as patient types and the length of their stays were transformed and the hospital population, in keeping with the rest of the population, got older and the conditions from which they suffered less amenable to treatment. New modern scourges – road accidents and cancer – replaced the old scourges of TB and the infectious diseases, creating demand for new skills and facilities as well as obsolescence. As will be seen, the ways in which Leeds and Sheffield developed their hospital provision in the early twentieth century was shaped by both general trends in demand and by the specific needs, capabilities and cultures of the two cities.

2 HOSPITAL PROVISION: VOLUNTARY AND MUNICIPAL

During the nineteenth century England acquired the hospital infrastructure which would form the institutional basis of the NHS. By 1861 there were around 65,000 hospital beds in England and Wales and this figure more than trebled to almost 200,000 by the outbreak of the First World War. Although growth slowed considerably between the wars, the stock of hospital beds had passed a quarter of a million by 1938 – a fourfold increase on the mid-Victorian period.[1] Development was most rapid in major urban centres like Leeds and Sheffield which saw the emergence of general and specialist institutions shaped by both the generic health-care demands common to city regions of an advanced industrial nation and the specific needs of the place influenced by socio-economic structures and political considerations. In particular, Leeds developed a single acute centre with extensive associated provision for women while Sheffield saw a more fragmented acute and specialist service with strong local authority institutions all focused on addressing the health needs of adult male labour.

Prior to 1929 hospitals were created by three separate agencies reflecting separate responsibilities and income sources. Acute care for the sick poor was provided by voluntary institutions which were maintained by subscriptions, donations, legacies and other non-public funds and staffed mainly by unpaid medical practitioners and professional nurses. As well as providing the main general hospitals, they were also the site of developing specialities, especially treatment for eye, ENT and skin conditions and for demographic groups such as women, children and ethnic communities. Hospital care for the poorest, especially the aged and infirm, the chronically and incurably sick and many women and children became the responsibility of the poor law guardians increasingly delivered in separate workhouse infirmary wings. Until 1914 these focused largely on care rather than cure but some were employing resident medical staff who undertook surgical operations and drew on consultants to treat more patients. The extension of maternity beds and minor surgery attracted non-pauper patients while the 1929 Local Government Act gave councils the opportunity to 'appropriate' poor law infirmaries (PLIs) as general hospitals and by 1939 around half of the major authorities were running such institutions.[2] Prior to 1929 council service had focused on the isolation and treatment of infectious diseases and TB. From the 1870s councils were obliged to make provision for the isolation of smallpox and other infectious diseases – especially typhoid and epidemic childhood conditions like scarlet fever and measles – while the National Insurance Act of 1911 provided funds for the development of TB sanatoria. Local authorities were also obliged to provide accommodation for mental health patients while some boroughs opted to establish their own maternity hospitals rather than subcontracting to other providers.

Historians have questioned the effectiveness of this method of developing hospital services to meet the needs of the local population, in particular the arbitrary nature of the location of voluntary hospitals which led Abel-Smith to assert that the 'pattern of provision depended on the donations of the living and the legacies of the dead, rather than any ascertained need for hospital services'.[3] Equally, Webster in his influential survey of the NHS pointed to the chaotic local authority contribution, highlighting south Wales where by 1945 ninety-three hospitals were under the management of forty-six different bodies.[4] However, a more subtle reading of these developments has emerged as historians drill down to look at how and why hospital systems emerged as they did in different localities. Although some, like Mohan's study of the north-east of England during the depression, confirm the older narrative of inadequate, disjointed provision, others point to the positive interaction of place and provision. Thus, Marland has commented that 'By looking closely at the functioning of medicine in a known locality, material for comparison with other communities becomes available ... which helps build up a picture of the development of modern medical services and the medical profession'.[5] Pickstone, Gorsky, Cherry and Doyle have added to this task with studies which place hospital services in their local context to challenge narratives of serendipity, chaos and inadequacy.[6]

As the statistics quoted above suggest, the nineteenth century was the era which witnessed the establishment and initial extension of many hundreds of institutions. From the 1870s, however, hospitals underwent two important changes. First was the rapid expansion of hospital medicine to embrace a range of new specialities and the inclusion of excluded groups such as women, children, the elderly and ethnic minorities and excluded conditions such as maternity, the infectious and the incurable. Second, this era saw a significant reorganization of the physical space of the hospital. Sturdy and Cooter have drawn attention to the application of new management techniques to institutions at this time but it is clear that this movement was also physical, demanding increased spatial specialization within the hospital separating both different classes of patient and the functions of the institution.[7]

To explore how, when and where these changes occurred this chapter will examine the development of the twenty or so hospitals operating in Leeds and Sheffield between the wars, paying attention to the growth of sites, buildings and bed numbers in the voluntary, poor law and municipal sector. The emphasis will be on the acute and general medical services and reference will not be made to the development of mental health provision as most of the institutional beds for this category of patient were provided by West Riding County Council (WRCC) outside the boundaries of this study.[8] Although much of the provision in this period – both voluntary and public – followed national trends, as will be shown below the nature and form of the institutions established in Leeds and Sheffield were influenced by the functions and fortunes of the local economy and the relative importance of the class and gender profile of each city. Furthermore, after 1918 class and gender issues were overlaid by competition and co-operation between the voluntary and expanding state sectors within a context shaped by increased patient demand, immense urban change and the challenges and opportunities offered by technological advances. This chapter will be divided chronologically into the periods 1850–1918 and 1918–48, and to aid organization the institutions have been grouped into four types: voluntary general and dispensary; voluntary specialist; local state general; and local state specialist. The key data for each of the institutions is provided in Table 2.1 and 2.2, which set out the founding dates, 'ownership', type and changes in bed numbers from establishment to 1946.

Table 2.1: Hospitals and bed provision in Sheffield by type, 1797–1948

	Founded	Control	Type	Beds on opening	Beds 1900	Beds 1918	Beds 1930	Beds 1938	Beds 1948
Royal Infirmary	1797	Voluntary	General	100		363	476	476	460
Royal Infirmary Convalescent	1914	Voluntary	Convalescent	24	0	24	24	24	24
Edgar Allen	1911	Voluntary	Physiotherapy OP clinic	0	0	0	0	0	52
Royal Hospital	1832	Voluntary	General	0	165 (1903)	236	340	392	301
Royal Hospital Annexe	1908	Voluntary	Convalescent	40			45	93	119
Jessop	1864/1878	Voluntary	Women/maternity	6	57	117	146	151	211
Children's	1876	Voluntary	Children	6	40	60	92	157	210
City General	1881	Poor law/municipal	General	365	643 (1906)		820	854	682
Nether Edge Gen	1865	Poor law/municipal	General				395/445	340	459
Lodge Moor ID	1888	Municipal	ID	156		434	540	416	508
Redmires	1925	Municipal	Smallpox				200	closed	
Winter St TB	1881	Municipal	TB	88		110	106	106	110
Commonside TB	1908	Municipal	TB.				43	42	40
Crimicar TB	1902	Municipal	TB	50		98	110	104	53
Nether Edge TB	1929	Poor law/municipal	TB				267	261	
King Edward VII	1916	Municipal	TB/orthopaedic children				130	136	140
Fir Vale Infirmary	1881/1929	Poor law/municipal	Chronic					787	1,083
West Riding Mental Hospital	1872	Municipal	Mental		1,600		1,972	2,122	2,089

Table 2.2: Hospitals and bed provision in Leeds by type, 1767–1948

	Founded	Control	Type	Beds on opening	Beds 1900	Beds 1918	Beds 1930	Beds 1938	Beds 1948
General Infirmary	1767/1869	Voluntary	General	27/320		469	527	571	
Maternity Hospital	1905	Voluntary	Maternity	16	0	33	108	140	
Hospital for Women	1853	Voluntary	Gynaecological/women	(1860) 40	(1903) 50	50	50	95	
Public Dispensary	1824/1867/1904	Voluntary	General OP	0	0	0	20	40	
Jewish Hospital	1905	Voluntary	General	8		8	32 (1932)	40	
Hope	1918	Voluntary	VD	0			28	28	
Cookridge Convalescent	1869	Voluntary	Convalescent	0				101	
Ida & Arthington	1888/1905	Voluntary	Convalescent	42/46	42	88	100	101	50
St James	1879	Poor law/municipal	General/maternity	0			1,278	1,300	1,679
St Mary	1918/1928	Poor law/municipal	General/maternity	4			245	239	213
Rothwell/St George	1903	Poor law/municipal	Chronic	0			356	338	
Wyther	1918	Municipal	Children	0			50		
Seacroft	1893/1904	Municipal	ID	407		489	489	480	
Killingbeck	1904	Municipal	TB sanatorium	0		180	220	242	
Gateforth	1901	Municipal	TB sanatorium	0			50	52	94
The Hollies	1921	Municipal	TB sanatorium	0			40	40	
City Smallpox	1904	Municipal	Isolation				20	22	
South Lodge	1879	PAC	PAI					215	
North Lodge	1879	PAC	PAI					91	
Marguerite Hepton Memorial Hospital		Voluntary municipal Jt	Orthopaedic	0					90

Voluntary General Hospitals and Dispensaries

The two largest and oldest hospitals originated in the eighteenth century as part of a general movement in most important cities.[9] The General Infirmary at Leeds (LGI)[10] was founded in 1767 for patients from city and county and acquired purpose-built accommodation in 1771, while the 100-bed Sheffield Royal Infirmary (SRI) began taking patients in 1797.[11] Admission regulations for these hospitals were characteristic of the period with patients recommended by subscribers and both institutions excluding the incurable, pregnant women, the infectious, the mentally ill and children under six. These institutions saw limited expansion in the early nineteenth century but the SRI was extended in 1843 and again in 1872[12] while the 150-bed LGI was replaced in 1869 by a new 300-bed neo-Gothic edifice in the most up-to-date pavilion style.[13] The failure of the general hospitals to meet the demand for appropriate medical care for the poor, led to the opening of public dispensaries in Leeds and Sheffield in the early nineteenth century.[14]

Public dispensaries offered more flexible treatment options, combining outpatient facilities and home visiting. The Dispensary in Leeds began in 1824 where its focus on prescribing drugs, home visiting and treating the casual sick in its outpatients department made it the poor man's general practice. It resisted opening an inpatient facility until the 1920s and despite numerous changes of location remained in the heart of the city in an area adjacent to some of the town's worst slums. The Dispensary in Sheffield, however, developed along different lines. Its formation in the city centre in 1832 with an open surgery and home treatment if resident within two miles of the parish church, owed much to straightforward medical competition.[15] In 1852 the honorary staff set up a casualty and operating ward, and in 1860 inpatient wards were opened with twenty-one beds, rising to fifty-one five years later, by which time it was known as Sheffield Hospital.[16] The decision to set up in opposition to the Infirmary owed something to a shortage of opportunities for a growing medical community as well as demand for additional inpatient facilities. Nor was it alone in setting up in competition to an established provider. For example, the Bristol General was established in 1832 while between 1860 and 1864 Middlesbrough gained two general hospitals although in the latter case religion and politics, as much as medical demand, motivated the promoters.[17]

Across Britain the last quarter of the nineteenth century saw a vigorous period of extension in the established general hospitals as demand grew steadily and classification and specialization emerged.[18] New building was often prompted by anniversaries, such as the centenary of the Sheffield Royal Infirmary in 1897[19] or by generous legacies like those received by the Sheffield Hospital in 1895 or the LGI in 1888 (which funded the hospital's first convalescent home). These extensions were focused on novel improvements to the facilities including general and specialist operating theatres, outpatient and ophthalmic departments and various ancillary buildings such as a laundries, mortuaries and post-mortem rooms.[20] Edwardian upgrading focused on the introduction of the technologies, management practices and infrastructure which would shape hospital provision up to 1948. In Leeds the Infirmary saw a major programme of works associated with the death of King Edward VII, incorporating new wards, operating theatres and outpatient facilities[21] while in 1908 a substantial donation of £5,000 provided a convalescent home at Fulwood for the SRH. Overall, these new additions aimed to provide space for better patient classification and treatment of outpatients along with spaces for new technologies such as X-ray departments and significantly improved operating theatres with electricity.

Thus by the end of the Great War, general hospital provision in Leeds and Sheffield had grown from around 250 beds at the beginning of the nineteenth century to over 800 supported by a further 120 convalescent beds. Moreover, Leeds offered a substantial free dispensary serving the needs of the poorest section of the city's population and easing the burden on the outpatient departments at the voluntary hospitals. Patients were organized in increasingly sophisticated ways with numerous specialist departments providing inpatient and outpatient treatment. New technology was increasingly evident while the growth in beds and patient numbers required commensurate increases in staff, especially nurses, to care for them. As a result a pressing requirement for most institutions between the wars was more and better accommodation for nursing and other staff preferably separately from the institution. Furthermore, this burst of growth left most institutions located in cramped inner city sites with little room to grow, prompting calls for the general hospitals to relocate to the suburbs. Insufficient space was a constant refrain of the interwar period – especially in Sheffield – and emerged strongly in the Ministry of Health reports at the end of the Second World War.[22]

Voluntary Specialist Institutions

The development of voluntary specialist hospitals was focused on patient groups and medical practitioners largely excluded from the general hospitals, particularly women, children and maternity cases.[23] By the 1860s some areas of specialist treatment, such as eyes, had been established at the general institutions. However, the importance of the professional, as well as the medical, imperative driving the creation of specialist institutions is demonstrated by the Leeds Infirmary for Eye and Ear cases (LIEE) founded in 1822 – a year before a similar venture in Birmingham.[24] Although the LIEE was incorporated into the new LGI in 1869, medics insisted that the current staffing of three surgeons 'are always retained in the Ophthalmic department'.[25] A hospital for diseases of the skin proved less successful and from 1901 dermatology was a specialist department at the LGI.

More significantly, hospitals for women were opened at Leeds in 1853 and Sheffield in 1864 – fairly early creations for this type of hospital, with St Mary's Manchester becoming a hospital in 1854 while the Women's Hospital in Birmingham opened in 1871.[26] Professional interest was a motivating factor in the Leeds Hospital for Women's (LHW) establishment, but socio-economic factors were also important. The hospital aimed to ensure specialists treated diseases of women, with particular attention drawn to the needs of the large number of women workers in the city. However, when a complete new hospital was begun in 1900 its focus was on gynaecology, the committee choosing to omit obstetrics and maternity to a few abnormal cases. Similarly, although the LHW included children in its original formation, they were never a central part of the work and in the Edwardian period their treatment was transferred to the LGI.[27]

The Sheffield women's hospital was promoted in 1864 to provide midwifery amongst the poor and relief of diseases peculiar to women but – like the Women's Hospital in Birmingham, which benefitted from the interest of Arthur Chamberlain[28] – its success owed much to individual philanthropy. In the later 1870s steel manufacturer Thomas Jessop contributed £30,000 to build a new 35-bed hospital known as the Jessop Hospital for Women[29] which, unlike the LHW, undertook significant maternity work.[30] The impetus for the Leeds Maternity Hospital (LMH) campaign, on the other hand, came from a group of women, reflecting their importance in medical services in Leeds.[31] When the 1903 redevelopment at the Hospital for Women failed to create new lying-in beds, the Leeds Women's Jubilee Fund Committee promoted a maternity home of their own. The 16-bed Leeds Maternity Hospital opened in 1905 and following the gift of a larger site, doubled in size in 1910. The committee behind the hospital was entirely female and unlike the LHW the institution had a policy of employing female surgeons.[32] Finally of the specialist institutions, 1876 saw the founding of an 8-bed hospital for children in Sheffield – rather later than similar institutions in Liverpool (1851), Manchester (1852) and Birmingham (1861)[33] – which by 1888 had 30 beds and an operating room. It ran a successful outpatient branch in the city's poor east end until 1916 and from around 1905 it developed links with the adjacent university.[34]

The emergence of specialist institutions raised the prospect of duplication but from an early date there was pressure to co-operate with the general institutions to ensure an efficient allocation of cases. Amalgamation between the LHW and the LGI was first mooted in 1885, reappearing in 1906 following the opening of the LMH when the division of the various types of female patients between the three hospitals was suggested, with the university pushing for a unified management and faculty to aid teaching. In developments similar to those in Manchester, a sophisticated delineation of roles developed as the LGI took on all of the children's cases, the LMH focused on normal – and increasingly abnormal – births and the LHW concentrated on gynaecology.[35] In Sheffield, however, the specialist institutions remained separate from the general hospitals – which both took children and some women's conditions. But in general the Jessop handled a growing maternity load and a range of gynaecological work, while the children's hospital focused mainly on older children – over three years of age – though from 1916 limited numbers of infants were admitted. Therefore, as in Manchester and Birmingham, more efficient voluntary services were developing with an increasing delineation of responsibilities encouraged by the medical schools' need for a range of patient types.

State General Hospitals

The institutions of the local state which emerged after 1870 were developed largely to serve those excluded from the voluntary sector. Public hospitals, both general and specialist, were initially created to treat patient groups who presented a physical or moral threat to the population.[36] However, from the turn of the twentieth century they were increasingly shaped as public institutions focused on curing rather than policing the infectious and indigent. How they developed and their particular focus was determined in part by the socio-economic environment, local party competition and the interests of the leading health officials.[37]

Efforts to provide general services for the very poor emerged out of boards of guardians' workhouses where managers began to separate and reclassify children, the elderly and the chronically sick and to adopt a more liberal attitude to those who were admitted due to ill health.[38] A separate Infirmary was designated at Beckett Street, Leeds in 1874, making it the first distinct infirmary outside of London.[39] The suburban unions also provided more or less distinct infirmary provision, St Mary's Infirmary at Bramley proving the most professional. In Sheffield, the Nether Edge workhouse acquired a hospital block in 1865[40] while the new city workhouse erected in 1878 included male and female asylums, a hospital block for 366 patients and a fever hospital, making it the largest hospital complex in the city.[41] Indeed such developments were common by the end of the century as boards of guardians sought to adapt their provision to their changing clientele. Middlesbrough opened a workhouse with separate infirmary around the same time as Leeds, while Salford guardians provided a hospital in 1882 to accommodate 880 beds.[42] However, the picture was less dynamic in towns like Norwich, where the minimal infirmary the guardians built in the early 1890s proved inadequate for anything but the most basic care.[43]

In Leeds and Sheffield the 1890s and 1900s[44] saw rapid expansion on all of the main sites and, as with the voluntary sector, the focus was on more and better accommodation for nurses and administration; improved laundries, kitchens and heating; and room for the more effective separation of patients. Thus at St James' in Leeds a nurses' home and new imbeciles' ward released space in the main infirmary for a further 600 patients.[45] At Nether Edge, Sheffield, small-scale improvements were effected regularly from 1891, including a nurses' home, maternity blocks and operating theatre lit by electric lighting[46] while at Fir Vale a children's hospital and a male sanatorium ward facilitated additional patient classification. When the hospital separated from the workhouse in 1906, blocks for administration, stores and a kitchen were added and medical facilities were improved by the addition of a dispensary, operating theatre, laboratory and mortuary.[47]

Thus, by 1914 general services had been developed by the boards of guardians as they sought to move beyond the stigmatized 'pauper'. New identities were fostered by name changes, the dropping of uniforms for patients, improvements in nurse training and attempts to provide non-pauperized treatment for the elderly and chronic sick. Thus, at Fir Vale a new classification system was brought in which designated the sick as 'those of any age who are temporarily or permanently infirm, and whose character is very good', assuring respectability and minimizing stigma.[48] Such developments were in line with changes elsewhere. In Middlesbrough, the 1910s saw a number of reforms including a name change while a new hospital – Southmead – was under construction in Bristol to a standard that would rival voluntary hospitals in many towns and cities.[49] Yet in other respects the institutions of Leeds and Sheffield remained residual in the facilities, staffing and treatments available. In particular, there were few resident medical staff or consultants utilized and nursing staff were grossly overworked, especially in the smaller unions of Leeds.

Local State Specialist Institutions

The specialist hospitals of the local state were created in four areas normally outside the purview of the voluntary general hospitals – infectious diseases (ID); pulmonary TB; maternity; and children's diseases, especially non-pulmonary TB. The most extensive part of this provision was the ID hospitals promoted by the 1875 Public Health Act,[50] yet these isolation hospitals have received little attention in the historiography beyond the excellent survey of Lancashire by Pickstone and the biography of Edinburgh City Hospital by Gray.[51] These historians demonstrate the contested nature of ID hospitals in the later nineteenth century but highlight the growing recognition of public health as a branch of medical knowledge, Pickstone concluding: 'General isolation hospitals, like other special hospitals, were an essential part of modern medicine, because modern medicine was increasingly based on specialisation and on hospital treatment.'[52]

Leeds, like Manchester, was initially served by a voluntary House of Recovery[53] but during the 1890s the council acquired land to the east of the city for new ID accommodation, a move prompted by local resistance to the siting of smallpox hospitals near built-up areas. Opened in 1904 as Leeds City Hospitals,[54] the main site housed the 452-bed Seacroft Hospital with accommodation for scarlet fever, diphtheria, enteric fever and isolation cases while the adjacent Killingbeck site was to specialize in smallpox cases. Together these institutions cost over £350,000 and were designed to meet the needs of the city for the foreseeable future.[55] Yet, as in many other towns and cities they had massively overestimated the future need for smallpox beds and by 1909 Killingbeck was empty most of the time. Sheffield Corporation opened a 100-bed ID hospital in the city centre at Winter Street in 1881 which excluded smallpox sufferers. However, a smallpox outbreak in 1888 prompted the acquisition of the suburban Lodge Moor estate where a permanent institution was built between 1902 and 1904 with a separate smallpox hospital adjoining at Crimicar Lane. There was little remarkable about either of these complexes – their delayed construction in response to severe smallpox epidemics reflecting a generally reactive policy amongst local authorities in the late nineteenth century.[56]

In tandem with the development of these ID facilities both cities established TB institutions, although in this case Sheffield's experience of 'grinder's lung' promoted a more active policy than that pursued in Leeds.[57] In 1905 Sheffield's Winter Street Hospital began taking TB patients, in 1908 a suburban sanatorium was opened at Commonside while the smallpox institution at Crimicar Lane was converted to TB cases, giving Sheffield over 250 TB beds with patients managed from a City Centre Dispensary opened in 1911. Mirroring Sheffield, Killingbeck was converted from smallpox to TB cases – a practice seen in Middlesbrough and parts of Lancashire[58] – supplementing the sixty beds provided by the voluntary sector at the rural Gateforth Sanatorium and at Armley House on the outskirts of the city.

In this period neither local authority provided specialist maternity beds, although the various poor law institutions were beginning to establish lying-in wards by 1914. Similarly, hospital accommodation for children was very limited, especially for TB-related orthopaedic conditions amongst the young. However, as a memorial to Edward VII Sheffield raised around £18,000 – bolstered by a significant contribution from the City Council and a donation of land from the Duke of Norfolk – to create a 120-bed institution for children disabled by diseases such as TB, rickets and poliomyelitis. The need for such institutions was made clear by Leeds's MOH, Johnstone Jervis, who noted in 1918 that cases of surgical TB constitute a large proportion of the surgical work dealt with at the Leeds General Infirmary, but to get successful results ... they must be kept in institutions for a long time, even up to twelve months and the General Infirmary cannot afford beds for that length of time.[59]

Despite this need no such institution had been established in Leeds by 1939, the council continuing to rely on access to beds at the rural Marguerite Hepton Home run by the Invalid Children's Aid Society and at a voluntary institution in Hampshire.[60]

By 1918 there were a large number of hospital beds across a variety of institutions and providers and covering a wide range of conditions and patient types. As a result, the interwar period was one of consolidation, co-ordination and refinement rather than new creations. Indeed, relatively few new beds were added to the main voluntary hospital stock before the later 1930s while much of the increased capacity in the state sector came from reorganization rather than new building. Moreover, where construction was undertaken it was likely to be focused on services, administration, outpatients, enhanced classification or new techniques rather than additional beds. This was the era in which new forms of management were deployed to increase throughput of patients, though these were as likely to require physical as administrative changes. Yet these physical changes to the environment of the hospital have been largely overlooked, especially how they may have delivered cheap improvements in patient throughput for some of the poorer or low spending municipalities.[61]

Voluntary Hospitals between the Wars

Growth in the voluntary sector was largely determined by the local economic situation, by the ability of the region to provide capital for building projects and equally by the ability of ordinary income to keep up with the cost of extension.[62] Leeds General Infirmary was already a very substantial hospital in 1919 with over 450 beds, the SRI had just over 350 beds and the Sheffield Royal Hospital (SRH) 285.[63] The specialist institutions, however, were still rather modest. Only the Jessop Hospital had more than a hundred beds while those in Leeds could accommodate fifty patients or fewer. Over the course of the interwar period all hospitals saw some increase in bed numbers, with particular growth in accommodation for women and children. The immediate post-war period saw some new building, mirroring activity in places like Leicester and Nottingham.[64] At the LGI a children's department was created partly funded to commemorate the marriage of Princess Mary to the hospital's president, Lord Lascelles.[65] However, this was to be the last addition for fifteen years, economy and a shift in emphasis to outpatients seeing bed numbers fall to below the 1921 figure by 1935. The SRI also undertook a major expansion in 1925 when the bed tally jumped by around 100 although again subsequent adaptations were to outpatient accommodation, staff quarters and medical and ancillary facilities. At the Sheffield Hospital developments were more gradual with new wards added in 1923 and 1928 while following an appeal to commemorate the Centenary, a new orthopaedic block and thirty pay beds were added in 1937 bringing capacity to almost 400. The late 1930s saw the situation improve at the LGI as reorganization and a new ward took bed numbers to 572 while a substantial wing for private patients and an outpatient department were completed in 1940.

The specialist hospitals, on the other hand, saw significant growth at three of the four institutions. Bed numbers at the Jessop rose from 117 to 151 between the wars – largely through reorganization – with a further major expansion embarked upon in 1938 which included private beds and additional maternity provision. Equally important was the acquisition by Sheffield Hospitals Council of the Norton Hall estate which was assigned to the Jessop as an auxiliary institution providing forty-seven beds for the treatment of puerperal cases and others in need of isolation.[66] The children's hospital acquired new wards in 1927 while the gift of a 20-bed convalescent home by the Alderman Graves Trust in 1937 brought bed numbers to 150. In the two women's hospitals of Leeds there was little development in the 1920s but from 1930 there was marked augmentation at the LHW with the addition of pay beds and a general ward bringing the bed total to 100, while the LMH saw bed numbers rise from 67 in 1927 to 140 in 1936, making it the second largest outside London.[67]

One way in which capacity did increase was through the introduction of pay beds. Historians have paid little attention to private provision in voluntary hospitals, Pickstone noting Manchester Royal Infirmary had 100 pay beds by 1938 while Reinarz suggests development was quite extensive in Birmingham with the city's nine voluntary hospitals collectively treating around 2,000 private patients by the outbreak of the Second World War.[68] George Gosling's more wide-ranging study contends that national statistics point to a greater preponderance of private beds in general, rather than specialist, hospitals and smaller rather than larger institutions.[69] Although his findings for Bristol tend to the contrary – with all of the city's specialist institutions offering some pay beds – he notes a significant supply of private beds in the general hospitals of Bath pointing to a regional market for private patients.[70] The evidence from Leeds and Sheffield tends to reflect the national picture, with substantial private units at the SRH and LGI and smaller provision in the LHW and the Jessop. However, pay beds made up a greater proportion of the establishment in women's hospitals and for women generally.[71] It would also seem that the substantial middle-class presence meant pay beds were becoming a prominent feature of Leeds hospital care.

Thus the LHW was the first in the running with six pay beds in 1930 doubled to twelve in 1937, Colonel Tetley, the President, explaining:

> We think there is a demand for this sort of accommodation ... because it is often difficult to find, outside a hospital, the facilities for diagnosis and treatment ... which the ordinary hospital patient receives at a voluntary hospital. Many people who are moderately well off ... now often feel that in times of sickness they themselves cannot obtain the modern facilities for treatment which they are helping to provide for the ordinary hospital patients.[72]

In a similar vein, the LMH noted in 1933 that they would like to add a pay block as:

> To the wives of young business and professional men living often in flats or furnished rooms the provision of a Pay-Bed block would be of the greatest value ... the Leeds Maternity Hospital will not be fulfilling its function completely until maternity services can be offered to all classes of citizens of Leeds.[73]

The SRH included a pay block with thirty beds in their new Miners' Welfare wing while the two big developments underway in 1939 included ninety beds at the LGI and thirty-two at the Jessop made up of twenty maternity beds and twelve for gynaecology, the former proving very popular by the mid-1940s.[74]

Not without reason, historians have tended to concentrate on the growth in bed numbers yet what really characterized change at interwar hospitals was improvements in ancillary services and especially: accommodation for nurses, medical staff and administration; extensions in outpatient and casualty facilities; additional isolation and research services; and modernization of domestic departments such as kitchens and laundries. Each new ward demanded more nurses, domestics, food and clean linen and space and equipment for treatment and recovery, all of which put severe pressure on hospital finances, forcing institutions to seek ways to treat more patients for less.[75] This included: better use of existing buildings; recruiting and retaining the best staff; classifying and managing patients; enhancing pre- and post-operative care through auxiliary sites and outpatient departments; and modernizing domestic services to increase capacity and cut costs.

The expansion of bed and patient numbers called for increased staffing, especially nurses. Yet hospitals had difficulty finding and keeping good nursing staff and increasingly managers looked to improved accommodation, leisure facilities and greater independence as recruitment tools. As the Jessop had noted of their 1938 nurses home:

> How to encourage a higher rate of recruitment [of nurses] is the problem being faced by the Hospital world generally. The Board are glad to feel that conditions under which nurses work and live at the Jessop Hospital now bear comparison with most modern hospitals.[76]

Developments in the 1920s had been largely piecemeal, so that, as late as 1933, nurses at the SRH 'were still housed in the home at the hospital; others in the old Theological Training College at Ranmoor and others in two houses at Lydgate Lane, which were formerly the Crookes Orphan Homes'.[77]

As a result, the 1930s saw a wave of new homes with facilities designed to appeal to modern young women. At the SRH's Tapton Court each nurse would have 'a separate bedroom with fitted wash-basin and wardrobe. Shower Baths and Shampoo rooms are also provided',[78] while externally there were gardens and a tennis court. In Leeds massive expansion saw new homes at the LMH in 1930, the Hospital for Women in 1934 and three new buildings at the LGI culminating in a fifty-room suite in 1940.[79]

Changing attitudes to patient management were a spur to improvements in outpatient and casualty facilities in most voluntary hospitals.[80] Outpatient facilities could free space for more beds, as at the LHW where the opening of a new outpatient department permitted the creation of an additional ward.[81] More impressive, however, were developments at the SRI which deployed modern patient management ideas to ensure efficiency and comfort:

> The Registration Department is an entirely new building adjacent to the Out-patient Department and consists of a commodious Waiting Hall and Registration Office for Out-patients, together with a suite of offices, modern in every respect, which accommodate the Almoner's Department ... each of the Departments ... (Surgical, Medical, Ophthalmic and Venereal Diseases) has been greatly enlarged, modernised and re-equipped. While in undertaking this reconstruction, the principal idea in the minds of the Board was to produce an Out-Patient Department of the greatest possible efficiency, another important object was to secure conditions for patients similar to those obtaining in the Surgery of the General Practitioner.[82]

At the SRH in 1927 a key aim was the separation of casualty from outpatients in the face of growth in both street accidents and patients attending day clinics.[83] Changes at the LGI not only allowed for more efficient management of inpatients and outpatients but they increasingly served as a clearing house for the bulk of those seeking treatment at any of the city's hospitals.[84] Thus, while scientific management and organization were prompted by the desire of doctors and administrators to increase patient throughput in an era of mass health care,[85] they may also have been stimulated by the financial hardship caused by the effects of the economic crisis. In particular, this reduced the capacity of the hospitals to appeal for capital until the later 1930s, encouraging them to seek other solutions.

Transformation was also seen in the increasing use of science and technology in the diagnosis and treatment of disease, prompting considerable investment in isolation wards, laboratories and research facilities. Although these developments were common to all voluntary hospitals[86] they were particularly evident in maternity and gynaecology units where the challenge posed by puerperal sepsis led to the creation of isolation facilities, such as the Jessop's Norton Hall annexe or the 4-bed ward built at the LMH.[87] Furthermore, the Jessop board announced in 1929 that they were opening a bacteriological laboratory at Norton to support 'organised research in relation to the complications of child birth', especially puerperal sepsis. The facility was recognized by the Medical Research Council in 1931.[88] In Leeds the LMH extended laboratory and research facilities in 1930[89] while in 1940 the movement towards closer working between the voluntary hospitals saw the LHW join with the LMH to extend pathology provision and employ a full-time pathologist.[90]

Laboratory and research capacity also grew at the general hospitals, underpinned by close links with the universities. The pathology work of the LGI was transferred to the university in 1918 while in Sheffield the professors of pathology and physiology were on the honorary staff of the Royal Hospital although much of the routine work for both the institutions was undertaken at the university.[91] As a result the hospital surveyors of 1945 commended the links between hospital and university, noting:

> It is most important that the medical teaching schools should be closely associated with all this pathology work. The seed of this already exists in Sheffield in the association between the laboratories at all the Hospitals of Sheffield itself and in some of the other neighbouring centres, with the University Department of Pathology.

They were, however, a little concerned about aspects of the relationship, commenting that the 'Sheffield instance is not entirely satisfactory because it appears to us that although the association is real in some hospitals it is nominal in others'.[92] As this suggests, the development of bench science as an integral part of the hospital regime was much more readily facilitated in cities with universities and medical schools like Manchester, Birmingham and Bristol where staff moved between the bedside and the laboratory. It was less advanced in the larger hospitals without academic support, like Derby or Middlesbrough, which had to wait until 1945 for a hospital-based pathology service to emerge.[93]

'Modern' medicine also demanded an increase in the scale and scope of technology devoted to diagnosis and treatment. Although electricity and various newly discovered rays had been in use before 1914, the interwar period was particularly characterized by the take-off in the use of X-ray as both a therapeutic and diagnostic tool, the widespread application of ultraviolet light and electric massage techniques and the slow distribution of radium in the 'war on cancer'.[94] Thus, at Sheffield Hospital, the new Miners' Welfare Block, a seven-storey construction of concrete pillars, brick and glass with furniture 'principally of the modern tubular steel type' included 'One floor ... devoted entirely to X-Ray and Radium treatment'. Moreover, scientific management was evident in the design of the building, a report on its early working noting that 'a block of seven floors is more conveniently worked than one of three or four', that it saved time, supervision was easier and 'The higher wards are quieter and the air is better'.[95] Similarly, at the LGI a new diagnostic X-ray department opened in 1940, along with operating theatres for paying patients and a radium centre. Developments at SRI were more modest. In 1939 improvements were made to the old and cramped X-ray department and there was also significant redevelopment of the operating theatre block,[96] while Sheffield Children's Hospital acquired a new operating theatre and isolation block.[97]

None of this was unique or unusual – operating theatres, X-ray suites and even isolation blocks were to be found in the smallest of cottage hospitals. But the need to keep up to date was essential for the leading teaching hospitals, Bristol General deploying 'Massage, Electrical and X-ray departments ... furnished with deep therapy and superficial therapy units, radiant heat baths, hot air baths, ultraviolet lamps, x-ray machines, electrical diagnosis equipment and a medical gymnasium'.[98] These were also objects favoured by benefactors and philanthropists, Lord Manton providing funds for the upgrading of the LGI's X-ray facilities.[99] Moreover, as surgery became the focal point of acute medicine hospital staff, boards, patrons and the public demanded facilities for excellent surgery. This was typified by the case of the fracture clinic which was enthusiastically promoted in the provinces if not in the voluntary hospitals of London.[100] Conversely, radium treatment returned some kudos to the physicians with the later 1930s seeing attempts to create discrete radium centres in both cities.[101]

Behind these well-known additions lay the need to modernize the dull but essential parts of the hospitals' work such as kitchens, laundries, canteens and recreation facilities – a development largely ignored by historians.[102] Given the volume of work involved in servicing 300 or more inpatients, considerable attention was paid to the work of the hospital laundry, both to increase efficiency and cut costs. Laundries were remodelled and re-equipped at the LGI, LMH and the SRI where the board were 'well satisfied that when the Laundry with its completely modernized equipment and facilities is re-commissioned ... it will carry out its work with greatly increased efficiency and stricter economy'.[103] Other improvements included new kitchens, dining rooms and accommodation for medical and domestic staff at the LMH and a room for medical records, facilities for a telephonist and new quarters for domestic staff at the Sheffield Children's Hospital.[104] These invisible services were vital to the increased efficiency of the hospitals, yet it was rare for benefactors to step in and aid in the upgrading of such services as they did for new technologies – though at the LGI former treasurer T. F. Braime did arrange the renovation of the workshops, gardens and Infirmary roads in the 1920s.[105]

Thus, interwar developments at the voluntary hospitals were concentrated on increasing beds for previously under-represented groups, including women, children and the middle class; providing the equipment and space for more scientific forms of diagnosis and treatment; creating space and systems for the more effective classification and organization of patients, especially through greater use of OP departments; and developing the ancillary services required to feed, clothe, house and entertain increasing numbers of patients and staff. So while economic conditions clearly limited the ability of the interwar voluntary hospitals to add to bed numbers, this was not a period in which they were marking time – but rather one in which other means were developed to increase throughput and ensure the more efficient care and treatment of patients.

Local State Provision between the Wars

There were no new additions to the stock of public hospitals between the wars but as with the voluntary sector these years were characterized by substantial restructuring of bed capacity and significant improvement to facilities. But local priorities varied depending upon the perceived service needs of the city and on variations in medical conditions and attitudes to particular classes of patients and institutions.[106]

The overall bed stock of the public hospitals saw little growth between the wars as most of the municipal and poor law hospitals were relatively new and had been built on good sites, with a generous bed capacity.[107] Where they did increase capacity their priority groups mirrored the acute hospitals – women and children along with the elderly. At the PLIs large children's wards were added at Fir Vale and St James's while new maternity suites were opened at Fir Vale, Nether Edge and St Mary's Leeds and the Leeds Infirmaries increased their capacity for chronic cases, bed numbers at St James's rising to 1,136 by 1934.[108] However, there were no significant alterations to the ID hospitals in the 1920s and only limited improvement to the TB provision. But administrative and political changes between 1929 and 1934 laid the foundations for a unified local authority hospital service. The process of transfer from the poor law and appropriation required major reorganization, restructuring and extension of the facilities.[109] The poor law hospitals of Sheffield were appropriated in 1930 although in Leeds Labour's plans were held up by the Conservative administration until 1934.[110]

Initial assessment of the 1929 Local Government Act tended to present a picture of failure to appropriate and missed opportunities amongst those councils which did bring the PLIs under Health Committee control. Powell, in particular, challenged this view, pointing to the success of a number of authorities (especially in and around London) and highlighting constraints such as financial stringency, poor facilities and other pressing priorities.[111] Although Mohan has reasserted the pessimistic position in his assessment of municipal developments in the northeast, others have pointed to a positive picture of improving environments and capacity.[112] Thus in Bristol, maternity care was expanded both by reorganization – moving chest and TB cases out of Southmead – and the building of new maternity blocks. Appropriation was quick in Manchester and Salford, but little new building followed, although both maternity and surgical work were augmented. Even in Norwich the Public Assistance Committee (PAC) built a new block at the end of the 1930s ahead of wartime appropriation.[113]

Appropriation in Sheffield saw Nether Edge and Fir Vale (renamed the City General Hospital) quickly brought up to hospital standard and closely integrated with the work of the voluntary and municipal institutions. Sheffield benefitted by inheriting good quality facilities which had been improved when the Sheffield and Eccleshall Unions were unified in 1926. Moreover,

> the two General Hospitals ... had been for years maintained entirely separately, with completely separate staffs by the Board of Guardians ... These hospitals had a staff of full-time Medical Officers, and had also a visiting staff of physicians, surgeons, obstetricians, etc., and were equipped with X-ray apparatus, laboratory facilities and had all the amenities of a general hospital.[114]

This analysis was a little optimistic as Nether Edge had only limited facilities for general hospital treatment, but following reorganization it specialized in TB, maternity and the chronic and incurably sick, while Fir Vale increasingly took on the mantle of a third general hospital.[115]

Reflecting the kind of developments already seen in Bristol, Middlesbrough and Manchester, the 1930s witnessed improvements designed to provide a complementary service to the voluntary hospitals and to allow the City General to take routine cases from their waiting lists.[116] In 1934 a suite of new buildings was opened that included three operating theatres, a maternity and antenatal unit, a much enlarged nurses' home, and a casualty unit to take accident cases from one-third of the city.[117] Further additions included a pathology laboratory, an additional maternity block and a new infants' ward. Moreover, a rearrangement of beds increased the surgical accommodation and allowed the transfer of some of the chronic medical cases.[118] Sheffield certainly benefitted from inheriting two good quality, well-managed and located institutions while the socialist administration – supported by the MOH and medical superintendent – was keen to develop a first-class local service, easily accessible to the city's population.

The situation in Leeds was more complex. The city could appropriate up to four institutions – St James's Hospital, the mixed St Mary's Infirmary, the infirm wards at Holbeck and the more up-to-date facilities at Rothwell. Although appropriation was delayed, some infirm and chronic patients were moved from St

James's and St Mary's to Holbeck and Rothwell allowing surgical work to increase at St James's.[119] Redevelopment focused on improving ancillary services with plans for a mortuary, improved antenatal department and an 'after-treatment' department; laboratories, a nurses' training school and additional accommodation for resident medical staff[120] finally begun following appropriation in 1934. Health Committee control led to further reorganization of cases with St James's focusing on the acute sick, infirm sick, children and mental health; St Mary's on maternity, TB and the infirm; Rothwell (renamed St George's) on male VD, children and the infirm; while the public assistance cases were divided between Beckett St and Holbeck. As with Nether Edge, the concentration of infirm cases in St Mary's and St George's was an acknowledgement that neither was suitable as a general hospital without 'entire remodelling and reconstruction', but that they were 'admirably suited for chronic cases'.[121]

Although delayed by financial constraints, a major programme of extensions and improvements at St James's was embarked upon and completed in 1940 with:

> its genesis in the rapid change in the amount and character of the work undertaken by modern municipal general hospitals ... Its aim is not to increase the number of beds ... but to improve the services, diagnostic and remedial, available for the patients.[122]

Costing £146,000, the changes were focused on similar concerns to those of the voluntary sector, including a substantial nurses' home with suitable leisure facilities, a nurses' training school, a physiotherapy department, an X-ray department, a pathology unit and mortuary block, and an operating theatre and electrical block.[123] In a conclusion which encapsulated the commonly undertaken changes at all acute hospitals in this period, the opening brochure explained that:

> The new extensions will enable the hospital to meet the exacting standards now demanded in the investigation and treatment of diseases, as well as in the provision of comfort for the staff, with the enhanced possibility of extending the all-round usefulness of the hospital.[124]

Clearly, in developing these services Leeds and Sheffield had considerable advantages over places like Norwich where the one PLI was swamped by infirm cases.[125] Indeed, even the larger city of Hull – which like Norwich was a Labour-controlled authority – was unable to develop an appropriated general hospital service because the city's two Public Assistance Institutions (PAIs) were unsuitable for hospital work even in 1945.[126]

In addition to creating a general hospital service, some work was undertaken on the ID institutions. The tendency to repurpose smallpox institutions as TB sanatoria was continued and developed. For example, at Killingbeck in Leeds changes in the treatment regime for TB patients – which saw average sanatorium stays rise from seven to twenty-eight weeks – necessitated a major extension and in 1936 an ultra-modern 100-bed block for women was opened. Stimulated in part by the weakness of the city's provision for female TB sufferers identified by the Ministry of Health surveyors in 1933 and partly by a desire to ensure women completed the extended treatment regime, the opening brochure observed that:

> In their new quarters the women patients will have greater comfort and the brighter surroundings will be an added incentive to them and to the staff to persevere in their efforts to bring the fight against disease to a successful issue.[127]

At Sheffield, a major programme of renewal took place at Lodge Moor in 1933–5 when the older wards were replaced by four 30-bed pavilions,[128] reducing the overall capacity from 540 to 420, reflecting the general retreat of infectious disease in the second half of the 1930s. Indeed this was replicated across the country, with Bristol concentrating all of its ID work on one site, Middlesbrough subcontracting beds to neighbouring authorities and even the relatively small institution in Norwich giving an increasing proportion of its capacity over to TB by 1929.[129]

War and Post-War

The outbreak of the Second World War both disrupted plans and created new configurations of services and facilities as central government became involved in directing hospital provision. The establishment of the Emergency Medical Service (EMS)[130] saw the redistribution of beds to accommodate the anticipated civilian and military casualties, evacuees, prisoners of war and even chronic sick from other cities. Moreover, bomb damage affected some institutions in Sheffield, while restrictions on materials and manpower stopped building plans and limited scope for routine maintenance.

In Leeds and Sheffield major developments were underway in the voluntary and local authority sector in 1939. The LGI's Brotherton wing was partially completed in 1940–1, with most of the pay-bed block opening in 1940 and the outpatients department the following year. An extension at the Jessop was held up until bomb damage at the main hospital closed a significant number of beds, making the completion of the new wing – with its additional maternity functions – essential.[131] Local authority plans met with less success. Although the St James's modernization was completed initiatives developed by Leeds City Council and the Joint Advisory Committee, including a 150-bed children's hospital and a joint Cancer Institute, had to be abandoned.[132] In Sheffield plans to build a new 600-bed municipal hospital; a 420-bed sanatorium for pulmonary TB to replace all of the existing provision and a 100-bed unit for surgical treatment of chest diseases were similarly abandoned.[133]

The outbreak of the war also led to massive reorganization of the hospital services of the two cities. EMS provision included city centre casualty clearing centres based at the general hospitals; and suburban institutions to treat military personnel whether sick or injured, as well as evacuees, civil defence personnel and prisoners of war. In anticipation of significant air raid casualties a proportion of acute hospital beds were kept free or accessible for emergencies leading to the extensive transfer of patients. Thus, in Leeds all maternity work was moved from St James's to the LMH which in turn took over part of the Cookridge Convalescent Hospital.[134] In Sheffield the allocation of emergency beds, combined with the instruction to close top-floor wards, reduced beds at the SRI to 250 in 1943[135] while the Royal Hospital had to make use of a convalescent home as a surgical unit.[136] In Leeds, even the small Hospital for Women had to allocate twelve beds for emergencies until 1943. Here and at the LGI the biggest effect was on the top-floor private wards and it is probable that hospitals allocated their private beds to the EMS, reducing pay bed capacity nationally by 1943.[137]

Municipal general hospitals were also brought into the EMS, leading to major shifts in patients. For example, in Leeds, St James's reduced the number of chronic male cases it admitted; TB specialization was initiated at St George's while St Mary's focused entirely on chronic and maternity services. Seacroft was transferred to the EMS while Killingbeck TB sanatorium was converted to ID use.[138] Beds at Seacroft were increased to 964, operating theatre, X-ray and physiotherapy units were installed and patient throughput was increased with the opening of a convalescent annexe. Sheffield municipal provision was less affected by the EMS and, overall, council hospitals contributed little, receiving no war casualties until 1944.[139] However, bomb damage did cause significant disruption, affecting Nether Edge, the Jessop and SRH directly and leading to the evacuation of the Children's Hospital for much of the war.[140]

With the end of the war approaching both the local authorities and the Ministry of Health conducted surveys of hospital provision.[141] In the latter case, the provision in Leeds was reviewed very favourably, especially the levels of co-operation between the voluntary and municipal sector and relations with the medical school,[142] while the assessment of Sheffield was far less complimentary, for though the fabric was deemed satisfactory, the organization of medical staff, management structures and relations with the university were all condemned.[143]

The Yorkshire surveyors were particularly interested in the physical fabric of the hospitals, medical staffing, levels of co-ordination (including with universities where these existed) and the scale and standard of specialist services. The Yorkshire team rated LGI as 'of a high standard', requiring no further comment on its professional capabilities. They were less impressed with the building which did 'not lend itself to the developments which are now required of a key hospital', recommending extensions to include accommodation for ophthalmology, orthopaedics, gynaecology (to be brought from the Hospital for Women), paediatrics, radiotherapy, thoracic surgery and clinical laboratories.[144]

Elsewhere, they commended the Leeds Public Dispensary (LPD) and deemed the work undertaken by the LHW excellent but felt the latter was too small for the demand. St James's was similarly applauded as 'it is obvious that the Health Authority are very much alive to what a modern hospital should be and are striving to their utmost to attain this object'.[145] About Seacroft they stated only 'This is a first-class infectious diseases hospital in every respect and needs no further comment on its equipment, staffing and organization'.[146] Even St Mary's and St George's gave a good impression as chronic case institutions, though their specialist maternity and TB accommodation was inadequate. Only the LMH attracted sustained criticism, the surveyors commenting they 'were not favourably impressed with this hospital. The building is not suited by its internal construction for good hospital work and administration, and the general effect produced upon the Surveyors was rather depressing'.[147] Further concerns included overcrowding, the absence of separate labour rooms, inadequate arrangements for isolation and no night nursery. Although they exonerated the professional standards of medical and nursing staff, their conclusion was:

> In the opinion of the Surveyors this hospital is out-of-date, and should be replaced by a modern institution of larger size. When this is done there should be considered the alternatives of providing either a separate maternity hospital or making it an individual unit or block of the extended LGI.[148]

The survey of Sheffield and the East Midlands was far less sympathetic, the strongest comments being saved for the organization and co-ordination of services. The United Hospitals (as the SRH and SRI were known following their amalgamation in 1939) lacked 'an effective common medical staff and the resulting duplication of special departments is wasteful'. Physically, the SRH was 'crowded on an inadequate site' where 'sound planning' was impossible while the Royal Infirmary's buildings were badly designed and 'ill arranged' so as to be inconvenient for administration.[149] The view of the City General was more favourable, for 'though handicapped by some old and unsatisfactory buildings, [it] takes a large share of the acute hospital work of Sheffield City'.[150] As elsewhere, the Children's Hospital was crowded onto an inadequate site while 'most of the buildings are old, ill-designed and overcrowded' and though the new Jessop Maternity Wing was commended, the gynaecology unit was located in the old buildings which were 'badly designed and have been damaged by enemy action'.[151]

As with the City General, comments about Firvale Institution were positive in the circumstances, and the surveyors were 'especially impressed by the system which is followed to prevent the premature classification of any patient as "chronic" and "incapable of treatment"'.[152] Lodge Moor, like Seacroft, received a glowing review with the design of the new wards 'admirable' and the general planning of the hospital 'excellent'. The TB hospitals, on the other hand, were 'unsatisfactory', especially Commonside, where 'the rooms are ill-adapted to use as wards for Tuberculosis' while the veranda wards were deemed 'even less suitable for the treatment of the disease'.[153]

Post War

Few physical changes were undertaken at the hospitals between the end of the war and the 'Appointed Day' when the NHS came into being. The main work involved moving units, such as the SRI's neurosurgery department, back to the main hospital centres from temporary wartime locations.[154] New provision included an Accident and Orthopaedic Unit at the Royal Infirmary, which opened in 1947 after considerable delay,[155] and a full outpatients unit at the Sheffield City General in 1945 while plans were approved for a new maternity unit at Nether Edge.[156] The situation was much the same in Leeds. The LGI developed as a regional hospital when it merged with the small Castleford and Normanton District Hospital while recognition as a National Radiotherapy Centre saw them open a Radiotherapy Unit at Hull Royal Infirmary.[157] St James's acquired the remaining part of Beckett St Institution, using it for chronic cases and some paediatric and dermatological patients. At St Mary's the war had seen the completion of a new maternity block raising the maternity accommodation to 106 beds while 107 remained designated for chronic sick, despite 'the immense difficulties which inevitably accompany the administration ... where two such distinct types of case are treated'. Concerns were also expressed about the TB unit at St George's, the Leeds A Hospital Management Committee lamenting the fact that 'owing to the admission of the more advanced type of case, the mortality rate is unduly high and this, along with the Poor Law stigma, has made it difficult to get treatable cases into these wards'.[158] Although Seacroft resumed its role as an ID institution, there was no longer the need for a 400-bed infectious diseases institution. As a result, 199 beds were retained for ID while the other 218 became a children's hospital, finally addressing a long-felt need in the city. Indeed the Ministry of Health surveyors had observed that the 'inadequacy of children's accommodation in the hospitals at Leeds is one of the most outstanding deficiencies',[159] although the decision to develop Seacroft did overturn a pre-war plan to build a new institution at Moortown.[160]

Conclusion

Relatively few new hospitals were built in England between the wars but those in existence grew significantly and, in particular, developed increasingly complex departments and facilities. Bed numbers in Leeds and Sheffield peaked in 1938 before the disruption of the war years and ensuing austerity reduced capacity across most institutions, especially the public hospitals. Between the wars growth in the voluntary sector varied from the sluggish – around 20 per cent increase in bed numbers at LGI – to enormous in the specialist institutions – 400 per cent at LMH. Conversely, few new beds were added to the municipal and poor law institutions but significant restructuring meant much more accommodation for acute and curative cases. In general the period saw a focus on services for women, children, the elderly and the middle class, especially in Leeds where maternity provision, gynaecology and private beds all flourished, reflecting the relative power of women and the middle class in the city's hospital politics. The period was also characterized by the creation of specialist departments and outpatient treatment which grew at a much faster rate than inpatient work. This required bigger, more efficient and effective outpatient and casualty units to admit, sort, record and treat the thousands of patients making hundreds of thousands of attendances each year.

However, the huge increase in the work of all of the hospitals created new challenges. The growing numbers of nurses and resident medical staff, along with the concomitant army of domestics, all needed to be housed, preferably away from the direct confines of the institutions. New technologies and scientific methods required space to accommodate X-ray and light departments, pathology and research laboratories and, increasingly, radium and radiotherapy facilities. Although both public and voluntary providers struggled to keep up with the demand for treatment and the ancillary costs of the massive expansion of patient numbers, it was the immediate aftermath of the First World War and the five years preceding the outbreak of the Second that witnessed the most growth in the hospital estate. This pattern was shaped both by the economic environment between the wars but also by the impetus given to hospital services by the 1929 Local Government Act which prompted upgrading at the former PLIs and stimulated action by the voluntary sector, sometimes in competition and sometimes in collaboration with their municipal partners. In particular, the emergence of the municipal general service, and the requirements of the 1929 Act that councils consult and work with the voluntary hospitals to avoid duplication, led to a more rational and efficient distribution of specialist services, which the next chapter will consider.

3 PATIENTS AND ACCESS

The provision of a modern and extensive hospital infrastructure, as seen in Leeds and Sheffield in the first half of the twentieth century, was intimately inter-twined with the growth and transformation of the patient population. Between the wars the general public acquired what one Leeds politician described as the 'hospital habit', with inpatient numbers increasing by about 35 per cent at the voluntary general hospitals, by around 300 per cent at the specialist hospitals and by at least 100 per cent in the municipal general institutions. By the out-break of the Second World War the cities' hospitals were treating around 58,000 inpatients – an overall increase of 65 per cent. Added to this impressive expan-sion was a growth of 50 per cent in the number of outpatients to 120,000 while casualties doubled to 80,000 and, most remarkable, outpatient and casualty attendances quadrupled to almost one million visits. Put another way, these combined figures were equivalent to one-fifth of the population of both cities receiving hospital treatment annually by 1938.

Inpatient and outpatient numbers rose across the country in this period[1] but the speed and shape of this growth in Leeds and Sheffield was determined to some extent by economic, social and political factors specific to the cities. Although there are clear signs that health care was becoming more democratic, this was not as yet a universal system and access to treatment was determined by a complex set of criteria. Securing a bed was governed by class, gender and age as well as the complexity or urgency of the condition. Moreover, the mix of factors varied from place to place with the shape and health of the local economy particularly important. In Sheffield strong unions in the metalworking industries developed a hugely successful contributory scheme with impressive employer support ensuring access for most working-class men. However, there is also evidence to suggest that women and children were major beneficiaries of the interwar expansion, especially in Leeds where, contrary to expectations, female patients were rather more likely to benefit from institutional care than men. This owed much to expansion at the existing specialist hospitals and to the development of a range of specialist services focused on meeting the needs of key social groups. In this, local political factors could be important, as council leaders, health committees and medical officers of health came to play a major role in the provision of general hospital treatment following the appropriation of the PLIs. In particular, their willingness to make the new hospitals accessible and their attitudes to working with the voluntary sector to maximize capacity were both significant in delivering growth.

But expansion also reflected general trends experienced across much of the country, including the decline of the traditional infectious diseases, the emergence of cancer and circulatory diseases as prominent killers and the changing age profile of the population, especially the increasing numbers of the elderly.[2] This chapter therefore will consider who the hospitals were for and how this changed over time; what criteria governed access; the growth of patient numbers; the shifting patient profiles across the sector as hospital treatment was democratized; the rise of the outpatient department; and the huge growth in casualty cases, especially as a result of road traffic accidents. It will suggest that while payment became the main condition for entry, thus opening up hospitals to a much wider range of the population, this was not at the expense of the traditional 'sick poor' who continued to secure treatment in both the voluntary hospitals and, increasingly, in the improved municipal generals.

Going to Hospital

Voluntary hospitals were focused on acute conditions which stood a good chance of being cured or 'materially relieved'. They were the main focus for accident and emergency cases in most cities while links to medical schools required a diversity of patients for training and research purposes. Initially they were charitable institutions established to provide free treatment to the 'sick poor' through the gifts of the wealthy and the unremunerated services of honorary medical staff.[3] As the 'hospital class' were unable to afford the services of a medical practitioner, access was restricted to suitable and deserving charitable cases. But this situation changed markedly after 1918 as more people secured non-charitable access by means of payment, forcing voluntary hospitals to adjust their mission away from a charitable gift to the sick poor to the voluntary delivery of a public service available to all.[4] This entry into the world of mass health care created financial, political and logistical challenges for the voluntary sector which were played out nationally in debates and policy decisions and on a daily basis in individual hospitals and their localities.[5]

Public hospitals were initially divided between the TB, infectious disease and mental health provision of the municipality and the poor law infirmaries operated by the boards of guardians until the 1929 Local Government Act.[6] Although neither body was obliged to provide hospitals they did have to make provision for the isolation and treatment of certain conditions and the priority they gave to these obligations varied considerably from place to place. Thus most public hospital provision in 1918 was residual, dealing with categories of patient eschewed by the voluntary hospitals. These included the infectious, the chronically sick, the infirm, the mentally ill, the tubercular, the incurable, the indigent, the 'dirty', the elderly – as well as respectable but difficult categories such as children and pregnant women. But these categories shifted as the number and type of infectious changed and as appropriation and reclassification saw poor law infirmaries transformed into municipal hospitals capable of treating a wider range of medical and surgical complaints.[7] Although the demographics of voluntary and public hospitals had not converged by the Second World War, the gap was certainly narrowing, yet a variety of factors still intervened to determine who received hospital treatment, where they received it and whether or not they had to pay.

Nature of Condition

Most voluntary general hospitals restricted admission with rules that classified both the objects of the institution and type of patient accepted. Derived from the eighteenth-century charitable foundations, like the Norfolk and Norwich Hospital, exclusions included paupers, those able to pay, the incurable, infectious, mentally ill, women about to give birth and small children.[8] In addition to these, as late as 1932 the North Riding Infirmary in Middlesbrough was still excluding patients more suited to other establishments, parochial relief or outpatient treatment and, significantly, those 'whose complaints are likely to be so tedious of cure as to preclude for a long time the admission of more urgent cases'.[9] Leeds General reflected these concerns and added epileptics, VD except those explicitly included, consumptives and those with 'habitual ulcers'.[10] The Sheffield hospitals, however, were more open, with a focus on need and income, the SRH targeting accidents and emergencies and 'persons who are unable to pay for medical attendance, and whose cases are found especially suitable for hospital treatment'[11] while the SRI declared itself 'Open to the Sick and Lame Poor of Every Nation'[12] – at least until 1929 when the hospital introduced an almoner department.[13]

The Leeds Public Dispensary (LPD) operated an open policy offering home visits for local residents in addition to a free service on an outpatient basis: 'To all poor persons who are unable to pay for medical assistance. Every applicant as qualified shall receive advice and medicine at the Dispensary or a branch at the appointed hour, without regard to place of abode.'[14]

Thus, general hospitals were not quite as general as they seemed, reserving their beds largely for the curable acute sick, with an increasing emphasis on surgical cases. The specialist voluntary hospitals were also restricted by demographic group – often those excluded from the general institutions – such as Sheffield Children's Hospital which treated children from birth to 14 years, and while 'no infectious cases are admitted', neither were letters of recommendation required.[15] The LHW admitted 'women suffering from diseases peculiar to their sex, if suitable cases' but emphasized that '**Ordinary medical and surgical complaints, common to both sexes are NOT ADMISSIBLE**'. Maternity cases were another problematic area for the voluntary sector. Prior to 1918 responsibility lay with the LMH and the Jessop Hospital for Women where maternity cases were admitted on income but after 1918 the public sector greatly expanded its maternity cover.[16]

Conversely, admission to a public hospital was more often required by local or national regulations, especially in the case of infectious disease or TB. As a result few local authorities charged although this did create anomalies where some infectious patients were admitted to the ID hospital for free and others ended up in the PLI and were charged for their care.[17] Moreover, patients and doctors had very different views of the purpose of a TB sanatorium and given the generally lengthy treatment regimes for TB, there was often resistance, especially among women, to these institutions.[18] Prior to appropriation, either the workhouse master or the relieving officer admitted most poor law infirmary patients. However, from the mid-1920s paying patients were seeking treatment at these hospitals, especially maternity cases and contributory scheme members. Manchester's PLIs had private wards in the 1920s, in Middlesbrough the PLI was popular as a maternity home and in Bristol around half of the admissions to Southmead were non-pauper patients.[19] Moreover, admissions were increasingly overseen by the medical superintendent of the hospital 'on direct application from the medical practitioners', or as transfers from the voluntary hospitals with very few coming through the relieving officer.[20] Some corporations were working with the guardians to develop integrated services, the socialist council in Sheffield funding the development of a new maternity unit at Nether Edge in 1927, while a number of boards of guardians made arrangements with contributory schemes to allow free emergency treatment for scheme members.[21]

Residence

In general, voluntary hospitals were open to residents from a wide geographical area. The proportion of 'country' patients could be as high as 45 per cent, as at LGI in the early 1930s, though usually the figure was somewhere between a quarter and a third, as evidenced by the 1945 hospital surveys.[22] In regional centres like Manchester, Birmingham and Norwich 'country' patients were a significant feature of the admissions, especially when specialist treatment was required.[23] This regional responsibility was a constant issue for hospital managers, leading Birmingham Women's Hospital to charge 'country' patients a fee and Newcastle RVI to make attempts to set a quota on the number of non-city admissions.[24] Leeds and Sheffield were clearly regional specialist centres, with their links to medical schools creating the demand for a range of cases to satisfy the needs of the medical degrees. There were some attempts to limit external patients, for example the LHW advising 'country' recommenders to submit their recommendation in advance to establish 'whether the case can be admitted',[25] but overall these institutions were open to all medically eligible patients.

Alternately, interwar local government finance prevented public hospitals from admitting patients from outside their administrative boundary except where arrangements for payment had been previously agreed. As such, the vast majority of poor law and municipal patients were resident in the towns under discussion with only a handful admitted from beyond the boundaries. There were some examples of arrangements to accept patients from other authorities, for example puerperal sepsis cases at Seacroft in Leeds, but the development of both specialist services and full co-operation with the voluntary sector were curtailed by the strict enforcement of these rules.[26] In Leeds by the later 1930s relations between the city council, WRCC and the voluntary hospitals were moving towards a regional arrangement of patients along agreed spheres of influence – but in Sheffield there is little evidence of similar developments.[27]

Patronage

By the turn of the twentieth century the subscriber-recommendation system was coming under pressure as new forms of income generation emerged. The recommendation system had been eased out in Newcastle and Middlesbrough before 1900 but it was still the norm in the hospitals of Bristol where workers' contributions were limited.[28] It continued in most hospitals in Leeds and Sheffield, though it was rarely advertised in the reports after the mid-1920s. At SRI, a complex tariff of privileges accompanied the various forms of giving, entitling subscribers, donors, clubs and societies and corporate bodies to recommend inpatients and outpatients, usually at a rate of one inpatient or four outpatients for two guineas.[29] At the SRH the privileges of subscription were less generous although firms, workmen, friendly societies and public bodies received 'all the privileges of individuals subscribing a similar amount'.[30] Only at LGI was the recommendation system definitely abandoned before the First World War. Moreover, by the 1920s very few patients presenting themselves to any of the hospitals relied on traditional patronage for access, most making some sort of payment. Although the majority benefitted from the coverage afforded by membership of a contributory scheme, a proportion, especially in the public hospitals, paid something towards their maintenance with the almoner emerging as a key figure in hospital access.

Payment

The interwar period is now recognized as one in which direct or indirect pay-ment largely replaced charity as the main non-medical criteria governing admission. Payment was already being utilized by some institutions before the First World War with hospitals for women and maternity institutions relying heavily on direct payment. Bristol Hospital for Women and Children set a five shilling fee for local patients,[31] a number of specialist hospitals in Birming-ham required patients to pay a registration fee, while in Leeds the Hospital for Women advertised that 'persons otherwise eligible, who are able to contribute towards their maintenance, may be admitted on such terms as the Committee may direct'.[32] Conversely, many children's hospitals, like those in Nottingham, remained free.[33]

However, as a result of the post-First World War financial crisis tariffs of charges emerged with patients assessed for their liability to pay. In the Sheffield hospitals a model for patient payment was introduced in 1922 by which:

> **IN-PATIENTS** – other than the necessitous poor (**who can at all times receive free treatment**), the Contributors to the 1d. in the £ Scheme, and their dependents, and children under 12 – are asked to pay a standard charge of 5/– per day towards the cost of maintenance. This amount may be varied upwards or downwards according to the circumstances of the patient.[34]

The LGI did not have fixed charges but used an almoner and a maintenance department to recover significant amounts from patients by the early 1930s. Income was also very important in the case of maternity hospitals, the LMH 'Rule 1' noting it was 'for the benefit of women unable to obtain the neces-sary attention at childbirth in their own homes. Each case to be investigated',[35] although the introduction of an almoner in the mid-1930s meant 'The cir-cumstances of patients shall be investigated with a view to ascertaining their suitability for admission to the Hospital and their ability to contribute towards the cost of treatment'.[36]

At the Jessop medical eligibility was largely absent from the published cri-teria for admission and although the free treatment of the necessitous poor remained central to admissions policy, complex arrangements were instituted revolving around the proportion of the National Insurance Maternity Benefit paid to the hospital dependent upon whether or not the patient was a member of the contributory scheme.[37]

The situation in public hospitals was complicated. Although there were exceptions such as Eastbourne that did charge,[38] treatment was free at Sheffield's Lodge Moor, King Edward VII Hospital, various TB institutions and the ID and TB hospitals of Leeds. Moreover, Sheffield's socialist authority opposed charging and though they appointed an almoner at Fir Vale 'in their opinion, the amount recovered does not render the procedure worthwhile'. Furthermore, the council was conscious of the anomaly whereby it was

> necessary to charge a patient suffering with pneumonia who is admitted to Fir Vale Hospital under Section 15 of the Local Government Act, whilst, on the other hand, a person admitted to the Lodge Moor Infectious Diseases Hospital and also suffering from pneumonia is not charged for maintenance or treatment.[39]

For the very poorest, treatment as either a charity or a public assistance case remained the main option, although in Leeds, 'Great use is made by poor persons of the Leeds Public Dispensary, whose Out-Patient Department deals with at least 30,000 cases annually. The Public Assistance Committee make a yearly subscription of £100 to the funds of the Dispensary.'[40]

This association between the PAC and the LPD was reinforced by Alderman George Martin, chairman of both bodies in the early 1930s, who observed patients at the Dispensary were from much the same class as those in the PLIs.[41] The role of this institution in supporting the city's hospitals was recognized by the surveyors of 1945 who reported that

> this Dispensary and Hospital fulfils a very valuable and useful function in the hospital service of Leeds and is a type of institution which might well be established in other large centres of population as a definite relief to the over-pressed out-patient departments of the general hospitals.[42]

In order to meet the cost of treatment and provide regular income for the voluntary hospitals, a range of schemes based on the small weekly contributions of workers emerged in the late nineteenth century and really expanded in the years following the First World War. Taking one of four organizational forms, the earliest were found in north-east England and parts of Scotland where accident hospitals in industrial areas saw workplace collections paid directly to individual hospitals. Where this type of funding predominated it was normal for the hospitals to abandon the recommendation system – as in Newcastle in the 1880s. Second were the Hospital Saturday Funds, town-wide workplace collections which distributed their income to the various medical charities of the locality proportionately on the basis of their expenditure. Hospital Saturday was widespread across the country by the First World War, though it was still seen as part of the charitable income of the institutions rather than as indirect payments.[43] The third form was the mutualist fund. Similar to Hospital Saturday, these were informed by concepts of self-help and mutual support rather than charity leading them to develop associational structures, including committees, branches and a range of social activities. Moreover, mutualist funds like the Leeds Workpeople's Hospital Fund (LWHF) acted in the interests of their members by supporting a range of health services including convalescent homes, ambulance services and district nurses.[44] Finally, contributory schemes emerged after the First World War as a response to the financial crisis. Merging aspects of Hospital Saturday and mutualist funds, the more successful operations were town wide, based on membership, developed forms of representation and set contribution rates and income limits for the membership.[45] By the later 1920s some were utilizing the Penny in the Pound method of collection pioneered by Sheffield where members saw a penny deducted from each pound of their earnings supplemented in some case by a contribution from employers. Collectively contributory schemes ensured free treatment when admitted to around 10 million workers and an equivalent number of dependents by the outbreak of the Second World War.[46]

Among those who had contributed to the schemes an expectation of entitlement to treatment developed along with a sense that they had made their contribution and should not be asked to pay again. Yet as Gosling and Gorsky, Mohan and Willis have shown, contributions did not buy an entitlement to treatment – only an entitlement to free treatment if admitted. The very success of the schemes in recruiting millions of members increased demand for services which in turn lengthened waiting lists and caused tension between members and hospitals.[47] The need to satisfy members' demands for treatment without additional cost prompted arrangements with the poor law and municipal hospitals to take members free of charge. Such agreements were operational in Manchester in the 1920s and in Burnley and Norwich by the mid-1930s, with the number of patients treated in the latter town rising significantly following appropriation of the PAI in 1941.[48] Arrangements were in place from the early 1920s in Sheffield[49] while a scheme was developed in Leeds in 1930 allowing LWHF members free treatment in the council hospitals. Although the arrangement was policed by strict rules, the numbers treated by the municipality increased from 350 in 1931 to over 5,000 by the end of the decade, ensuring quicker treatment for LWHF members and reducing the waiting lists at the voluntary hospitals.[50]

However, a particular issue dogging interwar institutions was the financial boundaries of the 'hospital class' and especially the upper limit for membership of the contributory schemes. The medical profession was anxious that treatment was restricted to income groups comparable to those covered by NI.[51] In the south-east the Hospital Savings Association (HSA) instituted strict limits on the earnings of members but in the big schemes of the provincial cities these were avoided and, as Gorsky, Mohan and Willis suggest, 'it seems that the better-off were simply trusted not to exploit the situation'.[52] In both Leeds and Sheffield the schemes avoided upper limits, the Penny in the Pound organizers claiming individual circumstances varied too much for a simple model to be fair. Clearly this was an unsatisfactory situation, leading to a major stand-off between the Sheffield scheme and its white-collar members at the end of the 1930s, although the opening of pay beds and the spread of provident schemes eased tension to some extent.[53]

Table 3.1: Source of patient maintenance, Sheffield voluntary hospitals, 1929 and 1938

1929

	Contributors to 1*d*. in £	%	Contributing towards maintenance	%	Admitted free incl. children under 12	%	Total
Infirmary	4,389	58.7	862	11.5	2,230	29.8	7,481
Hospital	2,414	48.4	309	6.2	2,261	45.4	4,984
Jessop	2,058	73.7	279	10	455	16.3	2,792
Children's	0		0		1,250	100	1,250
Total	8,861	53.7	1,450	8.8	6,196	37.5	16,507

1938

	Contributors to 1*d*. in £	%	Contributing towards maintenance	%	Admitted free incl. children under 12	%	Total
Infirmary	4,682	64.1	959	13.1	1,668	22.8	7,309
Hospital	3,709	61.5	666	11.1	1,654	27.4	6,029
Jessop	2,609	73.9	760	21.5	160	4.5	3,529
Children's					1,626	100	1,626
Total	11,000	59.5	2,385	12.9	5,108	27.6	18,493

Source: Sheffield Joint Hospitals' Council, *Annual Report*, 1929, p. 33; 1938, p. 47.

Contributory schemes were therefore central to hospital access and as Table 3.1 makes clear, a rising proportion of patients admitted to the Sheffield hospitals (though possibly fewer in Leeds) were members of contributory schemes or their dependents. Such figures compare favourably with trends in Bristol where those making no contribution to treatment fell to just 15 per cent at the Royal Infirmary by 1933 and around a quarter of admissions at the General Hospital in 1938.[54] Yet, despite the all-pervasive nature of the Penny in the Pound scheme and constant complaints that contributors were privileged over the sick poor, free patients remained a significant proportion of the city's admissions while direct payment at all but the Jessop was relatively rare.[55]

The Role of Almoners

Concerns about the boundaries of the hospital class, fears of 'abuse' of outpatient facilities, the need to establish who should pay and how much and a growing concern for the welfare of poorer patients encouraged voluntary and municipal hospitals to employ almoners in increasing numbers, especially after the First World War. The almoner is often depicted in popular histories as a heartless harridan who the grasping 'voluntary' institutions used to control 'means-tested access to beds' while in the post-1929 local authority sector it is claimed that in order 'to receive free treatment a patient was forced to undergo the indignity of a means-test conducted by a Lady Almoner'.[56] Yet Gosling's overview of the profession argues that almoners were in fact the key to the 'reciprocal economics' of the interwar voluntary system in which patients increasingly recognized their responsibility to contribute what they could in return for modern, disinterested hospital treatment.[57] This interpretation is broadly supported by the role of the almoners of Leeds and Sheffield. The LGI was one of the first provincial hospitals to employ an almoner – in 1910 – and by 1913 it employed three almoners, the number doubling by 1928.[58] The LMH made their first appointment in the early 1920s while the LHW did not employ an almoner until 1937. In Sheffield both the SRH and the Jessop made appointments in 1921 following the decision to levy charges while the SRI was rather slower, employing a woman to oversee the new After-Care Department instituted in 1928.

The almoner had a vital financial function, with most involved in interviewing the patients to identify whether they were eligible for treatment and if so whether they were required to pay. The workload could be enormous. At the Maternity Hospital in 1928 the almoner interviewed 5,435 outpatients while the team at the LGI saw all patients – assessing a total of 37,427 people in 1932.[59] By 1935 this had risen to over 50,000 following the decision to interview all X-ray and massage patients to 'ask for a donation from those able to give and who are not contributors to the Workpeople's Hospital Fund'.[60] At the Jessop the load was a little lighter for the single officer, who saw all 3,500 women admitted in 1938, while the new almoner at the LHW began by interviewing 250 patients a week though this fell to around 100 cases weekly in subsequent years.

Clearly, the almoner was intimately involved in policing the boundaries of admission. In 1938 the Almoner of SRI explained that her work included finding out how much a person could afford to pay and 'to prevent the abuse of a voluntary hospital' as it was 'to be remembered that the hospitals were charitable institutions to help those people who could not afford to pay for treatment'. But she was at pains to remind her audience that '"Penny in the £" contributors were exempt from payment for treatment when they needed it'.[61] Such statements could lead to a situation where 'Many are of the opinion that an almoner's duties consist of little but the extraction of money from unwilling patients' yet as the Secretary of the LHW went on to explain:

> in reality she may be of the greatest assistance to the patients and can facilitate their progress through the Hospital from their first attendance as an Out-patient to their discharge from the wards as a patient requiring convalescent treatment. It is hoped that all patients will regard her as a friend willing to help them in every way.[62]

Thus almoners were important in determining who was a suitable case for treatment in the transformed voluntary and public hospitals of the interwar period. Their front-line role was to establish, in the economy of reciprocity, what contribution a patient might reasonably be expected to make. In Sheffield this was relatively clear-cut as around two-thirds of patients treated were members of the Penny in the Pound scheme and a further 10 per cent were children. But in Leeds, and especially in the hospitals for women, the situation was more complex, entailing some close investigation of personal circumstances. But the interwar period also saw the almoner adopt a role much closer to that of the medical social worker, especially in Sheffield in the later 1930s, where the SRI's well-financed After-Care Department was providing services for thousands of patients.[63] Thus while their financial contribution was often fairly limited their overall contribution to the efficient operation of the institutions was becoming increasingly important.

The almoner was one manifestation of the changing social role of the hospital. The idea of the hospital patient as the object of charity or relief – the 'sick poor' or the 'infirm pauper' – was transformed in the later 1920s into a democratic ideal of hospital care by and for all. In 1929 the SRI abandoned its claim to be for the 'Sick and Lame Poor of every Nation', instead appealing for money on the basis that for 133 years it had 'served the needs of the Public as a Voluntary Hospital'.[64] Similarly for those raising funds to build a new hospital in Sheffield, ideas of charity had completely disappeared, the organizers observing that the 'great bulk' of the finance 'can only come from one source ... from the people of Sheffield and district ... from YOU'.[65] Similar trends were observed in other big cities. In Liverpool it was claimed that the effect of appropriation and changing public perceptions of poverty was to 'blur the once sharp line of demarcation between the voluntary and public hospitals' while the acquisition of the 'hospital habit' meant 'they are no longer places which the ordinary citizen avoids as long as he can', leading to a rapid growth in the hospital population.[66] In part this growth in patient numbers was determined by the shift from admission by patronage to the dominance of clinical criteria. As Gosling argues, once charity and pauperism were replaced by systems of patient payment, doctors asserted their right to admit to both voluntary and municipal hospitals on purely medical grounds, rapidly increasing the turnover of patients and changing the social relations between public and institution.[67]

Trends in Inpatient Numbers

Although the number of inpatients admitted to the hospitals of Leeds and Sheffield grew significantly between 1918 and 1948, this increase was not linear and equal for all of the sectors and was seriously disrupted by the Second World War. In the general voluntary hospitals (Table 3.2) the overall trend was an increase of just over 50 per cent in admissions between 1918 and 1938 with the number of patients rising from 19,500 at the end of the First World War to 28,000 on the eve of the Second World War. The biggest proportionate increase was seen at the SRH– a rise of 75 per cent – while in absolute numbers LGI reported the largest growth. Conversely, inpatient admissions were less than 20 per cent higher at the SRI. This pattern was similar to Bristol, where the Infirmary experienced a marked rise in inpatient numbers but growth at the General was notably lower.[68] Moreover, the trends were complex. Admissions peaked at LGI in 1928 – reflecting the absence of building in the 1930s – while the SRI reached maximum capacity in 1933. The Second World War disrupted admissions in Leeds but not Sheffield so that by 1947, the last year of full statistics, collectively the hospitals were treating 65 per cent more patients than in 1918.

Table 3.2: New inpatients at voluntary general hospitals: five-year intervals, 1918–47

	SRI	SRH	LGI	Total
1918	6,150	3,441	9,910	19,501
1923	5,445	3,631	11,253	20,329
1928	6,810	4,687	14,500	25,997
1933	8,012	5,140	14,154	27,306
1938	7,309	6,029	14,427	27,765
1943	7,796	7,891	14,279	29,966
1947	8,282	7,580	16,657	32,519

Sources: SRI, SRH, LGI, *Annual Reports*, 1918–47.

The incomplete evidence from the voluntary specialist hospitals (Table 3.3) suggests an even greater increase in usage.[69] Admissions more than doubled at all three hospitals for women between the early 1920s and the later 1930s – a pattern similar to that in Birmingham,[70] though modest in comparison to the huge rise in births at the Bristol Maternity Hospital in the 1930s.[71] Even the Sheffield Children's Hospital, where patients traditionally experienced longer stays, saw an increase of around a half between 1928 and 1938. Inpatient treatment was only introduced to the LPD in 1923, with the 336 admissions in the first year rising to 2,754 fifteen years later. These specialist services for women, children and the poorest were more adversely affected by the disruptions of the Second World War and by the emergence of local authority competition than was the case at the general hospitals.

Table 3.3: New inpatients at specialist hospitals: five-year intervals, 1918–47

	Jessop	Children's	LHW	LMH	LPD	Total
1918	1,502		901		–	2,403
1923	1,796		952		336	3,084
1928	2,761	1,176	1,175	1,908	1,009	8,029
1933	2,885	1,535	1,795	3,108	1,690	11,013
1938	3,529	1,626	2,165	3,984	2,754	14,058
1943	2,974		2,395	3,078	535	8,982
1947	4,015		2,778	3,064		9,857

Sources: Jessop, LHW, LMH, LPD and Sheffield Hospitals Council, *Annual Reports*, 1918–47.

From the early 1930s and especially in the 1940s, municipal providers emerged to meet the needs of many more patients (Table 3.4), with county boroughs averaging 42 per cent growth in admissions during the 1930s.[72] At St James's in Leeds and Sheffield's City General growth was rapid after 1930, admissions rising by about a third at St James's between 1928 and 1938 while at the City General comparable growth occurred in just five years. Mirroring developments in Bristol and Manchester, these institutions took patients from the waiting lists of the voluntary hospitals and developed casualty and maternity services.[73] Admittedly not all appropriated hospitals increased their admissions but where councils could appropriate more than one institution they were able to develop specialist services.[74] Thus both St Mary's and Nether Edge abandoned general hospital aspirations to concentrate on infirm, maternity and tubercular patients. As in the voluntary institutions, the war created diverse experiences for the municipal hospitals. At St James's numbers rose to peak in 1943 but then fell back while St Mary's became the council's main centre for maternity cases and took up some of the capacity lost by the maternity hospital from the early 1940s.

Table 3.4: New inpatients at public hospitals: five-year intervals, 1918–47

	St James's	St Marys	Sheffield City General	Total
1918				
1923				
1928	6,403			6,403
1933	8,090	1,497	6,754	16,341
1938	8,588	1,190	9,832	19,610
1943	10,925	1,003	10,590	22,518
1947	9,427	2,693	12,316	24,436

Sources: MOH Leeds, MOH Sheffield, *Annual Reports*, 1928–47.

However, not all hospitals experienced unbroken growth. The ID institutions (Table 3.5) saw a rather erratic pattern over the thirty years 1918–48. The unpredictable nature of epidemics notwithstanding, the period witnessed the disappearance of smallpox and wild fluctuations in scarlet fever and diphtheria. Moreover, many fewer cases of scarlet fever required hospitalization and when Seacroft reopened as an ID institution in 1946 almost half of the beds were permanently empty. Admissions for TB treatment followed a similar pattern in Leeds to other infectious diseases and with changes in treatment practices the number of patients admitted declined from the mid-1920s. In Sheffield, however, TB was taken very seriously and from the mid-1920s around three times as many patients were admitted to TB institutions than were treated institutionally in Leeds.

Table 3.5: New inpatients at specialist public hospitals: five-year intervals, 1918–47

	Leeds ID	Lodge Moor	Leeds TB	Sheffield TB
1918	1,778	3,770	699	839
1923	3,284		1,089	
1928	4,156	3,189	780	3,070
1933	5,387	3,176	583	2,988
1938	3,269	2,936	517	1,033
1943	2,674	4,255	305	1,090
1947	1,782	2,284	404	1,251

Sources: MOH Leeds, MOH Sheffield, *Annual Reports*, 1918–47.

Trends in Outpatient Numbers

The period under review also saw a notable rise in new outpatients, an enormous increase in outpatient attendances and a marked growth in casualty cases prompted by greater specialization and new diagnostic and therapeutic techniques which required little or no inpatient treatment. Voluntary hospitals had a rather ambiguous attitude to their outpatient departments. In the nineteenth century they had been the focus of conflict over 'abuse' by patients able to pay,[75] but increasingly institutions recognized that non-resident treatment could serve a number of important functions. For example, the OP department was an effective way of sorting and progressing patients through the mass health-care system now facing many large voluntary hospitals.[76] Furthermore, they allowed non-clinical staff to treat large numbers of patients using new techniques and technologies such as ultraviolet (UV) light treatment, massage, X-ray (for diagnosis and treatment) and orthoptics.[77] The growth in OP registrations nationally was substantial. The two Bristol hospitals saw 100,000 new outpatients and Liverpool's eight teaching hospitals registered 300,000 a year by 1938 while in Birmingham and Norwich the figure roughly doubled between 1918 and 1938.[78] Moreover, the number of attendances patients made, especially for conditions like VD, skin diseases and physiotherapy, could be significant.

New outpatients at the main general hospitals of Leeds and Sheffield (Table 3.6) grew by a little under 40 per cent between 1918 and 1938, a similar figure to inpatients. However, the pattern was rather different – with SRI seeing almost twice as many new outpatients by 1938, LGI increasing at above the average rate (66 per cent) between the wars and by more than 150 per cent by 1947, while at the SRH the change was scarcely more than 10 per cent with numbers at the LPD falling. Attendances, however, more than tripled to reach over 900,000 by the eve of the Second World War and, despite slight falls in Sheffield, remained at or above this figure on the eve of the NHS. Both proportionate and absolute growth was greatest at the LGI where there were quarter of a million more attendances while the figure more than doubled at the LPD. On the other hand they were flat at SRH, the institution which had seen the greatest inpatient expansion.[79] The voluntary specialist hospitals also developed outpatient departments but these were less extensive than the general institutions. At the maternity and women's hospitals new registrations grew slowly from around two to four thousand between the wars but at the children's hospital in Sheffield there was a sharp decline following the closure of their separate outpatient centre in the working-class east end – attendances halving from almost 100,000 in 1928 to less than 50,000 ten years later.[80]

Table 3.6: New outpatients and outpatient attendances, general hospitals, 1918–47

	SRI	SRH	LGI	LPD	Total
		New outpatients			
1918	21,699	28,157	17,622	14,146	81,624
1928	26,880	32,765	26,260	13,415	99,320
1938	40,486	31,372	29,362	13,593	114,813
1947	44,525	28,315	46,537		109,874
		Total outpatient attendances			
	SRI	SRH	LGI	LPD	Total
1918	63,032		141,915	74,336	279,283
1928	150,477	128,300	324,146	97,217	700,140
1938	228,113	138,530	390,338	163,325	920,306
1947	165,778	120,747	555,480		842,005

Sources: SRI, SRH, LGI, LPD, *Annual Reports*, 1918–47.

The municipal hospitals did not, in general, develop outpatient facilities before the coming of the NHS, though there were some departments created. Nationally, Powell's evidence shows outpatient attendances in municipal general hospitals rose from three quarters of a million in 1931 to two and a quarter million in 1938 – growth of 200 per cent. Yet, as the Liverpool Voluntary Hospital Commission explained, the city's municipal institutions 'have no out-patient departments in the proper sense of the term' although they did not 'neglect to "follow up" with advice or additional treatment any patients who require supervision after their discharge from hospital'.[81] Indeed most of the outpatient work was concentrated on servicing the needs of long stay, infirm and elderly patients rather than as an alternative, precursor or aftercare for the specialist departments.

In Leeds and Sheffield different policies were followed in relation to outpatients. In Leeds it was agreed that these would be concentrated at the LGI while St James's and St Mary's would only have 'follow on' departments to retain continuity for discharged patients needing further treatment or monitoring.[82] In Sheffield, however, the numbers involved were growing, at the City General, 2,000 outpatients made 10,000 visits by the eve of the war. On the other hand, both cities established non-institutional clinics for the management of antenatal and TB outpatients. Together these saw thousands of individuals annually and relieved the hospitals of much routine observational work and minor procedures.[83] Although not the full polyclinics imagined by Dawson, they did act as a central focus for municipal health care, with their focus on TB and maternity augmented by advice, welfare services and access to medical practitioners. Nor were these the 'prosperous' areas Webster claimed were the main beneficiaries of health centres, but cities struggling with unemployment and poverty.[84]

Patient Types

There has been very little in the way of detailed analysis of the gender, age and class distribution of hospital patients in interwar England. Yet a general consensus exists that women were disadvantaged, a recent general account claiming that the 'great majority of women, who fell outside the provisions of National Insurance, experienced little expansion in the facilities available for medical advice and treatment'.[85] It is often suggested that the general exclusion of both hospital benefits and women and children from National Insurance limited access to hospital beds and may also have contributed to women enduring long-term, untreated gynaecological problems.[86] Yet as we have seen, the main areas of growth in institutional provision between the wars were in services for women and children.

The evidence for Leeds (Table 3.7) reveals a surprising division between men and women. Although LGI normally admitted a quarter to a third more male than female patients, across all of the city's acute facilities there were around 50 per cent more women admitted by the 1930s. These differences are partly explained by the separate Hospital for Women taking all of the gynaecological work from 1933 and partly by the very high level of maternity admissions which accounted for a significant proportion of the women taken by St James's and St Mary's. Moreover, there were also a larger number of female admissions generally at both municipal institutions, whether chronic or acute. Indeed, it is possible that many of those admitted from the LGI waiting list through the arrangement with the LWHF were women.[87] There is, therefore, abundant evidence to suggest women benefitted significantly from the expansion of hospital provision between the wars, especially at dedicated institutions and in the municipal sector.

Table 3.7: Hospital patient admissions by gender, Leeds, 1918–47

	LGI	LHW	LMH	St James's	St Marys	Total
			Male inpatients			
1918	3,551					3,551
1923	4,700					4,700
1928	6,308					6,308
1933	6,514			2,980	421	9,915
1938	6,565			3,741	275	10,581
1943	5,826			2,843	171	8,840
1947	7,348					7,348

	LGI	LHW	LMH	St James's	St Mary's	
			Female inpatients			
1918	3,034	901				3,935
1923	3,800	952				4,752
1928	4,972	1,175	1,908			8,055
1933	4,715	1,795	3,108	3,949	960	14,527
1938	4,585	2,165	3,984	5,410	910	17,054
1943	5,527	2,395	3,078	5,299	813	17,112
1948	5,825	2,778	3,064			11,667

Sources: LGI, LHW, LMH, LPD, MOH Leeds, *Annual Reports*, 1918–47.

Unfortunately the evidence from Sheffield is not as detailed, but what exists suggests admission rates were broadly similar for men and women, with more men admitted to the general hospitals, especially for surgery and accidents, although this was balanced by the large amount of general work undertaken by the Jessop Hospital for Women. Moreover, the separate children's hospital freed beds for adults in the main general institutions. Evidence from the municipal hospitals points to more women than men being admitted, partly due to the maternity units at both the City General and Nether Edge which accounted for some of the 1,500 additional female admissions. However, as in Leeds there were also more chronic female than male patients, especially PAI bedridden and mental health cases.[88]

The needs of children were met effectively in Sheffield where there was a children's hospital plus beds in the general institutions and extensive accommodation for both early onset TB and non-pulmonary and orthopaedic cases.[89] Admissions increased by 50 per cent at the Children's Hospital in the 1930s, around 1,800 child TB cases were seen by the Health Department while almost all the patients at the Orthopaedic Hospital and the ID institutions were under sixteen. The situation in Leeds was less encouraging. Child admissions to the LGI rose from 1,800 in 1922 to a high of 2,850 in 1930 but stagnated thereafter, falling to less than a fifth of the total admissions during the 1940s.[90] The opening of St James's added significantly to capacity while the LPD taking on tonsils and adenoid work – a category sometimes transferred to municipal hospitals, as in

Barnsley – also made a difference.[91] Although ID provision was more than adequate most of the time, this was not the case for TB and in contrast to Sheffield
fewer than a hundred children per annum were treated in the 1930s. Provision
for non-pulmonary TB and orthopaedic work was similarly inadequate yet the
waiting list for institutional places for tubercular children of either type was
small.[92] In part this was due to more effective treatment, and the duration of
stay for children at King Edward VII's in Sheffield fell from almost two years in
1920 to around nine months just seven years later.[93] But the need for a children's
hospital in Leeds remained a priority, the lack of suitable accommodation for
the young being one of the few areas of weakness identified by the 1945 survey.[94]

Who attended which hospital was partly filtered by income, which was in
turn policed by the almoner. At one end was a small and declining group admitted to the public hospitals by the relieving officer.[95] Very different attitudes to
this group were evident in Leeds and Sheffield in the early 1930s. Thus, many
sick and infirm were still being admitted as public assistance cases in Leeds
despite the slowly changing profile of St James's. In Sheffield, as in Bristol where
the Health Committee declared the new hospitals would 'remove the stigma
of pauperism',[96] the council was seeking to limit, as far as possible, use of the
Relieving Officer in medical cases.[97] But after appropriation Leeds followed suit,
the first report of the Joint Hospitals Advisory Committee in 1936 explaining
that: 'The municipal hospitals ... have been developed ... for the treatment of all
classes of the community, the criterion for treatment being medical need rather
than destitution'.[98]

Moreover, the expansion of acute treatment in the public general hospitals
brought younger and better-paid patients into this sector[99] and although the
City General in Sheffield accommodated

> mainly medical cases and only a limited number of surgical cases, yet the turnover
> of the latter is considerable. It is anticipated that the development of the casualty
> work consequent on the opening of the new department will result in a considerable
> increase in surgical cases and notably of fracture work.[100]

Similarly, in Leeds a careful reorganization of the four council institutions available to the Public Assistance Committee/Public Health Committee allowed the
admission of many more acute and surgical cases to St James's and an increase
in the maternity work at St Mary's. Furthermore, in Sheffield, and to a lesser
extent Leeds, many of the unemployed were able to continue paying into the
contributory schemes and thus retain their right to free treatment in the voluntary hospitals – an option unavailable in Middlesbrough where public assistance
admissions increased in the early 1930s.[101]

As contributory schemes in these cities resisted fixing upper income limits for their contributors, the hospital class widened significantly between the

wars. The necessitous poor were still notionally those with first call but in teaching hospitals especially, medical need and diversity were more likely to govern admission than income. And despite a rhetoric which claimed the wealthier contributors to schemes were simply making a charitable contribution,[102] it is clear that by the Second World War all workers and many in the lower ranks of the middle class were eligible for free treatment in the big city hospitals.[103]

But this broadening of the hospital population created demand from some middle-class groups for hospital treatment.[104] As we have seen, almoner assessments attempted to determine ability to pay but a more practical response was the development of private wards.[105] These provided accommodation and nursing only, medical supervision being organized separately with the overseeing surgeon or physician. The Jessop claimed their new block would 'cater for all, from those who cannot afford full Nursing Home fees, but who can pay something, up to the patient who desires a private bathroom, etc'.[106] Women were a particular focus of early private accommodation with the first ward in Leeds at the LHW while extensive provision was initiated at the Jessop in 1938. Indeed services for women were in the forefront of paying provision, with the first private beds in Nottingham, Birmingham, Bristol and Middlesbrough all aimed at female patients.[107] In part this was because women, especially if unmarried, were less likely to be covered by contributory schemes while they were more likely to remain on waiting lists longer than men, encouraging the better off to seek private care.[108]

The Casualty Department

Accidents and casualty cases had always been central to the work of the voluntary hospitals. However, between the wars the role and demographic profile of the casualty receiving room was transformed by a number of factors including National Insurance, pressure from workers for better accident treatment – a case they could increasingly press given their prominent role in funding hospitals – and the dangers posed by the emergence of the motor car. With all of the voluntary hospitals seeing a marked rise in casualty admissions (Table 3.8), how they dealt with them and the extent to which a specialized service emerged varied by city and institution.[109]

Table 3.8: New casualty admissions and attendance: selected years, 1918–47

	SRI		SRH		LGI		LPD	
	Casualty	Attendances	Casualty	Attendances	Casualty	Attendances	Casualty	Attendances
1918	19,777	45,167	13,417		11,653		9,104	74,336
1928	27,355	77,219	18,473	80,190	16,513	46,711	10,165	97,217
1938	20,307	58,201	24,880	65,558	26,447	63,369	19,277	163,325
1947	25,237	63,574	30,690	63,747	24,961	48,077		

Sources: SRI, SRH, LGI, LPD, *Annual Reports*, 1918–47.

In Sheffield (including Children's Hospital and City General cases) new casualty patients increased by about one-third from 33,000 to 50,000 annually. In Leeds the proportionate growth was much greater – more than doubling from 20,000 to 45,000. Casualty attendances, however, peaked at the end of the 1920s and drifted downwards to a ratio of roughly two attendances per patient. The reasons for this growth are not clear. It has been linked to the National Insurance Act but the chronology is too irregular – with most growth in Sheffield in the 1920s and in Leeds in the 1930s[110] – although panel doctors may have had an incentive to push difficult patients on to hospital accident and emergency departments.[111] A sharp rise in the early 1930s may have been the result of the economic crisis, especially the loss of access to panel doctors for the unemployed – though evidence for this is contradictory. Hospital managers favoured road traffic accidents as a significant factor in the increase.[112] Coverage by contributory schemes, particularly for women, may have encouraged use of hospitals rather than general practitioners while a greater awareness of the risks associated with injuries may have led more people to seek help. Nor were Leeds and Sheffield alone in experiencing rises in receiving room demand as road, domestic and workplace accidents all contributed in different ways to a growing problem.[113]

The significant growth in casualty work after 1918 encouraged institutions to seek ways to rationalize entry and distribute cases – at first within the hospital but subsequently across the whole sector.[114] Thus in 1925 the LGI moved its casualty department to the outpatient entrance, making it 'the portal to all departments of Infirmary work'. Similar to the 'sorting room' at St Thomas' in London, minor cases could be treated at once, preventing 'the Out-patient department being overloaded with trivial cases'. An almoner was appointed for the receiving room to cut down on free riders.[115] In Sheffield the move was the other way, as the SRI separated the casualty and outpatient departments. The new block, completed in 1929, would 'liberate congestion in the old Out-Patients Department' and by focusing on casualty treatment and well-organized registration procedures, 'enable the Infirmary to deal more effectively and efficiently with the increasing demands'. Approximately 1,000 casualty and OP attendances daily prompted a similar response from the SRH who opened a new casualty department where it was 'hoped that with alterations to the Out-patient Department and the provision of a Registration Building, the efficiency of these departments will be further increased'.[116] Indeed it is possible that the large growth in casualty attendees in Sheffield in the 1920s was due to inaccurate recording of outpatient and casualty cases, with more efficient recording systems producing a sharp fall in the 1930s.[117] This was aided in 1934 by the reorganization of the outpatient department which placed 'the Infirmary in a thoroughly up-to-date position'.[118] These developments demonstrate the drive for the scientific management of patients emphasized by Sturdy and Cooter and was particularly evident in the Infirmary's new registration block which may have been informed by American hospital management practice.[119]

The modernization of casualty and outpatient facilities was accompanied by citywide organization of patient allocation and admission with local circumstances dictating how this was done. The plan devised for joint working in Sheffield saw a casualty unit at the City General as a central plank of the co-ordination of services, for

> the increasing number of street accidents requiring admission to the Voluntary Hospitals was a factor in swelling the waiting lists owing to the surgical beds being occupied by such patients. It was decided to provide a fully equipped Casualty Department at the City General Hospital which would not only reduce the number on the waiting lists but would provide improved facilities for patients suffering from accidents.[120]

Moreover it was proposed that 'the city shall be divided into three areas ... with the police ... drafting accidents to the appropriate hospital assigned to the area'. This arrangement was supported by the organization of all ambulances in the city under the control of the Hospitals Council and located at a central ambulance station.[121] As Pickstone notes for Manchester, the policy of zoning for casualties was important not just in increasing A&E capacity but also in raising the status of the municipal general hospitals with the hospital chosen being 'determined by geography not by the status of the hospital or the patient'.[122] In Sheffield the zoning of street accidents was commenced in 1935 but as the new casualty unit at the City General was under-resourced, it proved unable to meet its full obligation.[123] Yet by 1938 it was treating 6,000 casualties, around a fifth of the figure at the SRH, while accidents received at the SRI had fallen by the same number since 1930, suggesting some reallocation of the burden.[124] Moreover, by 1945 a degree of specialization had developed at the casualty departments of the city as 'Heavy industrial casualties tend to be concentrated on the Royal Infirmary and the Royal Hospital takes casualties from lighter industry'.[125]

In Leeds, where the LGI remained politically dominant, all new casualty and outpatients were admitted through the receiving room at the Infirmary to the most appropriate department or institution. For example, a proportion of accidents, suicides and emergency cases would be referred to St James's to relieve pressure at the LGI. However:

> Owing to the fact that there is as yet no casualty department at the latter hospital, it was decided that for the time being the Infirmary Casualty Department should serve the needs of both institutions, suitable cases being diverted to St. James's Hospital by the Receiving Officers.[126]

Once a casualty unit was set up at St James's it was expected that the city would be zoned for accidents. But as was the case in Manchester, progress was slow, the medical superintendent explaining in 1938 that the 'question of the Casualty Department has not yet received more than preliminary thought and might well be the subject of a discussion by the Joint Hospitals Advisory Committee'.[127] This was clearly not a priority for the Health Department, with no progress made in 1939, although around one thousand accident cases were treated at St James's in 1938, contributing to the growing number of operations recorded at the institution.[128]

Road Accidents

Although industrial accidents were an accepted part of hospital work, the increased speed and volume of road vehicles, especially cars, motor cycles and pedal cycles, put drivers, passengers and pedestrians at greater risk and placed a significant burden on the receiving rooms of the voluntary hospitals.[129] The road traffic accident crisis was intense but relatively short-lived, coinciding with the first boom in popular car ownership after 1924.[130] Comment and concern became commonplace from 1927 as the hospitals reported increasing numbers of cases but little or no income to meet the cost while the severity of the injuries was believed to lead to bed blocking.[131] As the SRH *Annual Report* observed, 'Motor Accidents ... occupy beds much longer than the average surgical cases do and this factor largely accounts for the number of patients who are awaiting admission to the surgical wards'.[132]

The number of road accident victims was higher in Leeds[133] than Sheffield, with the burden falling unevenly on the institutions. LGI received five times more street casualties than the LPD while in Sheffield the SRH saw twice as many as the SRI. Street accidents in Leeds rose from approximately 400 in 1924 to settle at some 1,500 annually during the early 1930s, with around half detained in the hospital for treatment. These figures were substantially higher than in Manchester where road accident victims admitted to the wards numbered just over two hundred in 1932.[134] The evidence for Sheffield is less clear-cut, with numbers falling in the early 1930s but then climbing from 1934. The LGI calculated most road cases stayed for around twelve days and collectively occupied twenty beds a day, with one surgeon claiming they blocked beds that might have been used to treat more worthy cases, like those suffering from cancer.[135] Although similar concerns were expressed in Sheffield,[136] the enduring disquiet was the cost of the patients and the difficulties encountered in recovering payment.

Anxious comments about the financial burden of treating road accidents first appeared in 1927, the Leeds Public Dispensary claiming that 'very many' of the additional 2,000 casualties seen over the preceding five years 'arise from motor accidents, and the expense thus thrown upon the Institution ... is causing the Board considerable anxiety. So far, no solution has been found for recovering payment from the parties at fault in this type of case.'[137]

Similarly, T. F. Braime of the LGI despaired that 'It seemed most absurd that people who owned motor cars, many of them with plenty of money, should put this hospital to a cost of £4,400, and yet reimburse the Institution to the extent of only £62. ("Shame")',[138] while the SRI added that:

> These patients in many cases were poor, and could make no recompense to the Institution for their treatment. Our enquiries show that many owners of cars concerned have been found to be uninsured and quite unable to compensate the injured patient when called upon to do so.[139]

The voluntary hospitals were further angered by the inequitable basis of existing insurance regulations, for while PLIs and nursing homes could claim against the insurance companies,[140] drivers or their insurers could 'escape liability, simply because the injured person is treated by a voluntary institution maintained by public beneficence'.[141] The hospitals mounted a national campaign to mobilize public opinion in favour of compulsory insurance on the motorists although they were in a difficult position as 'They could not, of course, threaten the Government to turn such cases away, because, unlike local poor law institutions, they were obliged to keep their doors open'.[142]

Institutions with casualty departments put much faith in the 1930 Road Traffic Bill.[143] However, despite Abel-Smith's suggestion that the voluntary hospitals benefitted financially as the Act 'compelled' insurance companies to pay the treatment costs of victims, in reality it proved to be a big disappointment as hospitals only received payment from the companies if 'a claim for damage is proved or accepted'.[144] Thus for the SRI 'the position is worse than before', with the hospital receiving payment in only 14 out of 94 claims to insurance companies,[145] a similar situation to Manchester where the Royal Infirmary recovered just one-third of the £1,095 spent treating 214 inpatients in 1932.[146]

Despite initial disappointment, there is evidence that more was being recovered to meet the cost of road accidents – at both receiving room and inpatient stage. SRI was able to reclaim more than three-quarters of the costs in 1932 while LGI announced that although the amount was still low it was 'an appreciable increase on the previous year and compares favourably with the experience of other Hospitals'.[147] Finally, the 1934 Road Traffic Act introduced payments 'irrespective of the question of liability, of 12s.6d. per case for Emergency Treatment, where first given at the Infirmary'.[148] As a result LGI were recovering almost 60 per cent of costs of the inpatients along with a further £500 from the casualty room by 1936. Furthermore, the Sheffield hospitals began to place an increasing emphasis on supporting the work of the Safety First campaign as the state increasingly focused on attempts to educate the population in the need for safer behaviour in all environments – although this may indicate the triumph of the wealthy car lobby over the poor pedestrian.[149] SRH applauded 'the increased attention which is being given to the toll of accidents in the streets, in the industrial establishments and in the homes'.[150] In 1935 they focused specifically on the roads, revealing that over the preceding five years, while fatal accidents averaged 58, non-fatal accidents had risen from 1,569 in 1931 to 2,025. Thus, 'As the Royal Hospital is the most popular receiving depot for Traffic Accidents the vigorous activities of the Minister of Transport are very welcome'.[151]

From this point, the Sheffield hospitals stopped worrying about road accidents but with the coming of war, blackout conditions led to a sharp rise in road accidents across the country, resulting in Leeds' highest number of casualties ever and the most inpatients since 1933.[152]

Conclusion

The thirty years between the end of the First World War and the inauguration of the NHS saw hospital inpatient and outpatient numbers rise inexorably. Despite the depressed state of the local economy all institutions, except those for infectious diseases, experienced significant growth. Admittedly this was not evenly spread between the hospitals, sectors or across time, but by the end of the Second World War it had markedly increased the opportunity of hospital treatment for most of the population on a fairly equal basis. The greatest beneficiaries of this change were women, especially in Leeds, with maternity services, as we will see, at the centre of this expansion – although it is evident that women's access to gynaecology and general medicine made notable advances. Children, though less well served in Leeds than Sheffield, also enjoyed increased access while the elderly and the chronically ill saw their experience of treatment as well as their likelihood of receiving it, improve. At the other end of the social scale the lower middle class were much more likely to gain entry to hospital wards and outpatient departments through their membership of contributory schemes, while those on the next rung up the social ladder were granted pay bed facilities which seem to have benefitted women disproportionately.

Much of this was similar to trends in other large towns and cities which also experienced expansion in the number of inpatients and outpatients seen, particularly strong growth in the better municipal hospitals and a falling-off in the need for isolation in ID institutions. But there were also elements which were more particular to Leeds and Sheffield, shaped by local economic and social patterns and political preferences. Thus, the prominence afforded to services for women owed much to the important role of women in the economy and local health governance. The depression clearly weakened the ability of the institutions to expand capacity, especially once the main efficiency gains of the early to mid-1920s had been effected. This was especially the case in the large voluntary general hospitals – though it also impacted on the ability of the appropriated municipal hospitals to undertake capital projects until the later 1930s. Like the voluntary hospitals in the 1920s, they concentrated on organization and efficiency in these early years of municipal control – increasing throughput, expanding surgery cases and redistributing patients across their institutions. In this they had the advantage only really available to the larger authorities of more than one site – although notably Hull, with two institutions, failed to develop a modern municipal service before the Second World War.[154]

It is also apparent that behind these figures there were a range of political considerations influencing outcomes. We have noted – and will return to – the place of women in the health politics of the two cities, but the impact of the labour movement was also important in creating and sustaining very different contributory systems. It also influenced the type of party politics played out in the council chamber, where the broader middle class of Leeds gave strength to a conservative party initially opposed to appropriation while the power of Labour in Sheffield led to early appropriation and an increasingly independent, competitive approach by the Second World War. But socio-economic factors also had an impact on the mix of services offered and the growth of hospital specialization, to which we now turn.

4 SPECIALIZATION AND THE CHALLENGES OF MODERN MEDICINE

As hospital patients diversified in the first half of the twentieth century, so too did the institutions and staff who treated them. New techniques and knowledge, medical markets and the desire to order and manage patients all influenced the emergence of hospital specialization and by the arrival of the NHS the population at large increasingly identified the hospital as a centre of specialist treatment. Moreover, as the population became healthier and wealthier their expectations of hospitals changed. They began to see them as places where modern medicine would cure or at least repair them while their financial contributions gave them a sense of entitlement to the best, most advance care. These new demands from a more affluent and democratic society produced variable responses, reflecting the effects of the economy and the relationships and hierarchies within the different hospital structures. They also added a new element to the stimulus to special services – local need. Rather than the diversity of specialist provision reflecting the failings of a system which had arisen without the benefits of rational planning, difference may have emerged from priorities shaped by specific economic and social structures and the ensuing political priorities. This chapter will consider the development of specialist services, especially those emerging between the wars, such as mental health outpatient services, and will then address two case studies which illuminate the influence of local economic, social and political factors in the shaping of orthopaedic and maternity services. It will show that while the development of new specialities was limited and not particularly novel, in these key areas of maternity and orthopaedics Leeds and Sheffield developed as important regional centres under the influence of both local need and national policy. In particular, it will demonstrate that by building on the gender structures of the labour market and society, Leeds produced more highly developed maternity services yet weaker orthopaedic provision than Sheffield.

Developing Specialization

As we have seen, the first half of the twentieth century saw a huge growth in the use of hospital services and their extension to almost every social and demographic group. The acquisition of the hospital habit both encouraged the development of medical specialization and forced hospitals to develop ways to accommodate the increasing numbers of patients demanding their right to treatment. As a result institutions subdivided their activities so that by the 1940s the general medical and surgical departments were supplemented by a wide range of specialities. Historians have debated the reasons for this, initially emphasizing the impact of scientific and technical advances;[1] from the 1980s the focus shifted to the interests of medical practitioners and individual philanthropists in the establishment of specialist institutions. In particular, failure in the competition for hospital positions and access to wealthy patients encouraged some doctors to carve a niche in the medical marketplace by setting up their own hospitals.[2] Subsequent research has tempered this view by highlighting the importance of funders as well as medics in the foundation, and especially the continuation, of specialist institutions.[3] Moreover, away from the competitive environment of capital cities with their wealthy patients, elite physicians and regulatory bodies, specialists were more readily accepted. Small specialist hospitals thrived in Liverpool, Birmingham and Manchester, though as we have seen they were less effective in Leeds and Sheffield.[4] Moreover, tensions between generalist and specialist could be eased by the introduction of specialist departments into general hospitals – especially when promoted by leading generalist consultants. In particular, the use of outpatient departments to initiate new specialities – and facilitate patient management – has been recognized as an important development of the modern period.[5]

By 1914 a fairly uniform system of patient classification had been established in the voluntary general hospitals where beds were allocated and outpatient departments created for general medical, general surgical, ophthalmic, ENT, skin and gynaecological patients along with a casualty department. These developments were intensified by the application of new techniques and technologies, especially X-ray, ultraviolet light (UV), massage and physiotherapy. However, some areas remained outside the voluntary general hospitals, such as TB, VD, maternity, the mentally ill, childhood orthopaedics and the 'incurables'. Their needs were met either by the local authorities or by voluntary organizations, including the early cancer hospitals in London, Manchester and Glasgow.[6] Specialist services provided a way to classify, manage and speed up the passage of patients through both the individual hospital and the wider hospital system. Moreover, they encouraged the development of specialist nurses and other allied professions, like midwives, radiologists and physiotherapists, who took responsibility for the majority of cases dealt with in the burgeoning outpatient rooms of the voluntary and municipal hospitals.[7] Yet Leeds and Sheffield had few specialist hospitals for cities of their size – Manchester, Birmingham and Liverpool all having six or more covering women, children, skin, eye, ear, orthopaedic and even the foot.[8] LGI proved effective at snuffing out competition from independent specialists by incorporating them back into the infirmary – as with skin and ophthalmic work which both secured specialist honorary appointments.[9] Only institutions for women survived, and even these were beginning to come into the LGI's orbit by the First World War.[10] Nor were there many more independent ventures in Sheffield beyond the Jessop Hospital for Women and the Children's Hospital, classic cases of medical and philanthropic self-interest driving institutional development.[11] However, there was some competition between the SRI and the SRH until the 1930s – mirroring the position in Birmingham, Bristol and Middlesbrough.[12]

Hospitals were, however, developing specialist sections under honorary staff. In Sheffield, dermatology was established in both hospitals by 1911 (under the same honorary surgeon, Rupert Hallam) but was not separated from the normal work of the physicians at Leeds until the 1920s. Conversely, LGI had a gynaecological section and had taken over the treatment of children by the time of the First World War. All general hospitals had eye and ENT inpatient and outpatient departments, some treated dental cases, SRI had a mental diseases clinic and LGI handled a small number of maternity cases. Radiology, massage and light treatment were also developing, the SRH having an honorary radiologist (again Rupert Hallam) from 1906.[13] Modern diagnostic and therapeutic tools were predominantly focused in outpatient departments and were taken up in some of the municipal general hospitals in the early 1920s. Following state intervention, VD treatment was commenced at the voluntary hospitals of Leeds and Sheffield by 1918 – supervised by paid medical directors.[14] These patterns differed little from the norm. Even where specialist institutions operated, most general hospitals also developed their own departments, as in Birmingham where Queen's had an eye specialist and the General ran a dermatology department despite the presence of both eye and skin hospitals in the city.[15]

The interwar period saw some expansion of separate departments and increasing specialization, although possibly less than might have been expected. Reflecting Sturdy and Cooter's contention that specialization was the handmaid of the generalist rather than a necessary form of separation, senior honorary physician, Dr Watson, noted of the LGI in 1936:

> Leeds has tended to become more and more a specialist hospital but when I speak of a specialist hospital I don't mean that it has become a hospital of special departments, it has become a specialist hospital in the sense that it has provided material and equipment for investigation of disease superior to that which can be obtained anywhere else in the district.[16]

This assessment confirmed the growing importance of the hospital and its staff as the centre of a sophisticated referral system which linked the general practitioner to the specialist skills of the new breed of consultants.[17]

In this context new departments were added and some reallocation of responsibilities between institutions was facilitated. In addition to the scientific departments which provided diagnostic support such as bacteriology, biochemistry and physiology (appointments often made from university staff), LGI formed a dermatology section in the mid-1920s while SRI appointed a gynaecologist in 1926. The early post-war period saw the separation of radiology from the electro- and radio-therapeutic section of the X-ray department, laying the foundations of a growing specialism in radium therapy at LGI,[18] while the SRH opened a diabetic outpatient department for the dispensing of insulin on the back of successful inpatient trials in 1924. This work showed an early link between university research and hospital based trials facilitated by the power of academics like Edward Mellanby and Arthur Hall to attract funding and opportunities from new bodies like the Medical Research Council (MRC).[19]

Although the hospitals were often accused of overlapping and duplicating services – a particular problem in cities with two general hospitals like Sheffield or Birmingham – there was an effort to minimize such duplication, especially in the areas of services for women and children. Both cities had specialist institutions for the treatment of diseases of women and although departments existed for gynaecology at both LGI and SRI, in the case of the former this was significantly reduced in 1933 when an agreement was signed which 'for practical purposes ... centralizes in the Hospital for Women the treatment of all gynaecological patients from Leeds and district' and, along with the creation of a unified medical faculty, effectively made the Hospital for Women a department of the LGI.[20] These developments followed earlier decisions to concentrate all voluntary hospital maternity work at the LMH and transfer all childhood diseases to the Infirmary.[21] Indeed, such reorganization was quite common between the wars. In Norwich, the Eye Hospital merged with the Norfolk and Norwich in 1925, while in Birmingham, Reinarz noted that, in the interwar period, relations between many hospitals, 'even those with no previous connections, would be characterized by ... co-operative efforts'.[22]

On the other hand, the culture of centralization meant paediatrics was slow to develop in Leeds. The city had no specialist institution for children, except the local authority-run Wyther Hospital for Infants which focused mainly on 'malthriving' babies, and where the 'chief object of the hospital is to deal with infants suffering from dietic disorders, malnutrition, &c, and its work is preventative as much as curative'. This prompted the MOH of Leeds to describe the situation as a 'reproach ... upon the city' and to urge the founding of a specialist institution for:

> At present only the merest fraction of the cases requiring hospital treatment can be admitted, the remainder being left to run the gauntlet of death or of permanent disablement in dwellings crowded, ill-lighted, ill-ventilated and anything but suitable for nursing the sick.[23]

This claim was challenged by the LGI, which in the immediate post-war period used its available funds to create a coherent infants' and children's department by new building and reorganization. At the AGM in 1920 Charles Lupton pointed to 100 children's beds and 1,100 admissions at the LGI while attacking those who wanted to initiate a separate children's voluntary hospital, not least because it would disadvantage the medical students and would, therefore, be bad for the children:

> We want to take advantage of all the skill and knowledge we have in the city and to give the benefit to the children just as much as the grown up people and I am sure it is impossible to do so unless this new work is grouped around the Infirmary.[24]

The LGI completed their specialist provision for infants and children in 1924 with the opening of an orthopaedic department and a range of agreements with local authorities to treat children identified by the education departments.[25] As a result the LGI was the main centre of paediatric care in the city although provision was extended when a 200-bed children's block opened at St James's in 1926. This remained the situation until the 1940s when 199 beds were allocated at the increasingly redundant Seacroft Hospital as an institution for children.[26]

Conversely, the presence of a specialist children's institution and a substantial orthopaedic hospital meant paediatrics was limited in the general hospitals of Sheffield. However, Sheffield Health Department developed a specialty in childhood pulmonary TB. By 1933 the city diagnosed ten times as many children with the illness as any other place, while a quarter of all children in the country with the disease were in Sheffield. Although the City's TB officer claimed the children were suffering from 'Minor Tuberculosis' and that a few months treatment at this stage prevented 'major' TB later, the Ministry of Health's Dr Donelan was unconvinced, stating it 'does not appear to me to be clear that these children are definitely tuberculous and I think to a considerable extent Sheffield is providing a good deal of convalescent home treatment for children under the title of anti-tuberculosis work'.[27] Despite this criticism the city continued to focus on 'minor Tuberculosis', claiming its low rate of adult TB was the result of this strategy of early intervention.

There were, however, few major changes to the basic work of the hospitals of Leeds and Sheffield between the wars. As in most general hospitals, surgery dominated in the voluntary sector – with around three surgical admissions to every medical case.[28] This owed something to the quicker turnover of surgical cases which were often discharged in under ten days, a little to the large volume of accidents, and a little to the generally higher success rate in surgical over medical cases. However, outpatient departments did see some change. Routine procedures involving massage, sunlight, X-ray and VD treatments swelled attendance, as did increasing specialization such as the extension of the orthopaedic department at LGI by the addition of a chiropody unit in 1932, while the following year ophthalmology acquired an orthoptics clinic for the treatment of squints.[29] This was followed by a similar development at the SRI where, 'ever anxious to keep abreast of the times', the clinic would utilize new equipment and 'specially trained staff' to reduce the amount of surgery required, cut costs and free beds.[30] Bigger changes were brought by the Second World War. Although a joint neuro-surgery department had been established between LGI and St James's in 1939, the war ensured rapid development of this specialty, as it did in Manchester where Geoffrey Jefferson led the way[31] – the SRI noting in 1944:

> casualties of war have provided neurological centres with much knowledge in the care and treatment of head injuries. These are common and disabling injuries in times of peace and the facilities which have been created for dealing with these injuries of war should in peace be maintained and developed.[32]

The conflict also saw the creation of jaw and plastic units at St James's while a peacetime plastic surgery department followed at SRH which claimed to be the first of its kind in a voluntary hospital for civilians.[33] Moreover, in Leeds these new specialties were being taken up in the municipal sector both in alliance with, but also independent of, the voluntary hospitals, putting the city in the forefront of collaboration and regional development by the end of the war.

One of the more enterprising developments of the interwar period was the creation of mental health outpatient clinics at the general hospitals. Institutional provision for mental health in Yorkshire saw a county-based board provide asylums at Wakefield, Wadsley and three other locations and while there were some mental health beds in St James's, in Sheffield's these were limited to the public assistance wards of Fir Vale.[34] However, Yorkshire was a pioneer in the outpatient treatment of mental health, with the first provincial OP clinic opened at Wakefield asylum in 1890.[35] Outpatient clinics were operating in both Sheffield general hospitals from 1920 – around the same time a department of psychotherapy commenced in Queen's Birmingham[36] – and a full OP department for mental diseases was initiated in 1927 at SRH under Gilbert Mould, Honorary Physician for Mental Diseases, working with two medical officers from South Yorkshire Mental Hospital. As the report explained, the co-operation with the County Mental Hospital would be

> [of] great value not only in the early treatment of many preventable cases of Mental disorder, but also in follow up cases needing a further period of care and treatment after discharge from the Mental Hospital. The scheme has been carried out at the

suggestion and with the approval of those responsible for the care of such cases and the Board is pleased to think that in this movement Sheffield has been one of the pioneers in carrying it into effect.[37]

The work of the Wadsley doctors included treating their own convalescent patients, advising on cases occurring in the wards and ensuring a 'considerable number are saved confinement in a Mental Hospital'.[38] A similar department followed at SRI in 1932 – the honorary physicians including the medical superintendent of Wadsley[39] – and at the LGI in 1933, around the same time as a clinic opened at the Clayton voluntary hospital, Wakefield.[40] Established under the supervision of two medical officers from Wakefield asylum, it was observed of the LGI department that 'In dealing with those patients who are suitable for treatment at the clinic as out-patients, it has been possible to get satisfactory results in a considerable proportion of the cases' though they noted that to treat more difficult cases they needed more staff and, especially, 'the help of a social worker in dealing with adverse home conditions'.[41] The work of all of the units grew until the war, during which both new patients and attendances doubled at the LGI.

The municipal hospitals also developed specialities, though in most cases these were by default. As in Manchester earlier in the century, the amalgamation of the poor law unions and appropriation provided an opportunity for the reorganization and extension of the work of the public hospitals. As early as 1926 a reclassification of patients in Sheffield saw the 'majority of the "House", mental and acute sick' transferred to Fir Vale PAI and Hospital while Nether Edge focused on the chronic sick, maternity and TB, an arrangement which continued following appropriation. Further transfers of the chronic sick and infirm to Nether Edge and the infirm wards at Fir Vale House followed while plans were mooted to adapt PAI accommodation to release 200 beds at the City Hospital. Such reorganization was eased by Leeds and Sheffield both controlling more than one PLI, allowing the establishment of at least one acute institution. This reflected developments in Bristol where patients were reallocated to ID and PA institutions as Southmead undertook more, and more complex, surgery.[42]

Routine surgery also took off at the municipal general hospitals partly through the appointment of visiting medical staff. In Leeds, St James's could boast an impressive array of consultants by 1933, including two general surgeons, three physicians (one paediatric), a dermatologist, ophthalmologist and aurist, an orthopaedic surgeon and two gynaecologists.[43] Moreover, in common with many of the larger municipalities, maternity work was significantly increased.[44] More unusual was the development of casualty treatment in Sheffield City General, which proved more effective than the stalled arrangement in Manchester.[45] As this suggests, co-ordination between the two sectors promoted specialization. In Leeds clear boundaries for each type of institution were set with LGI to operate as a clearing house for the majority of cases seeking admission in the city. In addition suitable accident, suicide and emergency cases admitted to the LGI casualty department could be diverted to St James's.[46] Yet despite ongoing discussions hinting at the development of more varied and specialist work for the municipal sector, including a casualty department at St James's, little changed in Leeds prior to the war. The agreement in Sheffield gave more to the City Hospital, including increased maternity work, access to the waiting-list patients of the general hospitals, and a casualty department which was dealing with around 6,000 cases by 1938. This underpinned a marked rise in surgical work which saw over 2,000 operations performed at the City General by 1935.[47]

These changes notwithstanding, the traditional sources of public hospital patients predominated throughout the 1930s, blocking their rise to full acute status. The general medical patients at Nether Edge were 'in the main persons suffering from chronic or incurable conditions for whom little or no benefit can be expected from remedial treatment but who require medical supervision and nursing care',[48] while even in the mid-1930s the medical work had 'varied little for many years'.[49] More frustrating was 'the great shortage of accommodation for infirm patients who are no longer in need of hospital treatment' which hampered the ability of the municipal hospitals to increase the amount of acute hospital work they could undertake. A worsening problem during the 1930s, it had become 'very serious' by 1935, for as they increased their accommodation for the infirm and chronic sick the result was 'that our permanent population has steadily risen, and the shortage of beds for acute cases remains as it was before'.[50] Thus waiting lists for hospital patients grew, attracting the attention of politicians and the local press, the latter claiming one reason for bed-blocking was greater longevity which meant 'People of mature years were lingering on in life, and although not sick, were infirm and partially helpless, requiring care and attention given in municipal institutions'.[51] As a result around 200 medical beds at the City General remained blocked by infirm patients well into the 1940s.[52]

Orthopaedics

The increase in casualties, accidents and motor accidents, along with a long experience of industrial accidents, encouraged the general hospitals of Sheffield and Leeds to develop services specifically for orthopaedics and fractures. This was a contentious issue in the early twentieth century, with generalist surgeons, especially in London, opposed to the fragmentation of surgery while those in the provinces or with experience of war surgery began to push specialization.[53] The reception of the 'new orthopaedics' in Sheffield and Leeds was eased by trade union and workers' contributory scheme support, sympathetic industrial management, a number of surgeons with wartime experience[54] and the prevalence of broken bones arising from employment in heavy industries such as mining, iron and steel and engineering.[55] Indeed it was their experience of the large number of casualties from the 'industrial battlefield' with broken bones and damaged joints which led provincial hospitals and their staff to focus in these areas ahead of changes in health policy in the 1930s. These changes saw the encouragement of services to combat long-term disability from accidents, a process accelerated during the Second World War.[56]

Prior to the First World War orthopaedics was associated with the treatment of congenital deformities, non-pulmonary TB and rickets, with most institutional treatment focused on children who occupied beds for months if not years.[57] At the late nineteenth-century Birmingham Orthopaedic Hospital afflictions of the legs and feet predominated, with relatively few spinal or paralysis cases, while there was an increasing focus on operative treatments, with many orthopaedic patients enduring 'repeated surgical interventions over many years well into the next century'.[58] The late nineteenth century also saw a shift in attitude towards 'crippled children', from sentiment to treatment. Central to this was the open-air therapy pioneered by Agnes Hunt and Robert Jones at the Baschurch Convalescent Home in Shropshire based on fresh air, rest, sunlight and conservative surgery in a peaceful rural location.[59] In part due to the success of this mode of treatment, the interwar period was characterized by the removal of many long-stay orthopaedic patients from acute hospitals to these new specialist institutions, with the Birmingham Orthopaedic Hospital, among others, adopting this model.[60]

Yet despite the enduring focus on the 'uncontested territory of disabled children',[61] there was an emerging recognition that the damaged bones of adults could have long-term implications for their fitness to work, prompting the creation of some specialist units which laid the groundwork for both physiotherapy and modern orthopaedics.[62] Robert Jones, leading exponent of the 'new orthopaedics' at the turn of the twentieth century was key here. Jones trained in Liverpool where he was surgeon to the Manchester Ship Canal, encountering a wide range of accidents and injuries. When appointed honorary surgeon to the city's Royal Southern Hospital he specialized in bone surgery and pioneered the use of teams in managing his caseload. He was appointed Director of Military Orthopaedics in 1916 and solidified the group identity of orthopaedics by helping to found the British Orthopaedic Association in 1918, redefining the specialty as 'the treatment by manipulation, by operation, and by re-education, of disabilities of the locomotor system, whether arising from disease or injury'.[63]

Although the new orthopaedics received a boost during the First World War when Jones promoted the treatment of fractures by teams working in the military hospitals,[64] Cooter has argued that these advances were marginalized after the war by the elite surgeons and medical schools.[65] Yet the evidence from a number of provincial centres, especially Sheffield, is more optimistic. At Manchester Royal Infirmary, Harry Platt developed a fracture clinic as part of an integrated service for the city that included the municipal and smaller voluntary hospitals,[66] and in Birmingham a fracture clinic opened at the Queen's Hospital in the later 1930s, transforming into a full accident hospital in the 1940s.[67] Although the link between casualty departments and specialized fracture treatment was slow to develop in Leeds and Sheffield, specialist orthopaedic departments and institutions did emerge. In Sheffield the opening of the King Edward VII Hospital in 1917 promoted the open-air approach to children's orthopaedics.[68] Treating non-pulmonary TB and severe rickets, the institution was managed by a medical superintendent, who held membership of the Royal College of Surgeons, and a resident house surgeon but no visiting staff. More significant, was the voluntary Edgar Allen Institute. Founded in 1911 with a donation from steel manufacturer, William Edgar Allen, it aimed to provide outpatient treatment for a range of 'morbid conditions' – damaged bone, joints and muscles; arthritic conditions; neuritis/sciatica; and orthopaedic cases – that required 'physical treatment'.[69] Although many of the activities were commonly undertaken in hospital outpatient departments, its founders believed a fully equipped and funded unit dealing specifically with therapy for bones, joints and muscles would aid the speedy return of injured workers to gainful employment.[70] Drawing largely on Continental, especially Swedish, ideas, staff and equipment, by the early 1930s it was treating the effects of injuries, diseases, congenital abnormalities and arthritic and rheumatoid conditions and in 1933 it became the second recognized rheumatism treatment centre under the National Insurance Act.[71]

Orthopaedic departments with fracture clinics modelled on those pioneered by Platt in Manchester were created at both Sheffield hospitals in the 1930s.[72] J. B. Ferguson Wilson, an honorary orthopaedic surgeon who also acted as medical assistant to the Director of the Edgar Allen Institute, R. G. Abercrombie, drove development at the SRH. Abercrombie was an expert in adolescent scoliosis, a painful curvature of the spine found mainly in girls.[73] Ferguson Wilson became interested in orthopaedics during the First World War, joining the British Orthopaedic Association at its formation and though appointed honorary surgeon at SRH in 1934, he maintained an interest in orthopaedics until his retirement in 1943.[74] The Infirmary appointed Frank Holdsworth as Surgical Registrar in 1931 and under the influence of the honorary surgeon, Ernest Finch, a supporter of the new approach, he developed an interest in orthopaedic surgery.[75] Ferguson Wilson and Holdsworth promoted fracture clinics in the mid-1930s, encouraged by technological developments and support from industry, especially mining. Initially stimulated by improvements which meant '[b]y means of the X-Ray screen it is possible actually to see the broken bone as it is being reduced into position and, in suitable cases, perfect results can be obtained both anatomically and functionally',[76] the SRI introduced a scheme for the 'organised treatment of fractures'. A clinic was established in 1935 with 'the necessary equipment provided, including X-ray apparatus and Dark Room', and over 1,000 fractures were dealt with in the first year.[77] A similar unit was opened at the SRH in 1937 under Ferguson Wilson, with a specialist first assistant and in both cases it was hoped the new treatment methods would reduce the patients' stay, to the benefit of patient and institution. Teamwork was added to technology to increase the volume of work[78] and in 1937 Holdsworth was appointed the first honorary orthopaedic surgeon at SRI along with an orthopaedic house surgeon and an allocation of beds.[79] This development had the support of the board, who were 'convinced of the importance and great value of this special branch of hospital service'.[80]

The creation of this specialty was also stimulated by support from industry.[81] Although hospitals had seen motor vehicle victims as a burden for whom no one was willing to pay, in Sheffield and its environs both employers and employees were interested in addressing the cost of accidents at work. As the *British Medical Journal* (*BMJ*) explained:

> the heavy industry of the town and surrounding districts led to a high rate of industrial accident. Thus orthopaedics and accident surgery became linked from the beginning, and Sheffield, Rotherham, Mexborough, and Worksop looked to Sir Frank Holdsworth for guidance and practical assistance.[82]

In particular colliery owners and employees, who had been important contributors to the Edgar Allen Institute, began to focus on more advanced treatment in hospitals. In a novel move a relationship emerged between the Miners' Welfare and the Sheffield hospitals to develop orthopaedic services.[83] Thus during the SRH Centenary appeal:

> The Miners' Welfare Fund was invited through the South Yorkshire District Committee to make a grant to our Appeal. A number of visits of inspection to the Hospital were made by the members of the South Yorkshire Committee, representatives of the Miners and the Miners themselves.[84]

This resulted in a contribution of £25,000 as core funding for the Miners' Welfare Block completed in 1937[85] and evidenced a link between the hospitals and the Miners' Welfare at an earlier date than suggested by Cooter. Indeed, by the later 1930s accident work was also receiving donations from the Derbyshire District Miners' Welfare Committee, providing 'further indication of the liberality of the mining communities to hospitals generally and to the Sheffield Hospitals particularly'[86] while the South Yorkshire Miners' Welfare Committee agreed to provide a regular grant for the work of both fracture departments.[87] In turn the hospitals emphasized the benefits to industry of improved orthopaedic practices which accomplished more and more work of inestimable value, not only to the patients themselves but to employers of labour and Insurance Companies. In a city such as Sheffield the loss to industry as a whole through fractures sustained by workmen and others must inevitably be considerable, and the Clinic's aim and achievement has been an appreciable reduction of this loss through the organised treatment of cases.[88]

In a similar vein the SRH observed that there was 'little doubt that the duration of sick leave will be lessened and the loss to industry reduced by up-to-date orthopaedic treatment of fracture cases' and like the Infirmary they drew the attention of employers and insurers to the savings made 'in the hope they will consider giving the Clinic some financial support'.[89]

The Second World War saw further important developments at a local and national level, including the spinal paraplegia unit at Wharncliffe EMS Hospital[90] and the rehabilitation facilities for miners developed by the Miners' Welfare Commission. By 1944 there were seven residential rehabilitation centres across Britain and six special hospital centres managed jointly by miners and mine owners and covering 90 per cent of all working miners.[91] These initiatives were accompanied by significant developments at the United Hospitals in Sheffield where a radical accident and orthopaedic unit to serve the region was in operation by 1945. As the institution observed, it 'cannot be emphasized too strongly that the Royal Sheffield Infirmary and Hospital provides an area service in its special departments ... a service which in terms of patients treated, is one of the largest in the country'.[92] Moreover, in a copybook version of the schemes described by Cooter,[93] the department claimed to be 'the first of its kind ... associated with a general hospital' providing 'a complete service ... for all accident cases from the time the patient is brought into the hospital to the time when the patient is fit to resume his normal occupation at home or in the Works'. This included treatment in the fracture wards by the orthopaedic surgeon, X-ray and operative facilities and rehabilitation following discharge so that 'they will have the personal supervision of the orthopaedic team and so ensure full continuity of treatment, as essential to good results' serving to 'lessen the time of incapacity arising from accidents both industrial and domestic'.[94] The teamwork in the clinic was complemented by increasingly sophisticated convalescent provision specifically for accident patients. Maintaining the link with industrial injuries, 'The bulk of these patients have been injured as the result of accidents in the mines and works and under the care of the Orthopaedic Surgeons have continued their rehabilitation under ideal conditions' the home receiving commendations from industry and the Ministry of Health.[95]

Thus, this was clearly an area in which service provision was shaped by local economic and social imperatives. As a result of the dangerous nature of the region's heavy industry, the financial support of steel magnates, colliery owners and industrial and mine workers and the initiative of members of the honorary and teaching staff, Sheffield had emerged by 1945 as a leading centre of the new orthopaedics.

This was not, however, the case in Leeds where orthopaedic and fracture services were slow to develop. Leeds did not have an orthopaedic hospital for children nor did the LPD take a particular interest in orthopaedics – though it developed a modern research specialism with the opening of an arthritis clinic that received well over 10,000 attendances by 1938.[96] Following an appeal and support from the MRC, research was conducted into the causes and cures of the condition, especially the effects of gold therapy.[97] Undertaken in partnership with the university and the Royal Bath Hospital in Harrogate, the results were 'published in the leading medical journals, and received favourable comments'.[98] More conventional lumbar TB cases were sent to the voluntary Marguerite Hepton Orthopaedic Hospital at Thorp Arch while some adult cases went to the Royal Bath Hospital in Harrogate which specialized in rheumatism therapy. Provision was therefore concentrated at the LGI which, in 1922, appointed S. W. Daw as honorary surgeon in charge of a traditional orthopaedic department.[99] Daw, an assistant surgeon and clinical lecturer in surgery, had acquired a practical academic record during the First World War, including service as a surgeon to the Special Surgical Pensions' Hospital, an article in Sir Robert Jones's seminal work *The Orthopaedic Surgery of Injuries* and a textbook on *Orthopaedic Effects of Gunshot Wounds and their After Treatment*. Although close to Jones, he concentrated on standard orthopaedic work, developing a specialism in feet and toes.[100]

The work of the LGI orthopaedic department was extensive, including 10,000 attendances in its first year and a significant quantity of lucrative work for local Education Committees which secured the appointment of a resident orthopaedic officer.[101] However, a more up-to-date service developed when Reginald Broomhead replaced Daw. Broomhead had trained in Leeds acting as house surgeon to Lord Moynihan who stimulated his interest in orthopaedics. He visited the clinics of Jones in Liverpool and Smith-Petersen in America before his appointment as assistant orthopaedic surgeon and full surgeon in 1934.[102] With his assistant he instituted a fracture clinic in 1935, the extra work requiring a full-time registrar for the department.[103] The later 1930s saw moves to create Yorkshire-wide services for orthopaedics and fractures informed by the Interim Report of the Interdepartmental Committee on the Rehabilitation of Persons injured by accidents.[104] The Leeds Joint Advisory Council commissioned a report by Broomhead on facilities for orthopaedics that recommended LGI continue to treat fractures and short-term orthopaedics with 'suitable cases also being referred to St. James's Hospital'.[105] As a result, St James's claimed a fracture clinic in 1938 treating 1,000 people while West Riding County Council was amenable to 'the principle of a joint fracture service for city and county cases, subject to agreement later on the financial details'. Moreover, in 1939 a joint committee of the Leeds and West Riding County councils and the Marguerite Hepton Memorial Orthopaedic Hospital agreed on an appeal for funds to build a new 200-bed joint hospital for long-stay cases.[106]

These plans were underpinned by the LGI's major extension which included an improved orthopaedic department to meet the needs of the 4,500 outpatients who by 1938 were making 23,000 attendances.[107] When the new facilities opened in 1946 new patients numbered 6,500 making almost 50,000 visits. Included in these figures were a large number of chronic chiropody cases regularly visiting the clinic begun by Samuel Daw in the early 1930s.[108] The orthopaedic and dermatological departments at the SRI launched a similar venture, leading the Infirmary's vice-chairman to hope that in the

> great many cases where people had been suffering year after year, a great deal of curing as well as palliative treatment would result from the collaboration between the scientific men and the chiropodists. This would be a very great service because nobody really realised the large proportion of suffering represented by foot troubles.[109]

Moreover, given the chronic nature of many orthopaedic conditions the departments recognized the need to fit treatment around the lives of the patients. Thus, in Leeds the chiropody clinics were run in the evening to avoid interfering with the working day,[110] while the Edgar Allen Institute began afternoon sessions in 1936 with the effect that:

> the working-class women living in the surrounding districts now attend in considerable numbers in the afternoons ... They are thus free to devote themselves in the mornings to their domestic duties, including the preparation of their husbands' and children's dinners, a very real contribution to the social economy of the neighbourhood.[111]

As this suggests, hospitals were much more attuned to the needs and lives of patients and the demands of society than in the era of charity, a change informed in part by the transformation in funding regimes.

Maternity

If modern orthopaedics and fracture work typified the adaptation of specialist services to Sheffield's economic and social structure, maternity provision in Leeds offers equal evidence of institutional facilities shaped by local need. While Leeds clearly had extensive general and specialist coverage for women,[112] it was the scale and utilization of institutional maternity services which was most remarkable. In line with national trends, around one in ten Leeds women had their babies in hospital in 1918 but by 1939 this had reached more than half, around twice the national average.[113] Admittedly it was not unique in seeing a rise in institutional births as both the state and voluntary sector extended their provision.[114] The 1917 Maternity and Child Welfare Act gave a prominent role to local authorities in the management of childbirth, but the pattern of antenatal services owed much to existing delivery, especially in the voluntary sector. In Edinburgh the maternity charities, including inpatient facilities, were central to the doubling of institutional births between 1912 and 1924.[115] Conversely the marked increase in hospital confinements in Bristol – from 21 per cent in 1925 to 46 per cent ten years later – was driven by municipal intervention, as were developments in late 1930s Manchester, stimulated by the Molly Taylor scandal, when insufficient maternity provision and service co-ordination was blamed for a patient's death.[116] Thus, while historians have often focused on the municipal sector when assessing change in maternity facilities after 1918, these examples show growth was based on expansion in both the voluntary and public sectors with a culture of joint working deemed important.[117] But to what extent did Leeds and Sheffield follow these patterns?

Reflecting on his thirty years as MOH for Leeds, Dr Johnstone Jervis highlighted 'the growing tendency among women to have their confinements in institutions or nursing homes', the number rising from 11.5 per cent in 1917 to just under 65 per cent in 1946 (Table 4.1).[118] Moreover, maternity beds had increased threefold, from 87 to 260,[119] with expansion in both sectors.[120] Contrary to the view that the maternalist Infant and Child Welfare Act and its clinics medicalized women, pushing them reluctantly towards institutional births, much of the growth in the 1920s was among those willing to pay for their confinement, either in a private nursing home or the PLIs which required payment from all but the relief class.[121] Following significant extensions, births at the Maternity Hospital almost doubled in the 1930s while there was a substantial increase in the use of the public hospitals. In 1923 just one in a hundred births took place in Leeds PLIs but fifteen years later the proportion was over one in five. As the numbers delivered in the voluntary and public hospitals began to converge tensions emerged, which were resolved by a complex series of negotiations around the allocation of patients.[122]

Table 4.1: Institutional births in Leeds by institution type, 1923–38

	1923		1928		1933		1938	
	No. births	% all registered	No. births	% all registered	No. births	% all registered	No. births	% all registered
Leeds Maternity Hospital	1,384	15.39	1,251	15.68	1,863	26.36	2,187	28.72
Leeds PLI/St James	87	0.97	440	5.52	799	11.3	1,149	15.09
Bramley PLI/St Mary's	5	0.06	158	1.98	309	4.37	475	6.24
Hope Hospital/ St Faith's	97	1.08	30	0.37	6	0.08	–	–
Other	26	0.29	21	0.26	10	0.14	5	0.07
Private nursing homes	170	1.89	290	3.64	325	4.6	309	4.06
Total	1,769	19.7	2,190	27.45	3,312	46.85	4,125	54.18

Source: MOH Leeds Report: Maternity and Child Welfare Table, published annually.

This rise did owe something to municipal promotion, especially by the maternalist Jervis. From 1918 until the mid-1930s the Leeds Health Department took a positive view of institutional birth, largely as an alternative to births in the city's poor housing, the MOH stating in 1918:

> This generally growing number of births taking place in institutions is all to the good, for there is no question that in a great number of the small houses ... there is not reasonable accommodation for the process of child birth under the best conditions for the mother and child; there is, therefore, room for expansion of maternity hospital facilities.[123]

The case was made more forcibly the following year when it was argued that hospital births were to be encouraged because 'the present day home is in many cases the most unsuitable place for a baby to be born'.[124] Demand continued to grow and outstrip supply,[125] leading the council to sign agreements – as they did in Bristol – with various hospitals to provide beds for needy or medical cases. Thus, in 1923, the Maternity Hospital agreed to reserve thirty beds for women recommended by the medical officers of the antenatal centres or midwives to improve facilities for 'difficult or complicated cases of pregnancy or labour or of cases which for one reason or another require hospital treatment'. In addition, poor law unions set aside eight beds for corporation recommended cases 'with indifferent or bad home surroundings or those whose financial circumstances render it difficult or impossible to make the provision necessary to ensure the comfort and safety of mother and child'. Contrary to pessimistic accounts, this policy was designed to minimize infant mortality and address maternal mortality and morbidity, as 'much of the damage done to mother and child is due to lack of skilled attention at the time of birth ... This extra hospital provision should have the effect of minimizing this damage.'[126] Relatively few of these cases were destitute, as almost three-quarters of the cost was recovered from the patients while the number of illegitimate birth in institutions remained stable, though the proportion fell.[127] These trends were summed up in the MOH *Annual Report* of 1928 which presented a hospital confinement as a pleasure for the mother and an advantage to public health:

> Mothers are gradually becoming aware of the advantages of having their confinements in institutions, where they are away from all domestic worries, and can have constant attention with skilled help always at hand. She is in better hygienic surroundings, and the regular feeding of the baby can be instituted more easily away from home.[128]

However, from 1933 the proportion of institutional births, which had passed 40 per cent, was beginning to cause alarm. Concerns were first expressed by Dame Janet Campbell, who commended the council for considering paying fees to midwives attending 'necessitous women' and concluded that if 'a woman can be confined fairly comfortably at home, it may be better to provide a midwife and a sterilized outfit than to send her to hospital'.[129] But, in general, Campbell favoured an expansion of the local state provision, and indeed anticipated the position adopted in 1936, when she suggested:

> The Voluntary Hospital is overcrowded (it serves the West Riding as well as Leeds), and the number of abnormal cases is high. The provision at the Public Assistance Hospitals should be considered with a view to improvement; the maternity wards are evidently meeting a need, especially for normal cases living in bad homes, at a very reasonable cost ... A greater number of normal cases might be encouraged to apply for admission here in order to relieve the Maternity Hospital.[130]

Campbell's opinion that women may be better confined at home anticipated emerging views in the city and in 1934 the MOH and Gladys Russell, the Assistant MOH with responsibility for Maternity and Child Welfare, expressed concern about the scale of institutional deliveries. The former addressed the issue in the preface to his report, observing that an institutional birth was 'becoming the rule rather than the exception' with the result that demand for beds was outstripping supply and would have to be resolved 'either by increasing the number of beds which means building, or by introducing a system of case selection which will eliminate all those not really in need of institutional treatment'.[131]

Russell, inverting previous thinking, came down on the side of selection, arguing beds were not 'being used to the best advantage and for the benefit of those whose need is greatest'. In particular, she pointed to the many normal hospital cases 'in comfortable circumstances with good homes' who 'could quite safely be delivered at home', concluding 'Moderately good conditions at home are always safer than overcrowded conditions in hospital'.[132] This line continued for the rest of the 1930s though with no noticeable impact on the rate of institutional confinement. Indeed by 1938 it had reached 54 per cent, prompting the introduction of selection, with the Maternity Hospital concentrating on first births and abnormal cases and municipal provision expanding to accommodate the bulk of normal deliveries.[133]

Institutional provision was supported by a mixed economy of antenatal and post-natal clinics run jointly by the M & CW section and the voluntary Leeds Babies' Welcome, ensuring a high proportion of women were supported through their pregnancies, possibly contributing to the increasing scale of institutional births.[134] But there were many other factors feeding into the rise of hospital confinement in the city. In the early 1930s Janet Campbell observed that there was an 'increasing desire on the part of the poorer women to enter hospital'. She attributed this in part to midwives using practically no drugs – their use of chloroform had been banned by the MOH – while 'there is an increasing desire for anaesthesia among patients, and possibly patients are less willing than formerly to engage midwives because no relief can be given'.[135] Moreover, contrary to the widely held view of historians,[136] both local and external opinion attributed falls in maternal mortality to institutional facilities, Campbell observing: 'The comparatively low rate in Leeds is possibly due to easily accessible facilities for in-patient maternity treatment and to a medical school, which not only ensures consultant obstetricians, but encourages a high standard of practice among private doctors'.[137]

The position of the domiciliary midwife was bolstered to some extent by municipal intervention and the 1936 Midwives Act with its provision for municipal midwives. This Act is often seen as a key moment in state involvement in the management of childbirth although many of its provisions were already in place in authorities like Leeds. Thus the Leeds Maternity and Child Welfare Department had been providing support to poorer women through subsidies to the domiciliary service of the LMH as well as giving support to mothers in the Infant and Child Centres located across the city.[138] This was strengthened in 1935 by the issuing of free maternity outfits for mothers having their babies at home, supplementing the distribution of free milk to pregnant women and nursing mothers.[139] However, the 1936 Act did see the municipality take over the management of the majority of the midwives operating in the city, employing twenty-nine domiciliary midwives directly and meeting the cost of seven operated by the Maternity Hospital. But they did not respond to the *Report on Maternal Mortality* which recommended the establishment of maternity 'Flying Squads' to provide emergency support for difficult cases delivered at home.[140]

The Second World War wreaked havoc with institutional provision as St James's maternity facilities were closed, forcing the Maternity Hospital to take the vast majority of cases. Stopgap measures, including an annexe at Cookridge Convalescent Hospital, proved inadequate while the depredations of wartime meant the fabric of the hospital deteriorated severely. To compensate, additional beds were opened at St Mary's Hospital which came to focus mainly on maternity work and the maternity unit at St James's was reopened in 1943. The overcommitment of the Maternity Hospital drew the fire of the 1945 surveyors who reserved virtually their only criticism of Leeds' provision for that institution.[141] As hospital births continued to grow all commentators were agreed that the accommodation was inadequate both numerically and physically, the MOH suggesting that three 100-bed units were required, while the Nuffield Surveyors recommended a new maternity hospital on the LGI site as a priority. Yet redevelopment was held up and the Maternity Hospital continued as the site for difficult and first births until 1983.

In contrast to Leeds, maternity services in Sheffield were less well developed and the proportion of children born in hospital was lower. Although forty maternity beds were available at the Jessop Hospital for Women – allowing them to deliver between 900 and 1,000 women per year from the mid-1920s – this was significantly fewer than the 2,100 in the 140-bed Leeds Maternity Hospital. Public provision did emerge to bridge the gap, with the socialist council opening a maternity unit at Nether Edge in 1927 which, though located at the Poor Law Infirmary, was operated through the Infant and Child Welfare Department. It proved popular, with the number of births rising from 239 in the first year (1928) to 761 in 1934.[142] Yet despite this, Sheffield had the second lowest proportion of beds to births of the five largest cities in England in 1933 (Birmingham was marginally worse), Dr Donelan noting: 'The supply of maternity beds in Sheffield is at present somewhat limited, though something has been done to improve the resources by provision of 32 additional beds at Fir Vale Hospital.' Moreover, he quoted the MOH's assertion that 'the voluntary hospitals (e.g. the Jessop Hospital) are not doing their share in providing for maternity work' and supported criticism of the Jessop for 'sending women home on the fourth or fifth day, even in complicated cases with considerable obstetric interference'.[143]

The anticipated extra provision at the City General was one of the fruits of a 1930 deal between the council and the voluntary hospitals[144] and when they opened in 1934 they increased maternity beds in the city to 165 – a total of 122 in the municipal hospitals and just 43 at the Jessop.[145] The new beds allowed for almost twice as many women to utilize the hospital in 1935 although demand remained dangerously high with the 'experience of the past year's working' proving 'the necessity for provision of still further accommodation for Maternity cases'.[146]

This marked rise in institutional births in the city had a significant impact on the work of private midwives. In 1923 private midwives had attended just over half of births and medical practitioners just over a third, while one in nine had taken place in institutions. Ten years later, the number of births had fallen by around one-third while the proportions had shifted so that less than 40 per cent used a private midwife while almost three in ten babies were delivered in an institution.[147] The decline in midwifery cases left most practitioners in severe financial difficulty, although the council had initiated a scheme to pay the direct cost of attendance for poor women. But as in Leeds, the problem was changing attitudes which saw women and health professionals prefer a hospital birth, for as the Donelan observed:

> The Council's scheme for assisted midwifery, whilst it can guarantee payment to the midwife for such cases as she does attend, and, through the medium of the ante-natal clinic, can to some extent encourage women whose confinements are likely to be normal to utilise the services of the private midwives, cannot compensate for a decline in the number of confinements which are considered suitable for the private midwife, either on the grounds of physiological conditions or satisfactory domestic environment, nor can it do much to counteract the desire of a woman to seek an institution for her delivery. That more beds are being provided at Fir Vale indicates that there is not likely to be a tendency to persuade a woman to have her confinement at home even though the circumstances be suitable if she prefers to go into an institution.[148]

Thus, it was clear that institutional confinement was on the rise but it was still some way behind Leeds and only a little above the national average. Maternity bed provision remained inadequate for a city the size of Sheffield,[149] although the later 1930s saw significant developments as the Jessop approved plans to build a 78-bed maternity block (including eighteen for paying patients) while the council pushed ahead with its plan to add a further 32-bed block at the City General. Yet there is evidence of tension between the council and the voluntary hospitals over the Midwives Act, with Asbury attacking the provision which gave the Jessop control over three municipally funded midwives.[150] In one respect, however, the city was ahead of all but Birmingham and Newcastle in setting up a maternity 'Flying Squad' in 1937. These were mobile emergency units designed to 'bring the hospital' to seriously ill maternity patients unable to leave their beds. The units included a hospital consultant, a midwife and a variety of pieces of equipment including blood transfusion facilities. The emphasis on extreme emergency meant that, like the unit in Birmingham, it was not widely used, being called upon only eight times in 1937. As a result the facility was extended to residents in the West Riding as well as the city of Sheffield.[151]

It is therefore apparent that not only was maternity an undervalued and underdeveloped service in the city, there were also tensions between the voluntary and municipal sectors – evident from 1930 – which meant a system which was competitive rather than co-operative emerged. Moreover, the centralized system of maternity clinics – there was only one until 1938 which was run entirely by the department and the maternity staff from Nether Edge – left no room for voluntary effort and was felt to deliver a poor service.[152] In fact there were two parallel maternity services in the city with the Jessop running a completely separate antenatal and booking system. Thus, while there was agreement on the allocation of beds and resources in the early 1930s this was not maintained nor did it lead to real integration of services, as was beginning to happen in Leeds by the end of the decade.[153]

Conclusion

In the thirty years prior to the inauguration of the NHS the hospital patient and his or her experience changed markedly. Capacity expanded to meet the hugely increased demand stimulated by prepayment provision and the opening up of the poor law hospitals to general use. Due to the financial climate, especially in Sheffield, the opportunities to build new hospitals and even add significantly to existing stock were limited. Demand had to be met by other means and in particular the more effective use of the buildings, staff and space of the hospital. Investment flowed not to open more beds but to increase efficiency. Medical staff focused more of their energies on outpatient departments and on team-work, while paramedical staff began to appear to undertake a range of routine procedures. Yet the increasing compartmentalizing of medicine was resisted and relatively few new specialties appeared at this time. Certainly some were consolidated and some, like radium treatment for cancer, became very significant developments. But in general the boundaries drawn at the end of the nineteenth century continued to contain most specialist activity which remained in the hands of generalist surgeons and physicians.

However, in the two areas explored in this chapter – orthopaedics and maternity – there is evidence that the prominence of these specialisms owed something to local demand shaped by local need. In Sheffield medical staff, hospital managers, industrialists, workers and prospective patients all promoted the importance of the 'new' orthopaedics in a region where accidents at work were common and the economic and social cost of long-term incapacity readily understood by both sides of industry. Equally, the key role of women as policy formers as well as consumers of maternity provision in Leeds ensured that the city developed one of the most extensive services in the country with both municipal and voluntary institutions developing rapidly. Local demand was therefore crucial, but so too was financial capacity and political leadership for the scale, quality and effectiveness of provision, and access to it relied heavily on the development of new modes of voluntary and public funding.

5 FINANCE

In the period between the end of the First World War and the inauguration of the NHS the demands on hospitals grew significantly: inpatient and outpatient numbers soared necessitating increased accommodation; new drugs and technologies were developed; and more, better trained and better remunerated staff were required. To meet these financial commitments voluntary hospitals had to diversify the source and increase the volume of their income at a time when social and economic changes were weakening traditional philanthropic giving. Provincial voluntary hospital income – after an initial crisis between 1918 and 1923 – did largely keep pace with expenditure, increasing by about 65 per cent between 1920 and 1938.[1] Moreover, most historians accept that they were not on the verge of collapse by the later 1930s as argued by Titmuss,[2] with many adapting to the increased demand for services. Certainly the inability of traditional voluntary sources of finance – subscriptions, donations, collections – to meet growing demand meant payment, either direct or indirect, was vital to the survival of the voluntary system but how this was achieved and its long-term impact remain the subjects of considerable debate. It has been argued that while mass worker prepayment schemes were essential to the economic viability and vitality of these institutions, this was at the expense of any philanthropic claims they may have made.[3] Others see workers contributions as retaining implicit and explicit voluntary elements bolstered by the hospitals' insistence that prepayment did not ensure treatment.[4] A third strand of opinion points to the vitality of voluntary sources of income, especially for capital projects, and to the wide range of community fundraising and gift giving which sustained both the fabric and ethos of these institutions.[5] One key element to emerge from these discussions is an awareness of regional and inter-urban differences.[6] How hospitals responded to the challenges of the period depended on existing cultures of giving, social and economic structures, class and gender, state involvement and whether the institution was specialist or general.

In Leeds and Sheffield ordinary expenditure increased by about 50 per cent in the voluntary general hospitals and doubled at the specialist institutions. Change in the 1940s was even greater, producing a fivefold increase at the general hospitals between 1919 and 1947 (Table 5.1). Most hospitals were able to match expenditure with income by diversifying and to some extent democratizing the social base of their fundraising (Table 5.2). However, as the organized contributions of workers came to meet much of the need at all institutions, different systems of income generation emerged. In Leeds hospitals drew on a complex mix of direct and indirect payment, donations and investments, while Sheffield institutions relied overwhelmingly on the proceeds from the Penny in the Pound scheme. Yet, payment for treatment did not replace voluntary effort entirely and made little direct impact on income for capital purposes, which continued to rely overwhelmingly on voluntary giving. Moreover, as Gosling has shown, the expansion of direct payment reflected the changing nature of the patient base as the 'sick poor' were replaced by citizen patients able and expected to contribute something to their treatment.[7] This broadening of the patient base to include the majority of the population encouraged a democratization of the pool from which donors would be drawn, the SRI noting in 1938 that

> There are few, if any, who do not share either directly or indirectly in the benefits of the hospital's work, and for that reason the Board feel they can make a just claim for support from every section of the community.[8]

In the light of these changes we will consider who gave resources to the voluntary hospitals of Leeds and Sheffield and how this changed over the period 1918–48. In particular, we will draw attention to the way the base of voluntary effort was widened to include the whole community, rich and poor, old and young, male and female; changes in the source of capital income, especially the growth of popular appeals; and the basis of local government hospital finance. It is clear that the socio-economic structures of the two cities impacted upon the shape of hospital funding, with the broader middle class of Leeds ensuring a healthy mix of voluntary and contributory elements while the dominance of large-scale industrial unions and employers of the metal and engineering sectors created corporate responses in Sheffield typified by the Penny in the Pound scheme, the Million Pound Appeal and the centralist social policies of the Labour-dominated council.

Expenditure

The extensive discussions of the transformation in hospital funding have not been accompanied by similar attention to the substantial growth in expenditure which drove the need for new sources of finance.[9] Indeed, there is no consistent data on the growth in expenditure patterns over the interwar period, although Pinker has estimated spending rose by 100 per cent in London and tripled in the provinces.[10] Local studies point to rises ranging from 65 per cent at the North Riding in Middlesbrough to 150 per cent in real terms at Bristol Royal Infirmary with most experiencing a doubling of costs between 1922 and 1938.[11] In the hospitals examined here (Table 5.1), interwar change varied from just over 50 per cent at the LGI through the doubling experienced at most of the institutions to almost 200 per cent at the LPD.

Table 5.1: Total ordinary expenditure, general and specialist hospitals: three-year averages, 1919–47

	SRH	SRI	Jessop	LGI	LPD	LHW
1919–21	39,218	49,843		97,782	7,071	8,466
1922–4	37,553	49,936	18,296	97,577	9,160	8,620
1925–7	47,367	59,764	19,184	104,451	9,379	8,642
1928–30	49,745	64,815	25,434	102,821	9,474	8,874
1931–3	45,345	63,709	24,857	104,664	10,821	10,797
1934–6	47,330	73,046	27,474	108,493	13,343	12,271
1937–9	61,454	86,485	33,173	123,485	15,071	15,426
1940–2	72,394	89,541		150,414	14,158	16,683
1943–5	105,602	132,243		217,441	18,234	21,453
1946–7	209,300	237,277		375,991		

Sources: SRH, SRI, Jessop, LGI, LPD, LHW, LMH, *Annual Reports*, 1918–47.

Table 5.2: Total ordinary income, general and specialist hospitals: three-year averages, 1919–47

	SRH	SRI	Jessop	LGI	LPD	LHW
1919–21	21,163	30,417	12,030	56,597	5,896	6,297
1922–4	35,292	47,616	19,363	67,922	6,691	7,763
1925–7	43,838	54,643	19,850	77,785	8,251	8,362
1928–30	43,447	57,647	23,467	80,928	9,595	9,683
1931–3	41,342	55,106	23,252	92,330	11,314	10,846
1934–6	48,910	69,477	29,136	104,495	12,482	13,640
1937–9	59,355	87,437	32,994	122,771	14,758	16,159
1940–2	78,065	122,751	42,914	147,716	14,928	16,709
1943–5	89,868	147,310	55,229	203,233	18,263	21,612
1946–7	96,924	160,849	54,323	274,064		

Sources: SRH, SRI, Jessop, LGI, LPD, LHW, LMH, *Annual Reports*, 1918–47.

These increases can be accounted for by the simple fact the hospitals did more – they treated more inpatients and outpatients, they had more buildings and staff, they increased facilities for staff and patients and they had more complex administrations.[12] In particular, rises mapped closely on to the expansion in patient numbers. Growth was greatest at LPD which began admitting patients in the mid-1920s and smallest at LGI where after a sharp rise in the early 1920s inpatient numbers stabilized until the Second World War. Yet closer attention to the trends in spending complicates this simple analysis, with most hospitals experiencing sharp increases immediately after the First World War, broadly stable costs from the mid-1920s to the mid-1930s and a steady rise from 1936. The Second World War produced different outcomes depending on the contribution to war service, ward closures or direct war damage. However, in its later years and immediate aftermath the general hospitals experienced inflation of 150–200 per cent between 1943 and 1947.

Table 5.3: Categories of expenditure: five-year averages
General and specialist hospitals, Leeds and Sheffield, 1919–47

	Provisions		Surgery and drugs		Domestic		Salaries and wages		Admin and maintenance		Specialist		Total ordinary
	£	%	£	%	£	%	£	%	£	%	£	%	
1919–23	41,721	23	33,179	18	37,696	21	46,814	25	24,214	13			184,040
1924–8	39,605	19	36,267	17	38,690	19	63,684	30	30,750	15			209,006
1929–33	35,803	16	36,355	17	37,342	17	74,973	35	31,000	14	1,253	1	215,742
1934–8	39,823	16	45,404	19	40,174	17	86,195	35	28,747	12	2,253	1	243,356
1939–43	45,187	14	55,834	17	49,547	16	128,138	40	38,971	12	3,347	1	319,264
1944–7	73,673	11	114,312	18	100,571	15	277,708	43	67,983	10	19,678	3	658,958

Specialist hospitals: Leeds and Sheffield, 1919–43

	Provisions		Surgery and drugs		Domestic		Salaries and wages		Admin and maintenance		Specialist		Total ordinary
	£	%	£	%	£	%	£	%	£	%	£	%	
1919–23	2,195	20	1,756	16	1,874	17	3,083	27	2,256	20	34	0	11,350
1924–8	2,516	20	1,746	14	2,365	19	3,805	30	2,031	16	43	1	12,486
1929–33	2,897	18	2,142	13	3,121	19	5,362	33	2,679	16	241	1	16,038
1934–8	3,213	16	2,984	15	3,701	18	6,875	34	2,969	15	376	2	20,449
1939–43	4,006	13	4,492	15	5,899	20	10,806	36	4,936	16	325	1	30,139
1944–7	8,811	13	7,717	12	13,367	20	27,503	41	7,186	11	2,231	3	66,815

Sources: SRH, SRI, Jessop, LGI, LPD, LHW, LMH, *Annual Reports*, 1918–47.

Table 5.3 provides five-year rolling averages for expenditure in general and specialist institutions under the standardized headings adopted by most hospitals from the mid-1920s. The clearest trends at the general hospitals are the steady decline in the proportion of expenditure accounted for by provisions and domestic costs and the sharp increase in spending on salaries. The First World War and its immediate aftermath produced marked inflation, the LGI reporting that 'The expenditure of the Infirmary has nearly doubled in the last five years, owing to the increases in the price of food, labour, drugs, and other requisites for running a large hospital'.[13] But following this peak the interwar period saw basic costs decline from 45 to 33 per cent and then to just a quarter of spending by 1947 – shaper than falls at Bristol Royal Infirmary, where domestic costs were broadly stable but less than Middlesbrough's North Ormesby which saw housekeeping charges drop from over half to around one-third of expenditure.[14] Conversely, salaries and wages rose from 25 to 43 per cent at the general institutions of Leeds and Sheffield, almost exactly the same as the changes recorded by Gorsky, Mohan and Powell,[15] while the two headings which might have been expected to see greater prominence as hospitals became more 'modern' – surgery and drugs and administration – remained stable. Certainly more was spent under these headings but even in the wartime inflation this was far less than the expansion of salaries.

Variations at the specialist hospitals were less dramatic. The basic needs retained a more prominent place in hospital spending between the wars, with provisions and domestic falling from 37 to 34 per cent, outlay on both administration and drugs and surgery actually falling while salaries climbed far less precipitously. In cash terms, however, some of the rises were more notable as the average wage bill more than doubled while spending on drugs rose by about two thirds. These findings owe something to the different patterns of care and treatment provided by specialist and general hospitals – the latter having fewer paid medical staff while treatment regimes were still shaped by nursing care and good food. Overall, however, it is clear that the biggest challenge facing hospital managers was meeting the rising cost of pay, especially nurses' pay, Webster noting that by 1938 nurses' low pay and poor conditions were hampering recruitment.[16] In response hospitals improved accommodation for their growing corps of nurses, the Jessop adding a 96-room home in 1938 while LGI had opened three new homes the previous year.[17] Moreover, there were sharp increases in the number of resident medical staff – up to fourteen at LGI by the Second World War – while specialist scientists and administrators like pathologists and registration staff were required to deploy the new techniques of scientific management.[18]

Income

What were the means used to meet these increasing costs? Table 5.4 provides five-year averages for ordinary income sources for the general and specialist hospitals (excluding the Children's Hospital). These demonstrate diverse responses, calling into question recent ideas about the strength and impact of contributory schemes[19] and highlighting the importance of an effective maintenance department in spreading the sources of income.[20]

Table 5.4: Sources of income, general and specialist hospitals: five-year averages, 1919–47

	Sheffield Royal Infirmary and Sheffield Royal Hospital, 1919-47										
	Subs, dons etc.		Workers and employers		Investment income		Patient payments		Other		Total ordinary
	£	%	£	%	£	%	£	%	£	%	
1919–23	20,179	31.9	26,151	41.4	7,374	11.7	6,645	10.5	1,964	3.1	63,214
1924–28	12,167	12.5	64,642	66.4	8,771	9	10,105	10.4	1,210	1.2	97,340
1929–33	11,378	11.7	64,927	66.5	9,798	10	10,624	10.9	942	1	97,632
1934–8	11,426	8.9	95,723	74.9	9,455	7.4	10,019	7.8	1,240	1	127,863
1939–43	10,976	5.6	157,438	79.8	10,757	5.5	16,933	8.6	1,175	0.6	197,289
1944–7	13,084	5.2	163,586	65.5	18,024	7.2	35,085	14	1,510	0.6	249,826

	Leeds General Infirmary, 1919–47														
	Subs, dons etc.		Workers		Employers		Investments		Patient payments		Public authorities		Misc.		Total
	£	%	£	%	£	%	£	%	£	%	£	%	£	%	
1919–23	17,362	27.8	21,739	34.8	4,908	7.8	7,149	11.5	3,191	5.1	8,062	12.9			62,411
1924–8	22,969	30.2	25,753	33.8	5,738	7.5	8,974	11.8	7,570	9.9	5,149	6.8			76,153
1929–33	21,902	24.9	32,672	37.1	5,505	6.2	10,152	11.5	12,092	13.7	5,764	6.5			88,087
1934–8	20,671	18.5	43,588	38.9	5,202	4.6	13,540	12.1	20,562	18.4	6,268	5.6	2,178	1.9	112,009
1939–43	20,082	13.3	51,853	34	9,763	6.4	14,428	9.5	46,636	30.6	5,371	3.5	4,409	2.9	152,542
1944–7	25,184	10.2	65,000	26.2	13,907	5.6	19,602	7.9	95,018	38.3	8,502	3.4	20,676	8.3	247,889

	Specialist hospitals Leeds, 1919–47												
	Subs, dons etc.		Workpeople		Employers		Invest		Payments for services		Misc.		Total
	£	%	£	%	£	%	£	%	£	%	£	%	
1919–23	2,275	31	1,840	25.1	388	5.2	1,086	14.8	727	9.9	1,020	13.9	7,336
1924–8	2,025	20.3	2,253	22.6	694	7	1,055	10.6	2,816	28.2	1,123	11.3	9,966
1929–33	1,822	13.6	3,300	24.6	612	4.6	1,489	11.1	5,408	40.3	786	5.9	13,417
1934–8	2,016	11.9	4,844	28.5	668	3.9	1,750	10.3	7,017	41.3	701	4.1	16,996
1939–43	2,121	10.7	6,303	31.8	1,117	5.6	1,757	8.9	8,343	42.1	158	0.8	19,799
1944–7	2,227	5.8	4,800	12.5	1,444	3.7	369	1	29,074	75.6	552		38,466

	Jessop Hospital for Women, 1922–47												
	Subs, dons etc.		Workers		Investment income		Patient Payments (inc VD)		Public authorities		Other		Total ordinary
	£	%	£	%	£	%	£	%	£	%	£	%	£
1922–3	3,353	17.6	9,584	50.4	1,287	6.8	2,322	12.2	1,371	7.2	1,083	5.7	19,004
1924–8	2,683	13.2	11,546	55.9	1,698	8.3	2,168	10.5	1,289	6.3	1,005	4.9	20,367
1929–33	2,339	9.9	13,724	58.2	2,078	8.8	2,648	11.2	1,820	7.7	906	3.8	23,591
1934–8	2,421	7.9	19,553	63.7	2,353	7.7	2,923	9.5	2,676	8.7	747	2.4	30,679
1939–43	2,142	5	31,313	73.5	2,593	6.1	2,834	6.6	2,991	7	685	1.6	42,564
1944–7	3,057	5.5	30,531	54.5	3,277	5.8	9,675	17.3	5,784	10.3	3,926	7	56,053

Sources: SRH, SRI, Jessop, LGI, LPD, LHW, LMH, *Annual Reports*, 1918–47.

Funding models varied significantly across the country with workers schemes dominating in areas with large conglomerations of male manual workers, while traditional sources held up in areas with more diverse economies, especially those employing large numbers of women. Thus, by the early 1930s Liverpool and Birmingham both operated citywide contributory schemes on the Sheffield model with significant employer input. As a result the ordinary revenue of the Merseyside hospitals increased by 17 per cent between 1927 and 1933 while the proportion of receipts from investments, patient payments and traditional voluntary sources fell by a quarter.[21] Birmingham's scheme was collecting £400,000 from its 700,000 members by 1938, equivalent to around 85 per cent of the city's hospital costs,[22] while workers contributed between two-thirds and three-quarters of funding to institutions in Middlesbrough.[23] Conversely, in Manchester no single source dominated. Here, proceeds at all hospitals rose by 80 per cent, with traditional sources remaining stable at 40 per cent of the total while payments from Saturday Fund, patient payments and public funds together only increased their share from 31 to 41 per cent.[24] In Bristol, workers' schemes were of limited importance although patient payment, including almoner assessed direct payment, made up between 40 and 50 per cent of income by the Second World War.[25] Leicester and Nottingham resembled Manchester, with workers continuing to give through Saturday Funds rather than contributory schemes while philanthropic income doubled at Leicester Royal Infirmary.[26] Obviously there were exceptions, like Norwich, a low-wage consumer economy employing many women, where the Norfolk and Norwich received more than half of ordinary funds from the contributory scheme by 1940 while direct payment remained static at 6 per cent.[27] But overall the model is robust and appears to fit the income distributions we can see in Leeds and Sheffield.

Subscriptions, Donations and Collections

Nationally, charitable income experienced a notable decline, a trend apparent here – although the experience varied between stagnation in Leeds and collapse in Sheffield. In Sheffield both subscriptions and donations fell sharply following the introduction of the Penny in the Pound scheme as workplace collections were reallocated.[28] For example, at the SRH, half the 1921 subscriber income had come from works contributions but this halved over the next five years as most of these switched to the Hospital Council's fund. In a similar vein, donations to Sheffield's two institutions were healthy in 1920, totalling £10,000, with many large donations coming from fundraisers like the student rag, the Sheffield Cinemas and the city's two football clubs – although there were few personal donations of more than £10 even at this date.[29] As with subscriptions, within two years of the Penny in the Pound scheme coming into full operation donation income had collapsed to just over £3,100 and remained low until the Second World War. Thus from the mid-1920s the vast majority of subscribers and donors were individuals pledging small amounts of two guineas or less. In part this weakness is explained by Sheffield's relatively constrained list of potential subscribers,[30] but more significant was the incorporation of a generous employer contribution into the Penny in the Pound scheme. Unlike most contributory schemes, Sheffield secured the agreement of employers to add one-third to the contributions of their employees. This resulted in a substantial input to hospital funding that masked the continuing engagement of the middle classes who had switched their status from voluntary subscribers to corporate contributors.

In Leeds, however, the subscriber list did not change so rapidly. As in Nottingham and Leicester, a number of works continued to contribute through the subscription list rather than LWHF.[31] These were usually businesses located some distance from Leeds or with head offices in other towns, such as the Manchester based Co-operative Wholesale Society, big railway companies, collieries and council departments, while subscribers included associations from Leeds and beyond such as political parties, working men's clubs and village charities. In total, corporate subscriptions, whether business, mutual or charitable, accounted for just under two-thirds of the £5,600 subscription income in 1938. Yet just over half of the subscribers were still individuals, including contributions from some of the old elite like the banker Henry Oxley (£100) and the brewers Riley-Smith (£138) and Tetley (family total £131).[32] Although the number of subscribers was low in proportion to the size of the middle class – a characteristic noted by Gorsky in relation to Bristol – the continuing role of prominent families challenges pessimistic accounts of urban withdrawal suggested by Gunn and others.[33] The trajectory of the LGI's donations was equally diverse, growing from a healthy base in 1920 to peak in the early 1930s. In contrast to Sheffield, the number of personal donations more than doubled up to 1938 although the value of the gifts tended to be small playing only a minor part in the general increase in money raised. That came from the expansion of activities organized by clubs, associations and works' socials, ranging from big events like the annual charity police football match to the ubiquitous whist drives and dances mounted by political parties, trade associations and the employees of city business.[34]

Although frequently criticized by the hospital management for not doing their bit, donations from the fundraising committees of the villages and towns of Yorkshire were equally significant.[35] Undoubtedly, formal town and village collections provided a decreasing proportion of donation income, falling from almost half in 1920 to around 30 per cent by 1938 as more workers joined the LWHF or paid in other ways.[36] Thus, in Knottingley the Infirmary committee's donation of £180 in 1920 had become part of a contributory scheme by 1938 when their £220 appeared in the patient payment column.[37] On the other hand, ad hoc fundraisers in the villages and towns, many organized by works' social committees, underpinned growth as they did in rural areas around Leicester and Nottingham.[38] Concerts were a common activity, reflecting the importance of brass bands and choral music in West Yorkshire although it was the whist drive and dance which became the mainstay with almost 60 events raising over £800 by 1938. These complemented traditional activities like village carnivals and large-scale public spectacles along with door-to-door collections, garden fêtes like the one held in the small town of Settle which raised £150, fancy dress parades and collections of bun pennies.[39]

Less robust were the Hospital Saturday and Sunday and street collections like the Alexandra Rose Day. In Leeds, Hospital Saturday had been abandoned before the First World War while in Sheffield[40] collections dwindled from £2,000 in 1919 to less than £150 by 1924 due to the 'great success of the "1d. in the £" Scheme' which had 'naturally interfered with this Voluntary effort'.[41] The Hospital Sunday, an annual church collection, held up better though its contribution declined in real and cash terms. Thus, in 1919 the Sheffield collection had provided 5 per cent of the income of the city's four hospitals[42] but by 1938 takings had fallen by around 40 per cent,[43] while in Leeds they were down 25 per cent by 1938.[44] Alexandra Rose Day suffered a similar fate. Hugely important during the First World War, by the early 1930s the SRI was reporting that although 'the entire Nursing Staff devoted their free time throughout the day to the selling of roses between the hours of 6.30 a.m. and 9.30 p.m', the total sum collected was just £167[45] while the nurses of the SRH added £106 – scarcely a tenth of the 1918 figure.[46] Indeed, flag days in general were treated with increasing scepticism by the general public and local authorities, Leeds City Council making street collections very difficult to organize for groups like the Leeds Voluntary Hospital Committee in the 1920s.[47]

Community fundraising also took on some new forms, adding a novel dimension to the traditional entertainment or street collection, especially the student rags mounted annually in Leeds and Sheffield. Usually featuring slapstick spectacles, fancy dress, processions and comic events, they relied heavily on 'a good natured and generous public' for their success.[48] Incorporating many of the features of the post-war student fundraiser, for the first event in Sheffield the medical students:

> promoted a Football Charity Match between the Students of this Infirmary and the Sheffield Royal Hospital. The match was played on the Wednesday Ground, Owlerton (very kindly lent), on the 10th November last, the Infirmary Students being the winners of a cup (an old beer barrel aluminium painted). The match was preceded by processions in costume around the City, and this match and the processions, together with the collections organised earlier in the year, resulted in £1,550 being collected for the four Hospitals.[49]

The following year was a little less successful, the football match and rag raising £428 for the SRI though the 'organisation and enthusiasm' displayed by the students, 'both ladies and gentlemen', 'was a credit to them and to the City generally'.[50] In 1923 the students presented an 'up-to-date Daimler Ambulance' to the Hospitals Council while in subsequent years both the SRH and the SRI placed the donations of upwards of £1,500 to specific projects including new research laboratories, X-ray departments and the SRH's accident and orthopaedic department.[51] In Leeds the Rag contributed an average £1,000 a year, totalling £19,000 by 1938 which, from 1926, was devoted solely to endowing beds in Ward 20.[52] Carol Dyhouse's study of the gendered elements of the interwar Rag has suggested that it was more than just a bit of fun, pointing to the exclusion of women at some universities and an element of disapproval from some university authorities. As the reference above to 'ladies and gentlemen' suggests, gender was less of an issue in Sheffield, where by the mid-1930s the rag committee included the College of Art. More problematic was the frequently 'inclement weather' and the enduring economic problems – from depression in the steel industry to disputes in the coal mines.[53] Moreover, there was also some hostility from the university, the Vice-Chancellor of Sheffield, Professor Pickard-Cambridge, stating in 1935 that although the rag had raised £10,000 in the previous seven years,

> It is a tremendous sacrifice to the students. It takes a lot of time from their work, and I know a number of students whose prospects have definitely been injured as a result of preparation of the 'Rag'. If they said it was more than they could face I would find it difficult to oppose them.

Although he did continue that 'personally ... I hope the University will do all it can for the hospitals'.[54]

The decline of traditional income at the specialist hospitals followed a similar pattern to the general institutions, falling sharply at the Jessop in the early 1920s, then settling for the rest of the interwar period, while for the Leeds institutions the experience was less precipitous, with a gradual fall to the early 1930s and then a slight improvement over the following fifteen years. But as with the general hospitals, the key difference was in the proportion of income drawn from this source. At the Jessop this more than halved from 18 to 8 per cent while in Leeds the decline was more stark – from almost one-third to just over 10 per cent by the Second World War. Thus, the cash value of traditional income sources in Leeds remained broadly constant – as it did in Manchester – while in Sheffield it experienced a sharp decline in the early 1920s before stabilizing in a similar way to other areas with mass contributory schemes.[55] What is clear, however, is that traditional sources were no longer capable of meeting the growing demand for funds and it was to meet this gap that new sources of finance were sought by the hospitals, producing rather different approaches across the cities and institution types.

Workers and Employers Contributions

For most of the hospitals, the core of this new funding came from prepayment by workers collected by highly organized contributory schemes which tapped into a range of earners and increasingly drew subscribers on a regional basis. However, the scale of the scheme, the way the funds were operated, the method by which income was collected and distributed and the levels of influence and independence varied significantly between the cities. Both the LWHF and the Sheffield Penny in the Pound Scheme have received attention from historians and as such only the broad outlines will be sketched here.[56] The Sheffield scheme emerged from a committee established to examine the post-First World War financial crisis at the hospitals. It recommended a workers' contributory scheme operated on the novel 'penny in the pound' principle and in the ensuing months support was secured from a broad range of interests, especially the trade union movement and employers.[57] Run by the Sheffield Joint Hospitals' Council with members represented by the Hospitals Contributors Association headed by Labour Councillor Moses Humberstone, it was an immediate success, signing up most industrial employees and employers by 1925.[58] Benefits included free treatment for members and their families if admitted as an inpatient or outpatient to a Sheffield voluntary hospital, convalescent care and free emergency treatment in the city's PLIs.[59] After deductions to cover these extra benefits, around 75 per cent of income was distributed among the four hospitals and the Edgar Allen Institute broadly on the basis of patients treated. The Hospital Council allocated additional income to the SRH when they opened a number of new beds in 1924 while in the later 1930s the general hospitals received subventions to cover their current account deficits. Further support came during the Depression when the contributors agreed to pay a penny for each pound and for any additional part of a pound. An attempt to secure a similar agreement in Liverpool in 1932 was unsuccessful.[60]

The LWHF was an independent mutualist body set up in the 1880s to raise money for the LGI.[61] Until 1930 it operated as a collection fund when it became a contributory scheme on a fixed-income basis – adult males paying two pence per week, women and youths less.[62] Although the largest part of its income went to LGI, it made contributions to all the other hospitals as well as running three convalescent homes (two for women), a fleet of ambulances, a dental scheme and some ancillary services. Although the LWHF had a near-monopoly in Leeds, it faced competition from schemes outside the city where collection committees continued into the 1930s. Indeed, Gorsky, Mohan and Willis have calculated that West Yorkshire had one of the highest proportions of members in England paying amongst the highest average contributions.[63] The *BMJ* noted in 1939 that one Yorkshire district had 'more schemes than days in the month, with uniformity neither of benefits nor of contributions'.[64] But the key weakness of the LWHF was its failure to secure integrated employer contributions. Expectations were raised in 1920 when the Leeds Employers Contribution Fund was established, based on a voluntary payment of two shillings per employee to the fund.[65] Initially projected to raise £10,000–12,000 per annum, after a satisfactory launch it stalled at £4,000 a year and began to decline a little after 1926.[66] The employers' scheme was joined in 1924 by the Leeds Voluntary Hospitals Fund to collect from non-industrial workers, professionals and the self-employed, but it also proved a disappointment. Moreover, certain groups of employers proved hard to reach, with mine owners making no contributions during the tough years around 1926 and maintaining a complex payment method based on productivity rather than a membership head count.[67] By the later 1920s these sources netted around £6,000 annually while the workers provided five times as much – a ratio short of Sheffield's three to one, though probably better than many other schemes.[68]

Once established, there were few organizational changes to the Sheffield scheme beyond the extension of the deductions to the part of a pound and the formal arrangements with Barnsley, Rotherham and Retford in the 1940s.[69] In Leeds, however, the interwar period saw the conversion of the LWHF to a contributory scheme in 1930 and its rebranding as the Leeds and District Workpeople's Hospital Fund in 1933. Although the scheme resisted adopting the Penny in the Pound collection method, it incorporated the employee element of the Leeds Voluntary Hospital Fund and recruited a growing number of members from outside the city so that by 1938 it was raising a £100,000 a year.[70] In the later 1930s the employers' scheme was renamed the Leeds and District Voluntary Hospitals Fund to attract professionals and 'embrace all who were not in the ordinary sense employed persons'.[71] By the Second World War it was raising around £10,000 per annum, though the chairman noted that

> a list of 939 subscribers for a city of the importance of Leeds to a Fund which has for
> its purpose the alleviation of suffering and the relief of pain among our less fortunate
> neighbours does not connote a high standard of citizenship.[72]

The war benefitted the works' based schemes as takings in Sheffield rose to over £300,000 while both the LWHF and the Voluntary Hospitals Fund saw significant increases between 1939 and 1943 when income for both peaked. In part this emerged from a failed attempt to merge the two schemes and convert to Penny in the Pound collection which encouraged the LWHF to raise the flat-rate contribution to three pence,[73] producing an increase of about 25 per cent for the works fund, while employer subscriptions climbed 50 per cent to almost £20,000.[74]

The schemes were hugely important to the financial health of the hospitals. The LWHF and employer schemes provided just over 40 per cent of LGI income until the mid-1940s and around a third at the city's specialist hospitals. The impact in Sheffield was even more striking, as contributions quickly accounted for two-thirds rising to four-fifths of general hospital income and a half to two-thirds of funding at the Jessop. Cash from workers and employers doubled at the Leeds hospitals and the Jessop between 1918 and 1938, while at Sheffield's general hospitals the growth was in the order of three and a half times. The war saw subventions to most hospitals peak in 1944 before a sharp decline caused by the end of war production and uncertainty around the government's health proposals. Moreover, the proportionate importance of the schemes was weakened by the rise in patient payments in Leeds – though much of this came from other contributory schemes prior to the opening of the pay-bed block in 1941.

Neither scheme was prompted by the Cave Committee of 1921 – as often suggested by historians. Indeed, few of the larger schemes were, with the Norwich fund established in 1919 and those in Birmingham and Liverpool in 1927–8.[75] The LWHF dated from the 1880s and was already contributing 40 per cent of ordinary income by 1923 while the Penny in the Pound scheme had been proposed in 1920 and launched in 1922.[76] Nor are the overall effects of contributory schemes on the broader funding mix straightforward – for example, they did not necessarily reduce income from traditional sources. Thus the dominance of workers' contributions in Sheffield owed something to the city's economy which, with its small middle class and severe unemployment problems, had a weakened voluntary base. But it also owed much to the employers' 25 per cent top-up, which meant they were contributing something in the region of £40,000 per annum by 1939.[77] In this case it clearly did crowd out traditional middle-class voluntary giving while the establishment of the scheme transferred traditional workplace income from the Hospital Saturday Fund and the sub-scription lists of the two general hospitals from the charitable to the payment column. On the other hand, evidence from Leeds questions the view that con-tributory schemes were the only solution to the interwar funding crisis.[78] As in Manchester and Leicester, overall income from the workers and employers together grew at roughly the same rate as total income. Moreover, the failure of the scheme to adopt Penny in the Pound collection limited its ability to take advantage of wartime wage rises while the reluctance of employers and profes-sionals to commit to regular contributions left room for continued individual giving through subscriptions and donations.

However, the successful contributory schemes were not only responsible for rebadging income from the voluntary columns of the accounts as patient pay-ment, they were also the continuing focus for important fundraising activities that did not appear on the hospital accounts as voluntary giving. In early 1920s Leeds, almost 25 per cent of the income of the LWHF (around £11,000) came from activities like fêtes, concerts and carnivals, the annual Hospital Gala, and collections in pubs and clubs. Although these sources suffered during the Depres-sion, a recovery by 1938 saw a total of £7,500 raised by the LWHF through voluntary efforts that appeared in the hospital accounts as scheme income.[79] In Sheffield the Hospital Council organized subscriptions, donations and special events which brought in £3,000 per annum and collected the income from the village 'demonstrations'. This income had previously gone to the individual hos-pitals but was now distributed as part of the patient payment grant. Clearly the schemes could mobilize extensive voluntary support and under-recorded giving, raising further questions about the instrumental reading of these organizations.

Investments

Investment income in the ordinary account was derived from the returns on the portfolio of savings, shares and rents the hospitals acquired largely from legacies and endowments. In most provincial English hospitals this was a relatively small part of the operating revenue, although in London and Scotland it was a signifi-cant source of funding.[80] In 1919 investment income at the LGI amounted to £6,500 per annum, similar to the Sheffield general hospitals, which each aver-aged £3,400 per annum. Twenty years later, LGI averaged £14,500, providing 10 per cent of ordinary income, whereas in Sheffield investment income had stagnated.[81] Overall, the interwar period saw the Jessop and the LGI (where there was little building in the 1930s) double their income from investments. The Leeds specialist institutions grew by around 75 per cent, while the Sheffield general hospitals enjoyed a rise of less than 30 per cent. The ability to enhance the value of liquid assets was determined by both the prevailing economic environment and by hospital policy. From 1918 to the mid-1930s overdrafts at the general hospitals left no surplus for investment while it was common to use free legacies to minimize the deficit or reduce borrowing. Moreover, in Sheffield the close interrelationship of the four institutions in the Hospitals' Council meant most large legacies were shared equally among the establishments with the Jessop and the Children's Hospital benefitting disproportionately, allowing their investment income to rise more quickly than the general hospitals. Despite this, assets excluding buildings and equipment almost trebled over twenty years at LGI while at the SRH they were static and at the SRI they actually fell.[82]

In part this was because investment income was largely ignored at the SRH in favour of fixed assets, the hospital authorities following a policy of 'build now, pay later', with the result that the value of their land, buildings and equipment more than doubled in the later 1930s. Though less ambitious, the SRI completed a range of small building works in the second half of the decade at a cost of £25,000. Moreover, the Sheffield institutions committed £15,000 each towards the purchase of land and the drawing up of plans for the new amalgamated hospital.[83] In Leeds, however, the opposite trend is apparent, as the LGI increased its investment portfolio by 25 per cent between 1934 and 1938, aided by balanced budgets and a short-term boost from the receipts of the appeal. Although investment income did grow in the 1930s at the specialist institutions of Leeds, the increase was slower than the main hospital, in part because they too chose to spend on buildings rather than stocks and shares.

Patient Payments

By the early 1920s most hospitals had introduced a scale of charges for maintenance or, as Webster dramatically phrased it, sought 'to exact charges from classes of patients hitherto treated gratis'.[84] Thus, Sheffield established a citywide scheme whereby 'in-patients other than contributors to the Joint Hospitals' Scheme, their dependents and the necessitous poor should be asked to pay a standard rate of £1 15s. 0d. per week towards the cost of their maintenance'. However, this charge could vary, with the average amount collected in the early 1920s being 19/10 per patient.[85] Explicit charges were not widely advertised at the LGI while the LPD rarely recovered any costs directly from its patients. On the other hand, the Jessop and the LMH were already securing significant direct contributions from both mothers and the local state. Thus, who paid differed from institution to institution.

Direct payment by or for patients in Sheffield hospitals was broadly stable until the 1940s, which was largely attributable to the wide coverage of the Penny in the Pound scheme, which included many black-coated workers and a significant membership in outlying areas.[86] In Leeds, however, the proportion taken directly from or for the patient was minimal at the LPD – just 5 per cent of income in 1938 – but rose sharply at the LGI, LHW and LMH. This money was collected in different ways. At the LMH, 30 per cent of income came direct from patients in 1928 along with a further 25 per cent from Leeds Corporation under the Maternity and Child Welfare scheme. By the Second World War, the hospital received 72 per cent of its income from patients, Leeds City Council and other local authorities, but just 5 per cent from traditional voluntary charity while the LWHF and employers provided significantly less than at the other institutions.[87] In a similar vein, Bristol Maternity Hospital saw patient payments rise to around 80 per cent of income following the reduction of its local authority subvention in 1934.[88] However, the LGI provides the most interesting case in relation to payment. In 1924, following five years of substantial deficits, Alderman Lupton controversially recommended charging all patients a standard daily rate for treatment and although this was accepted by the Weekly Board the plan was dropped, probably due to opposition from the LWHF.[89] Yet the idea did not go away and in the early 1930s the LGI adopted an aggressive policy towards securing payment for many of its patients, especially those from outside Leeds.

Although the hospital had employed almoners since 1911 and extended their work to various outpatient departments during the 1920s, they appeared to offer a diminishing return as they came to focus increasingly on their social work element.[90] In response in 1929 the hospital set up a department designed 'to afford an opportunity to In-patients to contribute voluntarily in accordance with their means towards the cost of their maintenance whilst in hospital'.[91] The following year the report attributed the £2,500 increase in patient contributions 'to the efforts of the staff in the new Maintenance Department'[92] who proved particularly adept at extracting payment from 'the various Contributory Schemes now operating in areas served by the Infirmary', local authorities for treating special surgical cases along with 'Hospital Funds' and 'Contributory Schemes connected with other Hospitals'.[93] Admittedly this was a controversial approach as many smaller schemes were reluctant to hand over their hospital's income to the big city institutions. But Leeds proved effective, for while payments by and on behalf of patients were stable between 1933 and 1938 at around £12,000, those from other contributory associations increased from just £600 to £9,000 and those from other local authorities increased from £500 to £2,500.[94] This success emerged from the separation of inpatient maintenance from the work of the almoners and by aggressive pursuit of direct payment from other contributory schemes, possibly on better terms than could have been negotiated by the LWHF[95] through the kinds of reciprocal schemes operating in Sheffield.

The third way hospitals obtained payment was through the provision of pay wards.[96] The first of these was at the LHW, which opened in 1930 and by the end of the decade was contributing £2,500 to funds – more than either subscriptions and donations or general patient payments.[97] By this time pay blocks were open or under construction at the SRH, Jessop and the LGI, the success of the latter ensuring that patient payments was the largest single source of funds by the mid-1940s.[98] Overall, for most of the period payment was closely associated with areas where the state actively contributed to costs – maternity, VD and childhood orthopaedics.[99] Women seem to have been the earliest users of private beds – though the LGI's Brotherton wing was less gendered. On the other hand, the Penny in the Pound scheme, with its lack of official salary limits and extensive reciprocal agreements, limited the scope for extracting payment for general patients while LGI pursued a determined policy of seeking maintenance costs wherever possible.

Non-Cash Gifts

At the opposite extreme to the payments of the private patients and offering a marked contrast to the image of increasingly commercial relations, was the wide range of gifts in kind which reduced outgoings, increased assets and improved the experience of patients and staff. Such gifts drew on the full range of potential donors, from the wealthy philanthropist to the village school child, and served to encapsulate the persistent and increasingly democratic 'hospital spirit'. The development of a nurses' home at Tapton Court, Sheffield – a gift from J. C. Graves – was underpinned by additional gifts in kind, including a grand piano and furniture from the wealthy, while unemployed men from an allotment society 'kindly gave their services in helping to recondition the gardens and grounds'.[100] In a similar vein, the LGI treasurer, T. F. Braime, oversaw the redevelopment of the Infirmary's workshops, calling on a wide range of local firms to provide materials, equipment and even labour for free.[101] Moreover, most institutions benefitted from the growth of corporate giving by national and local companies, Sheffield's general hospitals receiving all of their oxygen for free from the British Oxygen Company, as well as free Izal disinfectant and groceries from Robertsons and Batchelors.[102]

As significant were the wide range of smaller gifts and donations traditionally derived from wealthy individuals such as fruit, flowers, old linen and clothes, books and magazines, sweets, Christmas treats, toys and cigarettes.[103] However, the profile of givers and the items given changed markedly during the 1920s. Gifts and donations of fruit, vegetables and flowers relied increasingly on community responses from market traders, schoolchildren and clubs and societies,[104] prompting the Sheffield Infirmary to emphasize the 'real value' of donations from allotment holders and gardeners 'resulting as they do in a saving of many pounds annually'.[105] Mass collection campaigns were also instituted, especially for eggs and silver paper, bringing in a wide range of volunteers, mobilizing supporters in outlying areas and facilitating involvement from women and children.[106] Lady Harewood's Yorkshire-wide 'egg week' – one of a number of similar ventures[107] – collected 133,000 eggs for Sheffield hospitals in 1934 – while a similar haul was valued at £600 by the LGI.[108] Equally important in terms of civic mobilization, although of considerably less value financially, was the collection of silver paper which took off in the mid-1920s. This activity was well suited to mass involvement – it was ubiquitous, could be collected by anybody, cost nothing and lent itself to communal efforts, by workpeople, pubs and clubs and, especially, the young.[109] The capture of support for the hospital cause by the community at large was most clearly exemplified by the role of unemployed workers, especially in Sheffield where the Council of Social Services arranged for furniture and splints to be supplied by 'men who, although unemployed, are desirous of helping the Hospital'.[110]

The linen guilds that organized volunteers to produce substantial quantities of bedding and clothing for the hospital wards reflected the enduring place of older, gendered traditions of middle-class giving. These guilds were often the only space for female involvement in the management of the hospital. In many hospitals women were denied access to seats on the board or a role in the decision-making processes of the institutions – one hospital even told women that involvement in the League was sufficient and appropriate.[111] Indeed, the Linen League and the Samaritan Society were the only leadership opportunities for women at Sheffield's general hospitals, though they had a more prominent role in the hospitals of Leeds. Similar to associations in Birmingham and Nottingham,[112] these were extensive operations; the Linen Guild set up at Leeds General in 1929 began with 1,200 members and income of £500 and produced 1,949 garments in its first year. But by 1938 its membership had doubled and it was contributing 6,500 garments underpinned by an income of £900.[113] The SRH initiated a Linen and Clothing Guild in 1925, the board noting that 'the activities and generosity of the Guild members saves the Hospital very considerable sums annually'. By the later 1930s it was providing over 1,000 yards of various materials for sheets, blankets, quilts, towels and dressing gowns, supported by a fundraising campaign of whist drives and 'American Teas'. There was also a Junior League with 350 members which increasingly focused its attention on equipping the children's ward. At the SRI the pre-war Ladies Working Association provided garments for both the wards and the aftercare service, mixing the roles of the Linen Guild and Samaritan Society. It received income from subscriptions, donations and, in the mid-1920s, special matinees at the Empire Theatre, the board recognizing their work by commenting that 'many poor patients had reason to be grateful for the help given in connection with the loan of garments made by the members' and by the end of the 1930s they were providing 2,000 garments worth almost £300, helping to reduce the linen costs of the institution by around a fifth.[114]

The longest running gift to patients and staff was the provision of Christmas presents and other festive treats. Mirroring the fundraising environment generally, these gifts became both more democratic and more organized. In Sheffield their collection was taken over by the Joint Hospitals Council who raised around £350 per annum in cash plus gifts of fruit, handkerchiefs, books, cigarettes, chocolates, sweets and toys from traders while the making up and distribution of the more than 2,000 parcels became the task of the city's Rotary Club. In addition, all the nurses received a box of chocolates while large permanent toys such as rocking horses were sent to the children's wards.[115] Similar arrangements were seen at hospitals in Leeds although on a more ad hoc basis, reflecting a general situation nationally. For example, in Middlesbrough patients at the North Riding Infirmary received a visit from the mayor and gifts such as cigarettes and chocolate donated by the public following an annual appeal from the matron.[116]

The provision of gifts in kind became the most open and democratic of the contributions made to interwar hospitals. In part because they relied more on time than money, activities like collecting tinfoil or eggs or making garments for the Linen Guild could be undertaken by the young and old, and many of those involved were women and children. Similarly, the unemployed could give their time and their skills at no personal cost. For the middle classes, the new voluntary organizations formed during and after the war, such as the Rotary Club, were prominent in providing time, money and resources for the benefit of the hospitals, their patients and families. In Sheffield the Christian Toc H staffed libraries while the Rotary Club was involved in taking relatives of seriously ill patients to hospital, relieving pressure on the ambulance service by ferrying patients home, and bringing in blood donors at night.[117] These were all tasks which required access to the new symbols of middle-class status – the motor car and telephone – while providing a space for social engagement for the younger or arriviste members of the elite who dominated these organizations.[118]

Endowments, Legacies and Appeals

In focusing on trends in ordinary income, historians have tended to overlook the large sums of money most institutions received as gifts, endowments, legacies or proceeds of special appeals.[119] This money often did not appear in the ordinary accounts, frequently going 'straight to the balance sheet', as was the case with the £250,000 received between the wars by Sheffield's two general hospitals. Until the mid-1930s this money was utilized primarily to pay off substantial bank overdrafts. Even at the relatively wealthy LGI, the books were only balanced by continuous use of free legacies to meet the operating deficit, despite the desire of the board that such income ideally 'should either be invested or reserved for special expenditure'.[120] Of more direct benefit to the hospitals of Leeds and Sheffield, as in Nottingham and Birmingham, were the significant number of endowments they received.[121] Endowments, which had previously been the preserve of the wealthy to commemorate the death of a close relative or as a personal legacy, stimulated by the First World War, became a part of the collective giving by organizations, workplaces and communities which characterized the interwar period. In Leeds the 130 £1,000 beds and more than 50 £500 cots came largely from individual donors, including some substantial contributions from C. S. Weatherill, who funded thirty-four beds in 1905, and H. S. Birtwistle, whose contribution endowed thirty-six beds in 1936, although around one-third of the beds and a quarter of the cots were sponsored by business or community groups. Easily the largest single fundraisers for the LGI was the Student Rag, which endowed a total of eighteen beds. Many organizations, especially sports and social clubs and societies, contributed sums on an annual basis to help maintain a bed, including Leeds' two competing amateur dramatic societies and the boys of Leeds Grammar School.[122] Yet, once again, giving was less common in Sheffield. Together, the two general hospitals acquired fewer than half the beds and cots endowed in Leeds, almost all supported by individuals, although there were additionally annual payments for cots from the entertainments charity the 'Gloops Club'.[123] Such a disparity may have derived from the relatively small activist middle class or the stifling effects on voluntary activity produced by the Penny in the Pound scheme, although the hospitals of Middlesbrough, with a similar economy and social structure, also received very few endowments between the wars.[124]

Hospitals also benefitted from large and small gifts and bequests. Notable testators included the steel magnate, Alfred Bosher, who left £70,000 to the Sheffield hospitals[125] as did Robert Halliday, the Hospitals Council utilizing his bequest to acquire the Norton Hall estate for a potential united hospital while in Leeds the bequest of Mr Bartholomew established a children's department. In general, however, these did not match the munificence of the cigarette barons of Bristol and Nottingham or the Cadburys and Chamberlains in Birmingham.[126] Rather, it was large-scale special appeals that fuelled the growth of the fixed assets and provided the opportunity for the cities' elites to make their mark.[127] Major appeals in both cities at the end of the First World War aimed to clear accumulated debt,[128] allowing the Sheffield hospitals to settle their building fund deficits and make limited inroads into their substantial overdrafts while in Leeds the £27,500 raised, plus a gift of £50,000 from the soap manufacturer, Joseph Watson (later Lord Manton), helped briefly to reduce the LGI's overdraft. Yet just five years later a second citywide appeal was required to clear the collective debt of £200,000 amassed by the Leeds hospitals. Almost all of this income came from business or wealthy individuals and very little from community groups or even smaller individual donations.[129] However, subsequent appeals were more broadly based as the economy slowed and it became necessary to widen the pool of donors. When the SRH launched its centenary appeal in 1932 the committee thought 'few large contributions could be expected owing to the depressed state of the local industries'.[130] Instead, it aimed to approach 'every section of the community with a request that efforts of all descriptions should be started; such as Entertainments, Concerts, Dances, Garden Parties, Collections, and so forth'.[131] The two political parties and the Trades and Labour Council agreed to put their organizations at the disposal of the hospital to support a house-to-house canvass for donations.[132] Other contributing organizations included the Education Department, unemployed workers, Rotarians and the Boys' Brigade. A film was made to show the 'actual work of a hospital' and an air pageant was organized by the Sheffield Motor Organisations. Despite this the total raised was disappointing – just £21,000 of the £100,000 target. It did, however, elicit £25,000 from the South Yorkshire Miners' Welfare Fund to pay for a new block and the gift of Tapton Court and six acres of land as a nurses' home from J. C. Graves.[133]

Fundraisers in 1930s Leeds similarly cast the net wide to raise the £250,000 needed for future expansion. They did this by securing donations from the wealthy, those families 'who have for generations given of their best, both in service and money, when an Appeal has been made to them' but also through a rolling programme that mobilized new constituencies across the life cycle of the appeal.[134] Thus in the first year of the appeal there were 30 personal donations of £1,000 or more, 100 contributions of between £100 and £1,000 and a further 100 of £25–£100, plus substantial company donations. The following year the appeal benefitted from large numbers of ordinary citizens mobilizing through the 'very many social and other events held on behalf of the Appeal which have been the means of raising considerable sums'.[135] Approximately 80 per cent of the more than a thousand separate donations in 1934 were for less than £100, drawn mainly from clubs and associations, many linked to sporting events, schoolchildren and students. In the final phase the Million Shilling Fund aimed for a more socially diffuse approach to fundraising. Twenty-five local committees were formed across Leeds and the surrounding districts and over a thousand firms signed up to give two shillings per week through two savings card schemes utilizing an image of a dragon and the slogan 'Help stamp out disease'. In all, £32,000 was raised to complete the appeal. The chair of the fund, in emphasizing its democratic nature, noted: 'With an Appeal of this size one would normally expect something like 5,000 donors; the number on our list is 60,000'.[136]

The most ambitious campaign, however, was the Sheffield Voluntary Hospitals' Million Pound Appeal that followed from the amalgamation of the SRH and SRI in 1938. It sought funds for five building projects, including a pay-bed block at the maternity hospital, cancer research laboratories and, most notably, a new general hospital. It was based on a tripartite appeal to all sections. 'It is not healthy', the appeal launch argued, 'for any community to depend on one or two benefactors to provide the necessary money for its Hospitals; it is the duty of the community as a whole – it is YOUR responsibility'.[137] Like the Birmingham united hospital venture, which raised £625,000 in the mid-1930s,[138] it sought to tap into existing corporate fundraising mechanisms. Thus, the Ministry of Health was informed that 'The majority of local Firms are co-operating, subscribing £50,000 per annum for seven years'. Similarly, the 250,000 subscribers to the Penny in the Pound scheme were to be asked to give a further penny per week. The final third of the money was to be raised through private subscription, including several local authorities.[139] By the time the appeal closed in 1947, £500,000 had been raised, the bulk of the money coming from worker subscriptions, although there was also a sizeable contribution from both business and private individuals, Graves once more stepping in to provide £100,000 for the Radium Centre.[140] Thus, in Sheffield, which had generally found it difficult to raise money for expansion by appeals and fundraisers, salvation came through a bureaucratic scheme which drew heavily on the existing Penny in the Pound arrangement, with only limited input from the kind of broad-based charitable techniques developed in Leeds. The willingly given additional voluntary contribution by scheme members does, however, suggest they viewed their membership as more than simply insurance and that they had become accustomed to 'giving' in this manner rather than through the ad hoc activities found elsewhere.[141]

In the specialist hospitals patterns of extraordinary giving were reversed with the Jessop performing proportionately better than the other institutions in the study while in Leeds gifts varied markedly from healthy at the LPD to minimal at the LMH. Moreover, unlike the general hospitals – or indeed small institutions in other cities[142] – the specialist institutions rarely embarked on appeals of their own, although they benefitted substantially from the citywide activities in Leeds in 1925 and Sheffield in the late 1930s. The biggest disparity occurred around legacies. Between 1919 and 1940 the LPD received over £50,000 in bequests, raising the book value of their investments to over £70,000, producing an average £2,200 per annum. The £28,000 left to the LHW across the interwar years allowed some augmentation of the stock portfolio. However, this took a significant hit at the end of the 1930s when a revaluation wrote down most of the railway stock to less than half its purchase price. At the LMH, however, investments were minimal as the institution received next to no legacies, while its share of both LWHF allocations and city collections were the smallest by some way. As a result it held only £7,000 in stocks and shares and received just £300 a year in dividends. The experience of the LHW and Jessop – where the fall in interest rates in the mid-1930s reduced income – suggests that investing in stocks and shares was not always the best strategy and ultimately most hospitals preferred to have buildings, rather than cash, on the balance sheet.[143]

Municipal Hospital Finance

Voluntary hospitals, as a product of nineteenth-century subscriber democracy, produced extensive reports of the finances and activities of the institution to demonstrate their public accountability.[144] The local authorities, on the other hand, were less public or detailed in their accounting procedures, so that identifying what portion of the local budget was spent on medical, and especially hospital services, is rather less clear-cut.[145] However, using a combination of the reported figures collected by Levene, Powell and Stewart,[146] council reports and the findings of the Ministry of Health surveyors, it is possible to gain a picture of hospital spending in Leeds and Sheffield.

At the macro level of overall health spending both cities were medium to high spenders.[147] In 1922 Leeds had the fifth highest per capita expenditure on health services of all English and Welsh county boroughs – behind Liverpool, Bradford, Eastbourne and Canterbury – while Sheffield, at twenty-fourth, was just outside the upper quartile. Manchester and Newcastle were also in the top twenty while Bristol and Birmingham were twenty-ninth and thirtieth respectively. Over the following fourteen years, per capita spending on health approximately doubled across the 83 county boroughs as it did in Leeds and Sheffield, with the result that the former fell to twelfth overall and the latter to twenty-sixth.[148] Other major cities had varying fortunes with greater than average increases in Manchester and Birmingham, while Newcastle and Bristol fell. On the other hand towns with limited spending in 1922, like Norwich and Middlesbrough, moved up sharply to thirty-fifth and twenty-eighth respectively.

As Levene et al. have emphasized, boroughs prioritized some services over others. In the case of Leeds spending had been high on mental deficiency and infectious diseases in the early 1920s but stagnated while the commitment to TB services grew. The picture in Sheffield was similar, with a greater commitment to TB – which took the largest slice of health spending before the advent of general hospitals.[149] Most relevant for this study, however, was spending on maternity and child welfare and general hospitals. In the former case Leeds was in the top ten at the beginning of the period, with expenditure around 75 per cent above the mean, while Sheffield was firmly in the middle with a ranking of fortieth. However, over the interwar period the latter city caught up as its spending grew more rapidly than the average, while the former slipped back as growth slowed and priorities shifted to supporting institutional births in the city's own hospitals. Indeed, in both cities the general hospital service expanded rapidly. Though some way behind the highest spenders on hospitals – Salford, Manchester and

Rochdale, who all spent twice as much as Leeds and three times the figure for Sheffield – by 1936 expenditure on hospitals accounted for around one-third of all health spending in Leeds and a more modest 25 per cent in Sheffield.

The poor law and municipal hospitals had very different income streams to those of the voluntary hospitals. The core funding came from the rates (local property tax) levied by the city council which meant that the proportion allocated was under pressure throughout the interwar period from general increases in local authority services and stagnant revenue due to the Depression.[150] Both Leeds and Sheffield increased their rate base from boundary extensions and from the building of new estates but in Leeds especially, rates were a major party political issue. From 1929 local authorities also received more flexible block grant allocations from central government and these assisted in Sheffield, especially where the rate base was significantly lower than that in Leeds.[151] Moreover, the extent to which party played a part in shaping health policy choices remains unclear though how rate and block grant income was spent on which corporation services was ultimately a political decision as will be seen in debates around appropriation in Leeds.[152]

As the patient profile in municipal hospitals changed over the period so they, like the voluntary hospitals, came to rely more heavily on direct payment by patients. The source of these payments varied across institutions and by patient type. The infectious diseases hospitals, including Leeds and Sheffield, did not charge, as most wished to ensure potentially dangerous patients were removed for the protection of others.[153] Poor law or public assistance patients, however, remained chargeable by local authorities with an attendant obligation to recover the costs of treatment wherever possible from friends and relatives or in the case of patients with a settlement elsewhere, from their authority. In Sheffield a complex arrangement for securing payment for out of city patients was developed while in Leeds the Conservative council blocked appropriation in part because the chair of the PAC 'did not think the Public Health Committee would run the hospitals as economically as the Public Assistance Committee, nor would they be likely to recover as much in the way of contributions towards the maintenance of the patients'. His view received support from the Public Assistance Officer who 'laid considerable stress on the possibility of loss through appropriation in the case of patients who had settlements outside Leeds'.[154] There is some evidence that Bristol and Gloucester were quite effective in recovering costs from public assistance patients but Middlesbrough proved far less effective in this area, with a sharp fall in income from patient payments in the first years of appropriation.[155]

Yet despite enthusiastic pursuit of this source of funding in some cities, it was proving of marginal significance by the mid-1930s. Much more promising was direct payment from non-relief patients. As in the voluntary hospitals this came either as a contribution from the patient or from the contributory schemes. In the former case sliding-scale charges were set at levels a little below the voluntary hospitals. In Sheffield this was 25/– (the fee they charged the Penny in the Pound scheme) while in Leeds various charges were in place. Almoners or assessment officers carried out checks to establish ability to pay, Sheffield employing an almoner in 1930 to make assessments and collections from liable relatives to cover costs. Yet this was seen as a somewhat wasteful operation by Sheffield Health Committee who reported in 1933 that:

> the amount recovered is very small and the Corporation limits the definition of persons liable to maintain to those members of the family actually resident in the patient's home and, I am informed that in their opinion, the amount recovered does not render the procedure worthwhile.[156]

Indeed it was only the legal obligation enshrined in the 1929 Act which made them pursue patients and their willingness to take patients from the waiting lists of the voluntary hospitals for free suggests they were not too concerned about direct payment as an income source.[157]

More lucrative for the municipal hospitals was the increasing numbers of contributory scheme members admitted and despite early fears that either scheme members would not wish to go to ex-poor law hospitals or that transferred patients would be a burden on the schemes, by the end of the 1930s the Leeds Workpeople's Hospital Fund was paying £7,000 to Leeds Council for treatment of almost five thousand contributors. In Sheffield similar numbers were entering the City General and other institutions run by the corporation at a cost to the Penny in the Pound scheme of £4,700 in 1938 and following a major revision of the tariff this had reached £15,990 by 1946 – a charge of £3 per patient.[158] Similar arrangements were made in a number of other cities, including Manchester, Salford and Bristol,[159] though in Middlesbrough the transfer of patients was slow to develop, held up by suspicion on both sides.[160]

Leeds Health Committee also benefitted from the expansion of hospital births which usually carried an assured income of thirty shillings from the state maternity benefit. In Leeds, for example, the maternity unit at St James's took three patient types:

> Private patients who pay the full cost of three guineas a week;
>   Patients who pay 4/6d. a day, which is the full cost of maintenance, and who interview the steward with a view to admission
>   Necessitous patients who have to see the relieving officer.[161]

While still under PAC control, St James's admitted 39 private maternity patients in 1930, rising to 71 in 1932 at three guineas per week while women paying the standard charge increased from 32 to 200 over the same period. St Mary's only admitted those paying the standard charge of 31/6*d.* per week and relief cases, the medical superintendent stating the majority of maternity patients paid the standard charge.[162] In Sheffield, however, many of the poorer maternity patients continued to be treated under the poor law. The Ministry of Health surveyor noted that the corporation's claim to spend a fifth of the outlay of Leeds on maternity and child welfare owed much to the fact that

> as far as possible all the costs of confinements in institutions are recovered through the Public Assistance Committee. Apparently women unable to pay full cost of maintenance in the maternity wards at Fir Vale and Nether Edge Hospitals are sent in as public assistance cases through the machinery of the Relieving Officer and recovery is made from them under poor law functions, so that in this respect the intentions of the Local Government Act, 1929, are not being fulfilled.[163]

This kind of practice raises questions about the reliability of the Local Government Financial Services returns as a guide to Health Committee spending, and possibly explains the relatively low cost of hospital services in Sheffield recorded by Levene et al.[164] It is therefore apparent that, like the voluntary hospitals, the municipal sector was developing complex funding patterns which meant it was not simply dependent on the rates and the attendant political constraints to which that source could be subject. However, when it came to capital projects it was much more at the mercy of external factors.

In the late nineteenth and early twentieth century local authorities, including boards of guardians, invested heavily in public health infrastructure paid for by borrowing sanctioned by the Local Government Board.[165] During this time Leeds borrowed heavily to complete the substantial infectious diseases and TB complex at Seacroft and Killingbeck at a cost in excess of £250,000.[166] This left the city with a significant debt which prevented additional work in the 1920s and may have had an impact on its ability to embark on improvements at the former poor law institutions in the early 1930s. The guardians had also spent heavily in the 1890s and 1900s, over £50,000 being expended at St James's and £30,000 at St Mary's between 1894 and 1906, while the early 1920s saw projects at St James's to improve the nurses' home and the maternity facilities.[167] The situation does not seem to have been so severe in Sheffield where building was more piecemeal in the run up to the First World War. But in both cities it is apparent that capital projects were curtailed from the mid-1920s by economic conditions and the burden of existing borrowing.

With the 1929 Local Government Act the Ministry of Health became supportive of some authorities, including Leeds, urging them to undertake improvements to their new facilities.[168] This contrasts with the picture presented by Mohan who enumerates a number of examples of Ministry of Health caution or even opposition to spending, especially in urban County Durham. Levene,

Powell and Stewart also comment on the exasperation of Ministry officials with the grandiose plans of some authorities, such as Doncaster, who applied to build a large new hospital without exploring appropriation or partnerships with the County Council and the voluntary institutions.[169] But in both cities new work was deferred until after the worst of the Depression had passed. Thus in Leeds, a range of projects were approved in 1931, including a number designed to signify St James's separation from the Beckett St institution and emphasize its new hospital role. However, the work was delayed by the Conservative council who were reluctant to increase borrowing and had not been undertaken by the time of the Ministry of Health survey in the summer of 1933. Convinced by the medical superintendent that these works were urgent and concerned by the 'keen eye for economy' motivating the chair of the PAC, the surveyor was moved to suggest the survey letter might urge their completion. He also hinted to Alderman Martin that new staff accommodation and operating theatres were required and although 'quite prepared for this' the chairman hid behind the need to complete the 1931 proposals 'before other improvements were considered'.[170] In a similar vein the surveyors noted that residential TB accommodation was 'inadequate in amount and in some instances not as satisfactory as may be desired'. However, this was 'recognised locally and but for financial stringency would have been remedied'.[171]

In Sheffield the planned developments at the City General, which aimed to redistribute patients by increasing maternity, surgical and accident facilities, were also delayed in part by Labour's defeat in the 1932 local elections. A similar scheme was delayed in Manchester, though the purse strings were loosened following the Molly Taylor affair in 1934.[172] The Sheffield improvements were completed by the end of 1934 at a cost of around £50,000 and the council was keen to push ahead with further developments at the end of the decade when additional maternity accommodation along with a new TB sanatorium and a 600-bed general hospital were being planned.[173] Similarly, in Leeds a women's block at Killingbeck Sanatorium was completed in 1936 while building finally got underway on the improvements at St James's. Initially approved at a cost of £50,000 in 1935 by the Labour administration, the Conservative-dominated Health Committee gave the green light to an enlarged programme of works. The new facilities opened in 1940 at a cost of £146,000 and included the addition of 224 beds to the nurses' home and the technical, administrative and staff-centred improvements seen in the voluntary hospitals in previous years.[174] As this suggests, like the voluntary sector, municipal capital projects were severely constrained during the interwar period by local economic conditions as well as shifts in the political composition of the council, political priorities – like Labour slum clearance campaigns[175] – and the attitude of the Ministry to local borrowing. However, it is clear that in both sectors by the end of the 1930s the worst of the squeeze was over and major capital works were underway.

Conclusion

In the years following the First World War rapid inflation and rising demand saw the cost of hospital care rise very sharply. Although these costs began to stabilize from 1924 they had left both a significant burden of debt and a substantial gap in the finances of the voluntary hospitals. The approach to filling that gap in the two cities was rather different, with Leeds relying on an increasingly diverse range of income sources underpinned by a solid contributory scheme while in Sheffield the city's voluntary hospitals came to depend overwhelmingly on the income from the Penny in the Pound scheme. A superficial reading of the accounts of these hospitals would suggest that in Sheffield middle-class giving was replaced by working-class contribution while in Leeds the figures point to the growing significance of direct patient payment – both suggesting a decline in the voluntary hospitals' charitable income and purpose. Yet the figures mask important continuities in these institutions' resources. There was much renaming of income as sums moved from voluntary headings like subscriptions or donations to the contributory schemes pots. Conversely, scheme income included significant charitable elements gathered at fundraisers or pub collections while substantial sums were derived from business through the employers' contributions. Moreover, away from the current account charity continued to flourish. Legacies, endowments and gifts in kind supported capital projects and underpinned running costs by their contribution to investments. Egg weeks, tinfoil collections, linen guilds and Christmas gifts all reduced costs, improved conditions and sustained the 'hospital spirit'.[176] Most impressively, new building was permitted by mass popular appeals in the 1930s which saw voluntarism extended to every social group from bankers to schoolchildren. Least important – and often ignored in Leeds – were the street collections so often pilloried by commentators at the time and since. In most cases where charity continued it was about doing, not just giving.[177]

The experience of the state sector was more like that of the voluntary hospitals than might have been expected. The nature of their core funding changed as ownership transferred to the council and the cost of hospitals had to compete with other municipal goods – especially housing. Moreover, as with the charitable sector, council hospitals in Leeds developed a diverse funding base which drew on direct payment, support from the mutual schemes, national insurance and rates and grants. Conversely, Sheffield's corporation hospitals relied far less on direct payment, reflecting the attitude of the non-state sector. But across both cities economic conditions limited the ability to build and adapt to meet the rapid growth in demand from patients and new technologies and techniques. In particular, from the early 1920s to the mid-1930s capital projects were limited as neither provider could raise sufficient cash or meet the future commitments inherent in large numbers of new beds. But, as shown in Chapter 2, institutions did use this period to enhance their ancillary facilities, reduce domestic costs, improve conditions for staff and extend scientific diagnosis and treatment. Moreover, from the late 1930s there was expansion everywhere based on large-scale appeals and centrally sanctioned borrowing shaped by diverse approaches rooted in local conditions. In Leeds a traditional popular appeal drawing on the city's large resident middle class underpinned the LGI's ambitions, while the Conservative council borrowed only for updating and not to compete with the voluntary sector. In Sheffield, however, both sectors envisaged major new – possibly competing – hospitals. In the case of the Hospital Council this was to be funded by modern bureaucratic fundraising techniques borrowed from the Penny in the Pound scheme, which would mobilize the business community, a small number of very wealthy individuals and the mass of well-paid workers. Moreover, across the cities and sectors the pattern and form of fundraising owed much to local social, economic and political cultures and health needs and it is the way in which local political cultures, in particular, shaped provision and practice to which we will now turn.

6 THE POLITICS OF HOSPITAL PROVISION

Between the end of the First World War and the mid-1940s hospital provision became an increasingly politicized field of social policy. National debates were prompted by the financial crisis of the early 1920s, the introduction of the 1929 Local Government Act and the series of reports and surveys produced in the later 1930s which laid the basis for national state involvement. Central to these discussions were considerations of who should finance and who should control public hospital services and while general issues of state subsidy arose, it was the relationship between the voluntary hospitals and the local state which occupied the key area of debate.[1] In analysing these debates historians have usually looked to national sources and the positions adopted by leading pressure groups such as the BMA or the British Hospital Association, especially in the period from 1937. There has been a tendency to emphasize Labour hostility to the voluntary system and support for a state-run service under the control of the municipality as espoused in *The Labour Movement and the Hospital Crisis* (1922). Those on the right, along with the medical elite, are less clearly drawn but are seen to provide consistent support to the voluntary sector coupled to a fear of municipal control. The Ministry of Health attempted to maintain a neutral line in these disputes but seems to have become increasingly hostile to the voluntary sector and their supporters in the contributors' associations. Underpinning much of this analysis is a view of two very separate systems of delivery reinforcing and reinforced by two coherent political positions.[2]

Yet the politics of hospital provision in the localities or the ways in which political, social and medical elites and organizations negotiated the demands for efficient, democratic and high-quality medical care remain opaque. Important insights into the ways in which systems developed over the interwar period in a number of cities and regions exist, but with the exception of the work of Levene et al., John Stewart and Tim Willis, how local party politics and political ideas shaped service provision has received very little attention.[3] In particular, little attention has been paid to the potential of local social and economic structures and ideological cultures to produce diverse political approaches that may have influenced the services provided and the extent of co-operation.[4] Such difference were most obvious in relation to the decision to appropriate and extend general hospital services in the 1930s and more generally in the health spending choices made by local authorities across the interwar period.[5] Moreover, these decisions were not only subject to party political pressures but were shaped by the interest groups and individuals involved in the management and delivery of hospital services, including hospital boards, health committees, contributory associations and the medical profession both inside and outside the hospitals. Indeed, while historians of urban elites – such as Gunn, Morris, Trainor and Doyle – have often disagreed about the extent to which leading social actors 'withdrew' from involvement in the politics and social life of the city there is agreement, though little evidence, that social leaders remained more closely involved with hospitals for longer than any other urban institution.[6]

How did these issues work out in Leeds and Sheffield? Who did run hospital services in the two cities and were they discrete cadres concerned only with their own sphere or was there interaction and even sharing of leadership? What was the attitude of the labour movement to the voluntary sector? Did this differ between and even within the two cities? If so what factors determined divergent responses? How robust and unified was the defence of the voluntary system? To what extent did politics shape local provision? Did it lead to competition or co-operation? Did it affect issues like appropriation, the prioritizing of services or the nature of the delivery? This chapter will address these questions, suggesting that political cultures, shaped by economic structures, class and gender were central to the development of both voluntary and municipal hospitals but were generally less important in influencing speciality formation or the direction of spending.[7] These issues will be picked up on in Chapter 7 which will explore issues of integration and co-ordination and examine the extent of collaboration within and between the sectors. It will take some of the themes discussed here and assess their impact on attempts to bring the various elements of the voluntary and local state provision together and consider the role of organizations, individuals, ideology and finance on efforts to deliver citywide and regional services.

Many of the rigid distinctions presented in the established historiography – of distinct and hostile municipal and voluntary systems; an unquestioning commitment to municipal services within the labour movement mirrored by a defence of the voluntary sector from the right; stark contrasts between the interests and activities of salaried state doctors and honorary surgeons and physicians[8] – are challenged and finessed by an examination of operational experiences in Leeds and Sheffield. In the case of politics it is clear that the impact of the local economy on the shape of labour politics played a very important role in producing distinctive responses, with Sheffield Labour concerned with the improvement of working-class living and working conditions while the Leeds party was driven much more by an ideological socialism.[9] Moreover, party very clearly influenced municipal policy choices in both cities, especially in relation to appropriation, co-operation and competition, as it did in Barnsley and to a lesser extent West Hartlepool.[10] Yet equally, close study of these localities also reveals the messy nature of the relationships between the sectors, the overlaps in office holding amongst both managers and doctors, political battles within the council and hospitals between boards, doctors and administrators and the long-running disputes between the contributors, hospitals, doctors and even politicians over issues of access, accountability and control.

Who Ran the Hospitals?

Hospital management was divided by function and by sector with political, honorary, medical and administrative officials all playing a part. During the nineteenth century the traditional elite – whether landed, professional or business – had guarded their control over hospital management and finances and had attempted to maintain some authority on the wards. However, by the outbreak of the First World War many of their privileges had been undermined, as doctors demanded the right to control admissions and new funders and social actors, including women, began to make claims on power within the institutions.[11] Within the voluntary sector each of the hospitals had a board responsible for operational oversight, usually led by a chairman supported by a treasurer and a relatively small number of members – though in the north-east where worker governors were common, boards could be very large.[12] In most cases the management committees were given some institutional weight by the inclusion of representatives of the honorary staff – whose presence usually grew over the period, as in Middlesbrough.[13] These bodies were very slow to change; the Board of Management of the LGI, for example, saw six (of a possible fifteen) members serve for the entire interwar period, including Elinor Lupton from 1919 to 1948, Henry Barran from 1897 to 1942 and Charles Lupton from 1882 to 1935, including twenty-one of those years as chairman and treasurer.[14] Similar longevity was a feature of other institutions – Henry Oxley was treasurer of the LPD for over forty years, Sir Ronald Matthews chaired the Weekly Board of the SRI from 1924 until the inauguration of the NHS, while the board of the Jessop Hospital saw Lady Stephenson serve for more than thirty years. This situation was replicated in other towns, for example in Preston, where Alex Foster chaired the Infirmary Board from 1924 to 1937 or Nottingham, where leadership at the General Hospital was confined to three men between 1915 and 1942, including William Player.[15]

It has been suggested that this continuity owed something to the fact that members of the elite held on to their roles in medical institutions for longer than their other civic roles. In Bristol, the Willis brothers remained very active in the management of the general hospitals as did the Cadburys in Birmingham and the Players in Nottingham and the hospitals of Leeds and Sheffield certainly support such a pattern.[16] At the LGI, for example, the 1919 board showed significant continuity with the group who had promoted the building of the new infirmary in the 1860s, with two Luptons, two Kitsons and a Tetley as well as Henry Barran and Frank Gott, all from well-established Leeds families.[17] Twenty years later there were still two Luptons and two Tetleys, although the board was beginning to include those from less well-established city families.[18] At the LPD the board drew on newer social groups with a business, social and political base in the city centre, including Conservatives, like Alderman Penrose Green and Sir George Martin, Jewish leaders such as Victor Lightman and Alderman Hyman Morris, while Sir Montague Burton was elected a trustee in 1931.[19]

The most interesting aspect of these bodies was their gender composition.[20] Women were much more prominent in the Leeds boards than they were in Sheffield. Although the LPD had no female board members, at the LGI the first women, Elinor Lupton and Lady Sadler, were elected in 1919 and at least two women were on the board throughout the period, while the board of the LHW included Mrs Frank Gott and Mrs A. M. Richardson in 1919, rising to four of the fifteen members in 1931.[21] The situation at the LMH was a little more ambiguous. Like St Mary's in Manchester, the hospital was established by a committee of women and in 1913 the president, vice-presidents, treasurer and secretary were all female as were all but one of the twelve lay members of the board of management.[22] However, women were eased out of some of the leading roles and by 1928 the chair had passed to Austyn Barran, while four of the fourteen lay members of the board were male, including the treasurer. Yet by the standards of Sheffield women held a prominent position in the management of medical institutions. By the early 1930s Sheffield Children's Hospital had three women on its ten-member board while the Jessop had a similar number on its twelve-person committee for most of the period. None held any of the key offices. At the general hospitals their role was even more marginal. The SRH had no female board members during the interwar period while the SRI elected their only woman in 1925. Women's participation was restricted to the Ladies Committees where their work was mainly pastoral, covering visiting patients and activities similar to those of the linen guilds. In this profile Sheffield may have been closer to the normal pattern; in Middlesbrough women were marginal on the main boards of the hospitals while in Nottingham, although the Women's Hospital mandated equal representation (as it did in Birmingham) the Children's Hospital excluded women from the board, limiting their role to the Ladies' Committee.[23]

These boards were supported in their work by a growing body of professional administrators, headed by the secretary-superintendent.[24] Certainly a number of the lay members were engaged and energetic in their commitment to the hospitals. Chairmen like Lupton and A. P. Nicholson at the LGI treated it like a full-time job while the chairman of the SRI attended committee meetings daily during a particularly severe financial crisis.[25] Conversely, it seems unlikely that the octogenarian Henry Oxley, honorary treasurer of the LPD in the 1920s, did much work on the accounts himself. Rather it was the superintendent who undertook most of the daily oversight of the institution and by the 1930s he was acquiring significant power and authority. S. Clayton Fryers, House Governor and Secretary to the LGI, achieved national prominence as one of the Ministry of Health surveyors in 1945 (working on the report on the Sheffield region) while H. Eason from Wolverhampton undertook a similar role for the Yorkshire survey. Often very long serving, like John Gibson in Preston, they had to find daily practical solutions to problems and a number – including Clayton Fryers – were ·sceptical of the value of the contributory schemes and strong supporters of building up investment income.[26] Although rarely acknowledged in the public work of the hospital, like the town clerk or the MOH, they were increasingly the real power in the institution and shaped many of the decisions taken by the boards.

The honorary medical staff, whose professional standing and role in the delivery of care made them a further pillar of authority in the institution, played little part in the operational management of the hospital. In Sheffield the key role at the SRI was taken by the honorary secretary of the medical staff who held a representative place on most committees, while at the SRH five of the medical staff took part in the work of the management board and the house committee. In Leeds the whole of the honorary medical staff were given seats on the Board of Management of LGI and the LMH along with some subcommittee representation. However, when the medical staff did have representation they could dominate the decision-making, as was clearly the case in Middlesbrough.[27] Yet they did not always get their way, with the broader interests of the hospital – especially where finance was concerned – often prevailing.[28] This may have been a consequence of their atomized structures which saw vertically integrated teams rather than horizontal status interest groups develop from the beginning of the century.[29] Thus, it is clear that power in the hospital was diffuse, spread between the traditional elite in their voluntary roles, the growing administrative authority of the paid officials, the professional weight of the honorary medical staff and even the more or less important position of workers and contributory scheme members who could make occasional significant interventions, though often their impact was negative.[30]

There were similarly fractured structures in the municipal institutions where the elected council members, acting in committee, set policy which had to be executed by medical staff working under the administrative authority of the MOH.[31] Unlike the voluntary hospitals, power in the Health Committee – or the Board of Guardians and its successor the PAC – could change quite suddenly. In both Leeds and Sheffield, membership of the Health Committee changed markedly in the 1920s as the old guard gave way to both Labour members and new faces amongst the anti-socialists. Thus in Leeds only the Conservative GP, Charles Moorhouse, sat on the committee throughout the 1920s, chairing it when the anti-socialists were in power. The Labour landslide of 1926 led to a shake-out reinforced by the huge Conservative victory of 1930. However, the 1930s saw much greater continuity, with four members serving the Leeds Committee for the entire decade. Churn also occurred in Sheffield where more than half the members changed between 1928 and 1934, in part as a result of the anti-socialists' surprise capture of the council in 1932.[32]

Indeed, party politics on the committee was another area of difference between the two cities. In Leeds, despite significant ideological difference, committee membership was governed by strict rules of proportionality. Thus, for much of the interwar period the committee was closely balanced, with the incumbent party having the chairmanship and a slight majority of the members. The deputy chair was always from the opposition and some of the subcommittee chairmanships were allocated to the minority party. In Sheffield, however, Labour took a political view of committees, holding both the chair and deputy chair and maintaining a large majority of the membership.[33] Yet there was some continuity in leadership. The Leeds' Public Health Committee was chaired by Charles Moorhouse for parts of the 1920s, by Labour's Councillor George Brett for much of the period from 1926 to 1935 and by Alderman Martin after that date while the Conservatives' Aldermen Weaver and Elizabeth Booth and Labour's David Beevers held prominent roles throughout the 1930s. Sheffield's Labour group offered similar levels of continuity, with William Asbury chairing the committee for almost the whole period from 1926 to 1940.

Historians have emphasized that women's role in local politics was usually restricted to domestic areas, like health, though even here they are usually shown to have had limited power.[34] However, notable gender differences emerged between the Public Health committees of the two cities. In Leeds women played a very prominent role in the committee, dominating it for a period in the 1930s. From three of twelve in 1930, female membership increased to nine of the sixteen Labour appointees of 1934 – five Labour and four Conservative – while the Maternity and Child Welfare Committee was composed of five female and four male council appointees and seven female co-optees – although the chair was held by a man. The female presence was reduced under Conservative control but the 1938 committee still had six women amongst the sixteen members while there were female chairs for the Hospital and Cattle and Milk subcommittees. Of particular significance, especially to the growing importance of maternity beds at the city's hospitals, was the central place of women in the Hospitals Committee. When Labour formed the committee the majority of the twelve members were women and though they fell to a slight minority from 1935 the chair was a woman.[35] Conversely, in Sheffield the 1934 Health Committee of twenty-one members included just six females, four Labour and two Citizen Alliance representatives.[36]

Thus, the political committees offered a picture of increasingly stable membership along with the presence of some dominating figures such as Councillor Asbury in Sheffield and Alderman Martin in Leeds.[37] However, amongst the medical and administrative staff there was also significant longevity of service. The MOH has received relatively little attention from historians.[38] As with other local government officials, his role had evolved over the nineteenth century as boroughs acquired increasing responsibility for the sanitary health of their citizens. Up to the First World War, therefore, they concerned themselves overwhelmingly with controlling nuisances, tracking infectious diseases and only very latterly with personal or preventative medicine.[39] In the changed circumstances of the interwar period, Jane Lewis and Charles Webster have suggested most were weak and timid in the face of huge health problems – with a few heroic exceptions, like M'Gonigle in Stockton. Yet local studies of Leicester, Lancashire and Middlesbrough are a little more optimistic, pointing to the large amount achieved in very difficult situations.[40] The MOH occupied an ambiguous position in both Leeds and Sheffield, especially by the 1930s. The Ministry of Health survey of 1933 felt that Dr Johnstone Jervis in Leeds was being marginalized while in Sheffield the MOH, Dr Rennie, was seen as increasingly old-fashioned and ineffective. Jervis had taken up post in 1917 and served until his retirement in 1947, occupying a university chair in Public Health Medicine and overseeing impressive improvements in services and health indicators.[41] There was similar continuity in Sheffield where Dr Wynne was MOH until his death in 1930, being replaced by his deputy, Dr John Rennie, who had worked in the city since 1912 and remained in post until the 1940s. Rennie shared his power with the medical superintendent, and deputy MOH, Dr John Clark.[42] Clark, like the medical superintendent in Leeds, Dr Dick, was a central figure in the delivery of services and in many ways the equal of the MOH. Their role – which has attracted little attention from historians – combined the medical oversight of patients, a fair amount of surgery and administrative management of the council's general and specialist hospital facilities. Both Clark and Dick maintained good relations with the voluntary hospitals as well as operational control of a number of hospitals with many more beds than the voluntary sector. Admittedly, some superintendents could cross over between sectors, Harry Brittan Jones in Middlesbrough rising to senior honorary surgeon at Middlesbrough's North Ormesby Hospital as well as running the town's four hospitals, but most were paid officials of the council and as such had little autonomy, while the MOH could indeed be weak or inefficient.

This was brought home by the Ministry of Health survey of Leeds in the early 1930s which showed that the MOH had been marginalized by both his political masters and the other departments. The council's refusal to appropriate meant the MOH had 'entirely dropped out of the picture in relation to public assistance work. He says he is never consulted and I gather that he feels that his advice is not wanted'. The real adviser was Dr Dick who was 'freely consulted by the Chairman of the Public Assistance Committee in connection with matters of administration and policy'.[43] Although the MOH's position was attributed to his support for appropriation, there was also evidence that he did not have the confidence of his administrative colleagues and may not have been 'quite equal to the task' of 'single centralizing administrative head' of all of the council's health services.[44] Rennie's position in Sheffield was stronger. He controlled the main branches of the health system and though somewhat conservative, retained the confidence of the council. It was suggested he was: 'Disquieted by no anxieties as to the "divine rights" of university professors or voluntary hospital officials [and] has no hesitation in laying down the law as to what he thinks should be done in the administration of the work'. It was also feared, however, 'that he scrutinises with extreme care the expenditure', thinking too much about the cost and 'not sufficiently in terms of the results'.[45]

However, it was the medical superintendents who emerge as the dynamic force in health provision. Clark was praised as 'A man of very considerable clinical and administrative ability, keen on his work' while Dick was 'an awkward customer' but a 'first class administrator' who managed St James's well and had 'given a great deal of thought to the problem of making the best use of the institutions as a whole'.[46] Moreover, it was the superintendents who decided on the management and direction of their hospitals, the Leeds surveyor noting Jervis would do best not 'to interfere in the internal administration of the hospitals'.[47] As will be seen, these findings are supported by the prominent role played by the superintendents in the development of joint working in both cities in the early to mid-1930s.

Indeed, the existence of joint committees adds a further layer of complexity and interaction to the politics of interwar hospital administration. Although such bodies developed at different speeds and evidenced diverse powers, they created new foci for authority and conflict. Thus, Mohan is sceptical about the effectiveness of joint working in the north-east – there was no committee in Newcastle and the one in Sunderland was moribund. Yet the committee in Manchester once established – as in Leeds – was very dynamic as was that in Bristol, while the modest arrangements in Middlesbrough and Barnsley show what was possible away from the big cities.[48] In Sheffield three bodies developed to bring together hospital providers. The crisis of the early 1920s created the Sheffield Hospital Council, with a citywide membership. In addition to setting up the Penny in the Pound scheme, pooling the city's ambulances and arranging convalescent care in the early 1920s it facilitated the treatment of contributors in the poor law hospitals and, in its most ambitious project, led the acquisition of

Norton Hall for a new hospital. Yet by 1927 it had abandoned its aspiration to be a central policymaking body and concentrated on the administration of its existing schemes.[49]

Its policy functions were adopted by a joint committee of the four voluntary hospitals which included both lay and medical staff. The committee had some executive power, completing the city's influential submission to the Sankey Commission[50] and driving through the amalgamation of the general hospitals while the move towards closer working ensured that new building and public appeals became a collective responsibility, limiting the autonomy of the individual institutions. Although the Voluntary Hospitals' Council in Leeds was much slower to develop, it did acquire significant power from the member hospitals. In particular, it created a united honorary staff for the LGI, LMH and LHW and decided on the distribution of patients, acting to restrict the ambitions of the LMH to monopolize institutional deliveries.[51]

Advisory committees linking the voluntary and municipal hospitals also undermined institutional autonomy. Made up of the chairmen of the voluntary hospitals and representatives of the Health Committee, representatives of the honorary staff and the MOHs and medical superintendents, the Leeds committee also acquired members from the WRCC and co-optees.[52] Initially the Sheffield committee ran on a very co-operative basis but by the later 1930s this had broken down and a more adversarial approach emerged, with the chair of the Health Committee refusing to call meetings after 1938.[53] On the other hand the Leeds committee remained effective, drawing praise from the 1945 surveyors. Although only advisory, these joint committees offered a means for the two sides to discuss matters of mutual concern and make recommendations back to their management boards and committees. In early 1930s Sheffield this produced major policy outcomes while in Leeds the focus was on agreeing priorities and spheres of interest.[54] Thus these committees had the potential to diffuse and reduce the autonomous power of the individual institutions though as the case of the LPD's refusal to agree to the rules of the Leeds joint committee suggests, this was limited. Indeed the discussions around regional committees that followed the Sankey Report demonstrate the tension between co-ordination and independence with advocates of regional oversight shying away from compulsory powers and sanctions for non-compliance.[55]

As has been shown in a number of studies, leadership and decision-making was also contested by the representatives of the contributors, the universities and their medical schools, by the local BMA and by trade unions representing hospital employees and contributors, though their power seems to have been largely negative. Thus Gorsky, Mohan and Willis, in their exploration of a number of contributor associations, especially in the north-east, found their ability to shape policy was limited. However, evidence from Middlesbrough and Nottingham is more positive, showing extensive involvement in management, though even here ultimate power was largely negative. Furthermore, in both Bristol and Birmingham medical schools were essential in driving the amalgamation of competing hospitals.[56] Some workers' groups had access to decision-making, with contributors represented on all of the hospital boards, though the scale of their representation was a recurring issue in both cities – a contrast to Middlesbrough where direct works' contributions gave contributors substantial representation and even power on a range of hospital committees.[57] Medical schools were not directly represented on hospital management committees though they gained access through honorary staff with teaching appointments. In the 1930s a professorial committee was formed at the LGI to recognize the growing link between hospital work, teaching and research – and included three municipal doctors amongst its members. However, with the amalgamation of the Sheffield general hospitals the new court of management made representation for these interest groups explicit, with eight members directly representing the contributors, along with the dean of the Medical Faculty and the VC of the University and a representative of the Local Medical Panel Committee.[58]

The negative influence of these groups was particularly evident in the case of the contributors who were denied proportionate representation on management boards but could be very effective in blocking or reversing unpopular decisions. For example, in 1922 the Sheffield Contributors' Association secured a preferential rate for women admitted to the maternity department of the Jessop while at the end of the 1930s they resisted attempts by the Hospitals' Council to limit access for better-paid members.[59] Contributors could also secure concessions for other groups, especially trade unions, who became increasingly vocal in the voluntary hospital sector in the later 1930s.[60] Thus, by threatening to withhold their contributions one union forced the LGI to reverse a decision to employ non-union labour, a tactic seen on a number of occasions in Middlesbrough.[61] Pressure groups could also use persuasion and indirect influence, as well as being utilized by hospital insiders to promote policy change. Thus, efforts to unify the honorary staffs in Leeds in the early 1920s were presented as coming from the university while the Maternity Hospitals' centralization plan was promoted in the name of the Medical School.[62] Furthermore, external interest groups could actually clash over hospital policy, especially income limits for contributory schemes which pitted the doctors against the contributors with the hospitals left to find a compromise position.

Hospital power structures were, therefore, porous and flexible, the independence and autonomy of management boards, honorary staff and local authorities being mediated by competing pressures within institutions and sectors as well as by relations between sectors and with external partners. Contrary to established views of rigid autonomy, power was complicated further by the presence of a significant number of individuals who were involved in more than one institution, often across the sectors. The most remarkable was Alderman George Martin, who by 1930 held a number of significant positions including chairman of Leeds PAC, chairman of the LPD and a seat on the Weekly Board of LGI. In 1935 he was appointed chairman of the Health Committee with a seat on the hospitals subcommittee and the chairmanship of the Joint Hospitals Committee.[63] He was a frequent attendee at the AGM of the LWHF and often spoke, quite controversially, on hospital politics. Alderman Moses Humberstone occupied a similar position in Sheffield where he was chairman of the Hospital Contributors' Association, a member of the board of the SRI, having first been elected in 1920, and a Labour councillor, alderman and Lord Mayor, though he did not sit on the Health Committee. His role can be contrasted to that of Councillor William Asbury who chaired Sheffield's Public Health Committee from 1926 to 1941 with just one year's break. Asbury, like Martin, was also chairman of the PAC, though in his case this was to ensure co-operation between the two sectors rather than Martin's desire for separation. Asbury was briefly a member of the SRI board in the early 1920s and though he was co-chair of the Joint Advisory Committee he took little part in the management of the voluntary hospitals. The politicians were matched by some in the voluntary sector who held central positions in the management of the city's hospitals and sometimes held roles that overlapped the different sectors. For example, in Sheffield Sir Ronald Matthews took over as chairman of the board of the SRI in 1924, chaired the Voluntary Hospital Committee and co-chaired the Joint Advisory Committee. However, he was never involved in municipal politics and played no part in the direct running of the municipal sector. Conversely, Alderman Charles Lupton, who was a member of the LGI board for fifty years and the chairman for over twenty years, was involved in both municipal and voluntary delivery though he was never a member of the Health Committee.

There were, moreover, a significant number of other figures who could be found with dual roles in either more than one voluntary hospital, or even across both sectors. The LPD, in particular, had a significant representation from Conservative aldermen and councillors, some of whom also held roles in the LWHF, such as the dentist Alderman P. T. Leigh.[64] But it was not just Conservatives; Alderman Frank Fountain, who had chaired the Health Committee in the 1920s was a strong supporter of the LPD, chairing its AGM as both mayor and deputy mayor and appearing as a member of the public at its AGM in 1939. The opportunity of some committees to make co-opted appointments meant that the Maternity and Child Welfare Committee of Leeds council always included two representatives from the LMH – one usually being Mrs Austyn Barran. The link between the council and local services was also reinforced in the 1920s by the tendency in Leeds to appoint doctors to the Health Committee – in 1925 there were no fewer than five doctors (and a dentist) out of a membership of twelve. These patterns were seen in other towns. In Preston the trade unionist and Labour councillor and mayor, R. C. Handley, was a strong supporter of the Royal Infirmary and a leading light in the local contributors association. In Leicester, the Maternity and Child Welfare Committee co-opted former members of the city's voluntary Health Society, while in neighbouring Nottingham a wide range of individuals held multiple voluntary organization responsibilities led by Charles Seeley and William Player – though there is less evidence of crossover between the voluntary and municipal sectors.[65]

Such interaction was reinforced by the increasing appointment of honorary staff as consultants in the municipal hospitals. Although this practice was not vigorously pursued in Sheffield, the city hospitals had appointed around half a dozen voluntary hospital consultants by the mid-1930s. The surgeons were generally the most active although the cancer and VD specialist – Rupert Hallam – was a frequent visitor while the Maternity and Child Welfare clinic employed a consultant obstetrician. Scepticism was expressed about the effectiveness of these consultants but some of them did provide a link between the two cultures.[66] In Leeds, however, the system was well developed from the later 1920s[67] and by 1933 the consulting staff included an orthopaedic and two general surgeons, a paediatric and two general physicians, a dermatologist, two gynaecologists, ear and eye surgeons, pathologists and a radiologist. Six visited on a twice-weekly basis, the physicians having wards allocated to them, while the other specialists came either weekly or when required.[68] The voluntary hospital staff were supported by the appointment of the city's TB officer and VD officer as honorary consultants. By the end of the 1930s the council and the LGI were making joint honorary appointments, for example in neurosurgery, and in 1944 the appointments committee of the voluntary hospitals was extended to include appointments at the city hospitals while membership was to include the lay and medical staff of the Health Department.[69]

Similar co-ordination existed in Manchester by 1940, while in Bristol 1938 saw the 'unification of the staffs of the voluntary and municipal hospitals' with a range of consultants visiting daily.[70] This extensive network of medical interactions clearly challenges the established view of separate spheres promoted by Rivett and especially Webster. The latter, for example, claimed that the 'emergency hospital scheme introduced medical staff to public work on a salaried basis. Mutual distrust was broken down as hospital staff from the two sectors became used to working together.'[71] Yet paid posts involving regular attendance and even control of beds were the norm in Leeds as well as Bristol by the outbreak of the Second World War. Moreover, the appointment of Henry Collinson as regional controller for the West Riding EMS was entirely appropriate as he had fifteen years' experience of both sectors. As this suggests, both lay and medical staff had developed complex interactions within and between the sectors by the outbreak of the war, which served to confirm rather than prompt developments in this direction. But what was the role of politics in shaping local hospital policy?

A Unified Labour Movement?

Historians have built their expectations of the labour movement's position on hospital provision from policy statements by the party and unions in the early 1920s, revised and strengthened at the end of the 1930s.[72] Official policy favoured a state system, managed at a local level but with some central funding.[73] It was heavily influenced by the Dawson report and the financial arrangements which flowed from it, with their emphasis on the MOH's co-ordinating role. By the end of the 1930s the party had become more committed to municipal control, inspired by the London County Council and the Socialist Medical Association.[74] But the trade union movement adopted a less fundamentalist line on hospital ownership, as they sought a solution which would improve provision and incorporate hospital treatment into the National Insurance system.[75] Thus, there was the potential for differences between the Labour party, trade unions and contributors associations as well as between the labour movements of Leeds and Sheffield. These were overlaid with changes over time both within the movement and between the cities.

Moreover, local Labour parties were not always very successful in promoting municipal hospital services. Certainly London was a success but in Hull and Norwich, where the party held control from the early 1930s, development was notably limited.[76] Barnsley developed some services by the later 1930s but these were little different to Middlesbrough which had an anti-socialist majority, both councils working closely to develop a complementary system with the voluntary sector.[77] Some of the most dynamic councils were non-socialist – Liverpool, Birmingham, Bristol, Bradford – while in others with a strong Labour opposition, like Manchester or Newport, there is little evidence that the party's representatives made much impact on policy.[78]

Both the trade union movement and the Miners' Welfare were strong supporters of voluntary hospital services, if not necessarily the system, during the interwar period. Thus, when the Penny in the Pound scheme was proposed, Sheffield Trades' Council were initially sceptical and demanded a commitment from employers that they would make a substantial contribution to match that of the workers.[79] When this was secured, the scheme secretary, Sydney Lamb, was able to claim that 'the trade unions through their leaders and a large number of branches have given consent to the operation of this contributory fund'[80] and as a result membership rose rapidly as both employers and employees signed up, the figure reaching over 1,000 firms and 100,000 members by June 1922.[81] This success owed much to the work of Moses Humberstone, whose position as an activist with interests in the Labour party, the trades' council and the contributors' association allowed him to influence each of these structures and secure widespread acceptance of the scheme by 1925. Moreover, as has been seen, the Miners' Welfare became a prominent financer of projects related to the development of orthopaedic services in the city, funding research as well as treatment.[82] Thus the aim of the labour movement in supporting the voluntary sector was to provide the best services for its members and working people generally and it was recognized that the voluntary hospitals were already providing this. Furthermore, support could be a stopgap, for as Sydney Lamb explained in 1921:

> Thousands of workmen in Sheffield believe in a state hospitals' service but for the sake of the sick and suffering, the disabled and dying women and children in our midst, their sense of fair play and sportsmanship lead them without exception when they are told the facts to support the voluntary scheme of contributions in their works until they can succeed by legislative means in bringing about another system which, in their opinion, is more efficient.[83]

The Sheffield Labour party was also broadly supportive. There was some opposition to the contributory scheme in the early 1920s, typified by the contributor to the *Sheffield Telegraph* letters page, 'Fountain Pen', who was particularly concerned that membership of the scheme might provide privileged access to a bed at the expense of the sick poor.[84] Thanks to the strong position taken by the Trades' Council on the one-third employer top-up, by 1926 it was estimated that around 95 per cent of Sheffield employers were contributing and increasingly the problem was identified as resting with employers outside the city and especially the collieries. Once the scheme was established the Labour Party seems to have given it considerable support. Alderman Humberstone was President of the Contributors' Association from its inception until 1940 while the leadership of the organization drew on other Labour men including George Rowland, who also sat on the Health Committee in the 1930s. Alderman Bancroft was the Contributors' Association delegate to the Edgar Allen Institute while as late as 1938 Alderman Thraves, a prominent trade unionist, was elected to the Court of Management of the amalgamated general hospital.[85] Even critics of the voluntary system played a part in their management, William Asbury holding a place within the Contributors' Association and a seat on the board of the SRI between 1924 and 1926. Remarkably the Labour party went so far as to support the SRH Centenary Appeal by providing canvassers to deliver appeal letters – with only limited opposition from local activists.[86] Yet such support was not uncommon. In neighbouring Barnsley the Labour council had good relations with the voluntary hospital mediated by the contributory scheme, while in south Wales workers effectively ran many of the voluntary hospitals as they did in Middlesbrough.[87]

In general, however, it was Moses Humberstone who spoke for the labour movement in defence of the voluntary hospitals. Humberstone came from a Lib/Lab tradition but by the early 1920s he was well established as the leading figure in the Labour party's council group. He was elected mayor and raised to the Aldermanic bench in 1926, retiring from the council in 1932. His support for the Penny in the Pound scheme in 1920 symbolized the joining up of the mutualist, industrial and political wings in support of the Sheffield scheme but he was also opposed to the subjugation of the voluntary hospitals to the local authority. Thus, while speaking favourably of close co-operation with the municipal system, he asserted in March 1933 that 'the Hospital Contributors' Association would never be agreeable to the hospitals going on the rates'.[88] Rather, he saw this work in moral terms, as a way to provide access to medical care for all without the stigma of charity or the poor law, declaring himself: 'in love with the movement'.[89] As such he was critical of insurance solutions, claiming Sheffield was not an insurance scheme 'and I hope that it never will be. I trust we shall all of us look upon this as a great humanitarian effort, and, come what will, those who are "down and out" shall be assured of treatment.'[90]

But there is evidence that the support from the Labour party was weakening by the later 1930s. In 1937 the council pulled out of the deal with the voluntary hospitals to take their waiting list patients, the town clerk making references to 'certain views expressed when the question was under consideration' – a comment implying significant criticism of the voluntary system.[91] William Asbury, who chaired the Health Committee at this time, had been critical of the voluntary hospitals since the 1920s, arguing in 1931 that

> Voluntary hospitals, although they had done much useful service in the past were now on their last legs. We had got to the state when the working classes would no longer be ignored, and accommodation had to be provided for them.
>   The sooner the hospitals were put on a municipal basis the better it would be for the community.[92]

By the later 1930s he had become much more direct in his attacks, declaring in 1939 that: 'The only satisfactory approach to the problem was for all hospitals intended for the acute sick to pass into the control of local authorities singly or jointly, as the particular circumstances might justify'.[93]

Yet not all Labour men were moving in this direction. Traditional figures like party leader E. G. Rowlinson retained a respectful position on the voluntary sector as shown when he chaired the visit of the Duchess of Gloucester which launched the Million Pound Appeal.[94] Even amongst contributors a less deferential approach was discernible from around 1930 as the Contributors' Association persistently pointed out that the Penny in the Pound scheme – and thus the working class – had saved the voluntary hospitals. Overall, by the Second World War, the labour movement in Sheffield was drifting away from its earlier accommodation with the voluntary hospitals as the party on the council asserted its socialist credentials over the traditional Labour right like Humberstone and Rowlinson.

In Leeds, however, the relative weakness of the trade unions meant that the political movement was the dominant force. Moreover, the party was strongly ideological, following a path much closer to that of the party nationally than the movement in Sheffield, especially in the 1920s. Opposition to the voluntary sector was voiced in a variety of public and private forums. In the early 1920s the Labour group had expressed concern about a council grant to the medical charities' appeal, for while Councillor Arnott supported the grant he challenged the Conservative leader's claim that 'voluntary hospitals were better than municipal hospitals' and in giving his backing to municipalized hospitals he asserted that 'the present voluntary system was unable to cope with present day public demands'.[95] When a similar grant was proposed four years later, Councillor Armstrong supported the subvention reluctantly, noting that

> some of us feel that the institutions which are so essential to the welfare of the people should not be subjected to charity. He did not wish to belittle charity but looked forward to the time when the municipalities and government would see to it that all such institutions were maintained from public funds.[96]

Opposition could also be practical. In contrast to the situation in Sheffield, attempts by the Leeds Voluntary Hospitals Committee to secure support from the parties for a flag day were unsuccessful: 'The Political parties would take no active part – the Labour party refusing assistance of any kind' noted the minutes. Alderman D. B. Foster wrote to say

> Sorry I do not feel like helping re Flag Day. I am so thoroughly convinced of the necessity, and wisdom, of Hospitals being maintained by public funds that I cannot be interested in efforts to continue them on charitable lines.
> I am very sorry to disappoint you but must be faithful to myself.[97]

Foster was a frequent advocate of municipal expansion, even in largely apolitical settings. Labour mayors were often speakers at the annual meetings of the medical charities and their comments were generally supportive of the work of these organizations. However, during his year of civic office Foster took the opportunity to raise questions about the effectiveness of the voluntary system. At the AGM of the LPD he urged public control to ensure greater equity through:

> a linking up whereby the organised beneficence of the public – the whole strength of the community – should be available to assist institutions such as the Leeds Public Dispensary ... and not to let the great work rest wholly upon those who had heart enough to sacrifice their time and money to it.[98]

His message was a little more guarded for the workers gathered at the LWHF meeting, who he told:

> Everybody ought to support the hospital ... There ought to be some means of insuring that the reserves of the city should be at the disposal of the needs of the city ... Public help must not lessen private charity. The ideal thing was to co-operate with the public funds of the city so that the magnificent private efforts of the charitably disposed persons might be supplemented. (Applause)[99]

From this it was a relatively short step to advocating public aid – both to balance the books and spread the load:

> I think the time is opportune for agreeing that, while we will continue the voluntary method in connection with our hospitals, we will nevertheless, be willing to accept some public help ... We want to give the voluntary system every chance to succeed, but this everlasting debt is intolerable.[100]

Foster's views were in line with Leeds Labour's strong support for the municipalization of the hospitals. A range of local and national features in the city's Labour newspaper, the *Leeds Citizen*, made this position clear. These included articles by local activists like Health Committee member Florence Hutson extolling the virtues of the PLIs[101] or speeches like that by Councillor Winifred Shutt condemning council aid to the voluntary hospitals which indirectly subsidized treatment of West Riding patients at the expense of Leeds ratepayers.[102] Commenting on the grant to the Medical Charities in 1924, the paper asserted that: 'The voluntary system in Leeds is a failure' as the 'people who should contribute liberally fail in their obligations and the only way to meet the situation is by spreading it out equitably as a rate charge'. They went on to claim insufficient hospital accommodation and chronic ill health fell mainly on the poor but could be eased if a 'municipalised service in Leeds could utilise the hospital accommodation in the Poor Law institutions' as was done in Bradford.[103]

The extension of local state provision funded in part by direct charges on non-pauper patients was a campaigning position at the 1924 Board of Guardians elections. The party's manifesto proclaimed:

> The fullest provision should also be made for patients who – apart from their illness – would not come under the Poor Law. Such provision would be a great boon to working people who, in general, cannot get the necessary treatment in their own homes, whilst many of them would willingly pay for adequate treatment provided under the public authority.[104]

This policy was followed, paying patients were admitted and by late 1927 St James's and St Mary's were said to be full. But this raised problems for ordinary workers as it:

> appears to be that we have adequate accommodation for the sick poor, and something
> approaching that standard for those who can afford to pay for institutional treatment
> but the majority of cases on the Infirmary waiting list do not come within either of
> these categories and it is to the needs of these people that our Public Health Service
> must pay some attention.

To meet this need they urged Parliament to empower and aid 'the local authorities to provide accommodation for institutional operative and surgical treatment in the same way that they provide for infectious diseases and tuberculosis'.[105] Although permitted in 1929, the 1930s in Leeds saw significant debate over the appropriation of these poor law institutions, but by 1937 the long-time Health Committee member, Councillor Beevers, was applauding their success as municipal hospitals contending: 'There is no doubt that Labour Party Policy, which was so long opposed by the Tory Party, has been justified and done much to relieve suffering by abolishing the long waiting lists for beds in the crowded voluntary hospitals'.[106]

But while support for municipalization was a crucial element of Labour policy, not all party leaders were hostile to the voluntary institutions. Some of the older members were willing supporters of both the LWHF and the LPD. Although their engagement with the contributory schemes was not as prominent as Labour involvement in Sheffield, party members participated in branch committees while Labour mayors attending the AGM praised the work of the LWHF and drew attention to its roots in working class radicalism.[107] As Labour mayor, John Arnott, pointed out in 1925, they were

> in the nature of a mutual insurance, an effort to pool resources, so that a person who
> did suffer from misfortune should have not only his own personal provision to help
> him in need, but that of his fellows who cooperated to help him.[108]

Moreover, John Badlay, who had attended meetings as an ordinary member, developed the theme of independence, suggesting that:

> When men now go to the Infirmary they don't go timidly to the back door, they go
> there as a right, feeling that they have paid for what they are going to get and have
> assisted others to obtain the same services. (Applause).[109]

Support for the Public Dispensary also recognized its central role in keeping the poor off the poor law, recasting it as a public service rather than a charity. Alderman Frank Fountain chaired the AGM twice when he emphasized the self-help elements of both the LWHF and the LPD. In referring to the contribution of the LWHF to the LPD in 1919 he noted that 'His old workmates were in the habit of attending the Dispensary in times of accident and other emergencies, and it was right that they should do their bit – and they had done it well',[110] while three years later he underlined the collectivist aspect of the workers' support both by those who had received treatment and from 'those fortunate enough not to require them [Dispensary services] to give a helping hand to their comrades'.[111] More generally Arnott claimed 'no better work' was being done than at the LPD which was 'not only commendable from an ethical standpoint but also from a commercial standpoint, as the health of a nation is its greatest commercial asset',[112] while Badlay asserted that of all the meetings he had chaired 'none ... had given him greater pleasure than the meeting of this wonderful Institution whose aim was to minister to the sick and needy, and give back health and happiness to all who came under its care'.[113] But the affection and support was not just ceremonial, the AGM in April 1939 was attended by two former Labour mayors, Aldermen Hemingway and Badlay.[114] Such encouragement underlines the importance of collective action in working-class support for voluntary institutions as in Nottingham, where backing for the Saturday Fund created a sense of ownership rather than insurance.[115]

Overall, the role of the labour movement in Leeds hospital politics was more conventional than that in Sheffield. There was less of a crossover between the sectors amongst Labour activists, even within the mutualist LWHF, and few politically active Labour men or women were involved in the running of the voluntary hospitals. Indeed only Councillor Lizzie Naylor, co-opted onto the board of the LMH, was a consistent Labour presence. There was also no distinctive trade union position or presence in either the workers' fund or the hospital boards, which served to strengthen the clear ideological stance taken by the representatives of the working class with leaders like Foster, Brett and Beevers consistently arguing for municipal control and questioning the continued role of the voluntary hospitals. Admittedly, as there was evidence of a growing challenge to the consensus in Sheffield in the later 1930s, equally there were those in Leeds Labour who displayed support for both the LWHF and more obviously the community role of the LPD which for the working class representatives of the party was an essential part of the fabric of city centre life. Indeed its voluntary nature was downplayed and it, like the LWHF, acquired a mutualist air which distanced it from its charitable origins.[116]

Defending the Voluntary Sector

In contrast, the proponents and defenders of the voluntary sector offered a unified position in both Leeds and Sheffield adopted by Conservatives, Liberals, the voluntary hospital elite, the press and many civic leaders. The primary venue for supporting the voluntary system was the medical charity AGM but it could also be found in private committees, council meetings and the correspondence columns of the press. Various tropes were expounded to justify the system, in particular that it was intrinsically good, that it was morally good, and that it was efficient.

The work of the voluntary hospitals was often highlighted as Christian and morally good – the LPD emblem was the Good Samaritan – and most meetings included speeches by representatives of the various religious faiths, typified by the opinion of the vicar of Leeds, Rev. Thompson Elliott, that the 'work of the voluntary Hospitals was a truly Christian one and deserving of the highest praise'.[117] Moreover, this Christian impulse was to be contrasted with the amorality of state services, Ronald Matthews contending 'There existed in voluntary hospitals a spirit of hopefulness and Christianity which they would not find in State-aided or municipal institutions',[118] while a few days later he pointed to its 'moral aspect, the fact that it provides an opportunity for large numbers of people to make personal sacrifices, both in time and money, for the benefit of others'.[119] This moral superiority was picked up by Harold Crawford, a stalwart of the LPD, who:

> deprecated the general tendency of relegating all social duties to the state or the Municipality. It was argued that it was only just to make every member of the community contribute, but ... voluntary deeds ... [were] productive of good in far reaching ways, and that mercy was an even finer thing than justice.[120]

The morality of the voluntary system underpinned a belief that the charitable approach was intrinsically good, something recognized by the general public who held voluntary hospitals in high esteem. Indeed, public support for the voluntary system remained high on the eve of the NHS while in cities like Leicester and Nottingham the broadening of the donor base reinforced links between the hospitals and the general public.[121] Thus, in 1919, at the height of the hospitals' financial crisis, the *Sheffield Telegraph* had contemplated the possibility that the Ministry of Health would 'compel the Corporation to provide adequate hospital accommodation, which would mean the end of the voluntary hospitals and the municipalization of the whole service'. However, in a trope which would become familiar in the coming years, they added that 'we doubt whether the community generally would quite like that or whether it would really make for efficiency and improvement'. Such a view was confirmed by Matthews who observed in 1928 that

> some people thought voluntary hospitals had had their day. To such a view he could not for a moment subscribe. He believed that apart from the financial considerations involved, the voluntary hospitals were too deeply rooted in the affections of the people lightly to be destroyed.[122]

In part this was due to the selflessness of volunteers, the Leeds Liberal C. G. Gibson emphasizing the superiority of public service over paid work:

> There was no phase of human life which called for more praise than that in which men and women did what was in their power to lessen the sum total of human misery

and physical suffering and more particularly when such help was given disinterestedly, and unselfishly with no thought of fee or reward, except the satisfaction that came from voluntary service.[123]

But for Matthews they also needed to be realistic about the attitude of the state and to recognize that 'their future is assured, provided they show that they are willing to co-operate in the great forward movement which is now taking place in the national health services'.[124] These themes of co-operation and intrinsic good were echoed by George Martin in a speech praising the way LWHF support had helped the LPD to avoid civic control, for while the 'Dispensary was on friendly and helpful terms with the authorities ... he did not think it would be a good thing for the citizens of Leeds if all their hospitals were municipally run and owned'.[125] Men like Martin and Matthews recognized the need to work closely with the local authority, but this had to be on a complementary basis and it was 'essential, of course, that they should retain in full measure their independence; that nothing should be done to dry up the streams of private benevolence'.[126]

As this suggests, it was often support for what it was not, a state system with the associated evils, which underpinned voluntarist discourses. Thus, the qualities of the voluntary system were most often expressed in contrast to those of its 'other' – state control. Addressing delegates to the British Hospitals Contributory Schemes' Association conference, Sheffield's Bishop stated that 'he was opposed to the idea that the voluntary system should be abandoned for compulsory State-aid' as 'red tape' would 'interfere with the freedom and the instinctive helpfulness which characterized the voluntary system'.[127] In Leeds, Conservative activists like Charles Lupton, P. T. Leigh and especially Sir George Martin, used the meetings of the LWHF to champion the voluntary system, attack state control and link the Fund to the preservation of the voluntary hospitals.[128] For example, in a characteristic assault prompted by the introduction of the Local Government Act, Martin praised the Fund:

> as a sort of bulwark against the municipal control of the voluntary hospitals of the city. However excellent municipal control might be, however painstaking, he was satisfied it would not be to the advantage of the hospitals to come under the municipality. It would be a very bad day for those who required the help and beneficent care which a hospital could give when such institutions were regulated and controlled by the municipality. (Applause).[129]

If the loss of 'beneficent care' was one possible consequence of state control, increased cost was another. Despite their constant financial crises, voluntary hospitals presented themselves as efficient, and undoubtedly the institutions of both cities retained low costs per bed throughout the period. But the voluntary system still had to prove it was better than the alternatives.

> To me [Matthews stated] it is clear that only so long as by voluntary means we can provide those services – medical, surgical and nursing – at a cost cheaper than, or at least equal to that of a State or municipal hospital, that the voluntary institutions can hope to survive.[130]

This he believed they could do, as:

> from the business point of view I am satisfied that under no system of State or municipal hospitals could the same services be provided as are being provided in our voluntary hospital system, especially here in Sheffield, at anything likes so cheap a cost.[131]

This was in part due to the contribution of voluntary workers who saved the hospitals significant sums each year. For example, the honorary staff received no remuneration directly for their work, Alderman Blanchard pointing out that 'Sheffield had been fortunate for many years in its production of many distinguished physicians and surgeons, and still more fortunate in the fact that those gentlemen placed their services readily at the disposal of that and like institutions'.[132] Indeed, the contribution of the honorary staff was crucial to the image of the voluntary system for they both saved a significant cost and ensured that the poor could have access to the services of the best medical practitioners in the city. As the *Sheffield Telegraph* commented during the 1919 crisis, it was hoped they could:

> retain a system which has done so much to alleviate pain and suffering and has brought to the very poorest in the community skill, knowledge and attention equal to anything the richest could purchase with their many guineas.[133]

Conversely, an expanded or complete municipal system would abolish the honorary medical staff, it was claimed, so that 'It would be a sad day for the poorer people of large cities if Hospitals and Institutions of this kind came under State Control, for they would not reasonably expect these gentlemen to give their valuable services gratuitously'. Moreover, the extensive interchange of honorary staff between the voluntary and municipal sectors provided evidence of the potential cost of paying the consultants – two sessions a week at St James's commanding a salary of £200 per annum.

The voluntary hospitals also saved on administration – a significant amount of the management was undertaken by the chairmen and sometimes their colleagues on the boards. In Nottingham, one chairman estimated his commitment at two days a week while others visited their hospitals daily.[134] Similarly, the major source of finance, the contributory scheme, was run on a shoestring by a tiny paid staff and an army of unpaid collectors.[135] Moreover, a significant proportion of income still came from subscriptions, donations, legacies and appeals (as well as the small street collections) and this would be lost to a state system.[136]

As such it was possible for supporters to claim complete municipal control would lead to a significant increase in the rates. For example in 1927 Matthews estimated that 'if the working of our hospitals was taken over by the municipality, it would mean an increase in the rates of at least 1s. 6d. in the £'.[137] Yet defence of the voluntary system involved some difficult decisions around what state support it might be appropriate to accept.

The post-First World War crisis seemed to make state involvement inevitable, Sheffield activists, Philip Wake of the Royal Hospital and H. H. Bedford of the SRI sharing the view that the state or municipality should provide some additional funds to meet the chronic deficits and support capital projects in exchange for 'a certain amount of joint management'. But even in those trying times, both were 'convinced that the present management can carry on the institutions better and at less cost than either State or municipal management would' and that 'the voluntary system is the most economical'.[138] In considering 'how far the State or the Municipality should contribute to the finances of the hospitals, and what share in the control that would entail', the press also struggled to balance a preference for the voluntary ideal with the evidence that it seemed no longer to deliver: 'Can the voluntary system produce the hospital we require? If not, it must be scrapped. Though, for our part, we hope a way may be found to save us from State or Municipal hospitals.'[139]

In the end municipalization was avoided and nationalization amounted to a small grant from the Onslow Commission. More significant was the refusal by the Treasury to provide support to capital projects, a theme which recurred in Sheffield in the mid-1930s as Ronald Matthews made a number of calls for government grants in aid of major building plans.[140]

Not everyone on the right supported the voluntary hospitals uncritically. In 1919 the treasurer of the SRH, J. H. Doncaster, felt nationalization or municipalization was coming and he broadly welcomed it for the same reasons as many on the left:

> it would ensure everyone paid their share for the benefit they received either in treatment or in the advance of medical knowledge; the existing hospitals could not meet the growing demands of medical science and public health from voluntary sources; and state control would deliver more effective coordination of institutions through a central authority.[141]

More interesting, however, was successful Leeds businessman, Montague Burton. Burton was continuously criticized for his limited engagement with the demands of the voluntary hospitals. Throughout the 1930s the Employers' Fund highlighted the negative impact of the failure of his firm to contribute the expected employer top-up.[142] This came to a head in 1937 when, following considerable pressure from the committee, Burtons agreed to an annual covenanted contribution of £50 (equivalent to £62) although this was regarded as 'totally inadequate for the importance of the firm' by the Fund.[143] Burton's attitude may have been linked to the tendency of Jewish employers to support the Herzl Moser Jewish Hospital, and to a lesser extent the LPD. Indeed, Burton was appointed a Trustee of the LPD in 1931 but at the AGM he announced:

> Some contended that Institutions like the Dispensary and the Infirmary should be subsidised by the State. He personally, had a certain amount of sympathy with that view, but would not have that sympathy if every Institution was so ably and efficiently managed as the Leeds Public Dispensary.[144]

Such dissent was relatively uncommon, though by the later 1930s some other voices were providing a critique of the voluntary system from within. J. Sanderson, a leading lay member of the LWHF, echoed comments from Sheffield when he asserted that 'it was obvious that had it not been for the working people of the city the voluntary hospitals would have been in a very bad way in the last ten years'. Moreover, in:

> paying a warm tribute to the efficiency of the medical work and the nursing at St James's Hospital, he said that the Workpeople's Hospital Fund had done a great service for the people of Leeds when they made arrangements for the patients to be received and treated at that institution.[145]

In a similar manner, the Liberal, Charles Boyle, used his mayoral speech to the LWHF in 1940 to claim workers 'had not got full independence yet. They still had to rely to some extent upon the State and upon charities, which was a thing Englishmen abominated'. Although he did hope 'that some day, perhaps not far distant, they would pay every penny of the cost of medical services in the City'.[146] Yet these tendencies were relatively few and far between and in general the freedom, virtue and independence of the voluntary sector was a touchstone of non-socialist members of the community.

Appropriation and Competition

These broad ideological positions informed the specific policies followed by hospital providers in both cities – and elsewhere across the country – especially in response to the 1929 Local Government Act and more generally as demands for hospital treatment increased in the 1930s. The foreshadowing of the 1929 Act prompted both sides to imagine what a unified system might look like. Furthermore, the opportunity to appropriate hospitals to the Health Committee brought municipal and voluntary into contact and conflict while the need to co-operate created opportunities and tensions which were neither linear nor expected. At each stage ideological positions informed the decisions taken to a greater extent than has generally been accepted. Certainly the decision to appropriate or not was based on a complex amalgam of factors of which ideology was only one, with socialist councils like Norwich failing to take over the infirmary while conservative administrations in Birmingham and Manchester developed large and expansive municipal hospital systems.[147] However, in Leeds and Sheffield party played an important role in the progress of the municipal hospital system, both at the initial stage of appropriation and in subsequent service expansion.[148]

The decision by Neville Chamberlain to scrap the poor law and permit the transfer of institutions to borough and county councils prompted significant debate about the implications at a local level, with both sides asserting their authority in the post-reform system. In a number of speeches Ronald Matthews claimed overarching control for the voluntary sector stating:

> It seems to me that the spear head of our hospital services must be the out-patients departments of our general hospitals. From the out-patient department it must be possible for patients to be sent either to the beds of the general hospital or of the municipal institution.[149]

This would ensure that while making clear that they were 'prepared to co-operate whole-heartedly with the local authorities in the co-ordinated health services' they had to retain their independence[150] and safeguard 'for ourselves that position of leadership to which I say unhesitatingly we are by our record entitled'. In particular, he rejected placing overall responsibility with the MOH, suggesting instead:

> The ideal scheme to my mind ... would be to hand over the administration of the new municipal hospital to a voluntary body drawn from the boards of the voluntary hospitals, say the standing committee of the four boards, with adequate municipal representation, and of course subject to municipal veto in matters of finance. This would make for complete homogenity of policy, and for the freest transfer of cases, and so obviate the possibility of the municipal hospital being made the pawn of contending politicians.[151]

He agreed with those on the left that transfer to the municipal authority would 'considerably' improve the status of the poor law infirmaries 'because the taint of pauperism, which undoubtedly has a retarding effect on their development at the present time, would be removed'. Yet he also pointed out that

> so far as Sheffield is concerned, that question hardly applies, because Firvale is so admirably managed and provides such excellent services that it stands out among the Poor Law infirmaries of the country and has, I think, to a large extent rid itself of the pauper taint.[152]

These latter views could be shared by Labour politicians – though for them such developments heralded an opportunity to supplant the voluntary system. In Leeds the chair of the Board of Guardians Infirmary Committee told an audience in early 1928 that St James's was 'gaining a reputation for excellent treatment' and given there were pay beds and a private ward, the poor law 'stigma' was disappearing: 'We have in the institutions of this kind the foundations of municipal hospitals and if and when poor law administration is taken over by the municipalities, we may hope to see the breaking up of the voluntary hospitals'.[153]

But for the Labour party the bigger issue was pauperism, the 1929 Act offering the possibility of helping the 'great masses of people because they need it and without them having to prove destitution'.[154] As such they supported appropriation first and foremost to remove the taint of pauperism then to promote administrative efficiency.[155] Although it is worth noting such views could be found in cities without socialist administrations, such as Bristol.[156]

With the passing of the Act the socialist councils in power in both cities prepared schemes for appropriation based largely on a main general hospital and ancillary institutions mixing maternity, TB and chronic services.[157] Both schemes were approved by the Ministry of Health at the end of 1930 and were in the process of receiving final backing from the council at the time of the municipal elections. The Sheffield scheme was adopted but in Leeds the council changed hands and appropriation was scrapped by the new Conservative administration. Conservative opposition was based on three factors: a perception that a system run by the Health Committee would be more expensive; an administrative concern that a specific Hospitals Committee should oversee the new institutions; and the deep-seated opposition to the idea of municipal hospitals held by Alderman Martin.[158] As he told the Ministry surveyor in 1933:

> The ordinary avenue of admission of non-urgent cases to the Hospitals should be through the Relieving officer. He does not approve of making it too easy for people to obtain benefits at the public expense or of too much 'spoon feeding' of the populace.[159]

Conversely, appropriation went through smoothly in Sheffield, even attracting guarded support from the medical staff who saw opportunities for a more effective distribution of patients and an easing of the waiting lists at the voluntary hospitals. Indeed the council and representatives of the voluntary hospitals had met as early as 1929 with co-ordination well advanced when the Act came into force in 1930.[160] As the ruling Labour party explained at the elections of 1932, the policy of appropriation was 'in accordance with our policy of limiting to the smallest possible extent the operation of the poor law in the City'. Furthermore, in sharp contrast to Tory Leeds:

> With the exception of persons and/or their dependents in receipt of relief, all cases are admitted as sick inhabitants, the payments, if any, to be made towards the cost of their maintenance being assessed by the Almoner. The reason we admit those in

receipt of relief as Public Assistance cases is to avoid duplication and overlapping in records and services.[161]

However, in Leeds debate over appropriation continued to sour relations between the parties in the early 1930s. Labour activists condemned the Conservatives as 'reactionaries' who were 'determined to continue the hospitals under the old pauperising system',[162] although by 1933 they were once again singing the praises of the institutions themselves, while continuing to attack the administration's PAC policy.[163] Martin remained obstinately attached to PAC control, informing the Ministry of Health surveyor 'quite bluntly that so long as he was Chairman of the Public Assistance Committee none of the hospitals or institutions would be appropriated'. His main objection was the potential cost, though he was also concerned that appropriating St James's and St Mary's but not Rothwell and Holbeck would 'interfere with … freedom of transfer of cases from one to another'. This obstinate opposition was confirmed by Conservative Alderman Weaver, Health Committee chair and consistent supporter of appropriation,[164] who informed the surveyor that 'the question of appropriation had not been considered by the Health Committee and he does not intend to raise the matter while the constitution of the Council remains as at present, as it would be useless to do so'.[165] However, soon after the survey the Conservatives were defeated and Labour quickly dusted off the 1930 plan and implemented appropriation against rather feeble opposition from Martin and the Tories.[166]

Hospital policy remained an important, though possibly never central, campaigning issue for Labour in both cities. In Sheffield it featured prominently in material produced for their unsuccessful council campaign of 1932 and was a notable feature of the 1945 council elections. In 1932 the party claimed that:

> The excellent health record of the City, as a result of our forward policy, has made possible the admission into our municipal hospitals of hundreds of patients who were waiting for admission to voluntary hospitals, but who could not be accommodated there.[167]

Meanwhile, the 1945 publication highlighted the huge increase in patients treated in municipal hospitals – by virtually 50 per cent – all 'under the Public Health Act and *not* under the Poor Law'. It also drew attention to the building of three 32-bed maternity units along with an outpatient department, operating theatre and children's department while plans were in train for a further maternity unit with all 'modern equipment'.[168] Leeds Labour also took credit for the expansion of municipal hospital services, Councillor Brett highlighting appropriation as 'undoubtedly the big achievement of the year … **It must be remembered that the Tories could have done that in 1930 but preferred pauperised hospitals'.** In addition, the party facilitated the transfer of PAC doctors to the Health Committee as 'we will never do away with the poor law taint as long as we have poor law doctors'.[169] Later in the decade, as they sought to regain power, they pointed to their successes in hospital policy and their plans to improve the service. As in Sheffield, they re-emphasized their responsibility 'for turning the Leeds Poor Law Hospitals into Municipal Hospitals' and claimed that an 'Efficient Municipal Hospital Service for All is Labour's Aim'.[170]

But positions were not fixed and the later 1930s saw some change as Alderman Martin softened his opposition to the hospital service while Councillor Asbury adopted a more belligerent stance in relation to the voluntary sector. With the Conservative return to power Martin became chair of the Health Committee and also the leading figure in the Joint Advisory Board. Yet despite his leadership roles in the voluntary hospitals, he fought hard to develop the municipal service. He led the fight against Austyn Barran's attempts to monopolize maternity provision in the city[171] and saw through the extensive and expensive redevelopment of St James's as a modern general hospital. Moreover, in an interesting incident that suggests that voluntary hospital doctors were right to be wary of municipal control, he asserted the primacy of the politicians over the medics. In 1938 the Leeds Voluntary Hospital Committee decided to propose a meeting between the Joint Faculty and Medical Officers from the municipality to consider the implications of closer collaboration between the voluntary and municipal hospitals as:

> such collaboration in order to be wholly effective, requires considerable re-orientation in medical policy, this Council recommends that the Advisory Committee request the Faculties of the Hospitals concerned to prepare a report upon the medical aspect of hospital policy with a view to its representatives placing such report before the Joint Hospitals Advisory Committee for its consideration.

However, Alderman Martin blocked the move, the Voluntary Hospitals Committee learning that at the Leeds Joint Hospitals Advisory Committee:

> The City Council representatives considered it inadvisable for their officials to serve on a medical Committee such as was proposed as it was not in accordance with the policy of the Health Committee to permit their officials to consider questions of policy until they had first been decided by the Health Committee. It was, therefore, agreed that no action be taken in the matter, it being understood that any report prepared by the Faculty and submitted to the Committee would receive careful consideration and that opportunity would be given for additional medical representatives to be present when the report was under discussion.[172]

Yet, equally, Martin retained his personal preference for the voluntary sector. In 1938 he pointed out to the annual meeting of the Leeds Voluntary Hospital Fund that if the employers did not support it the result would be a municipal system which would add £175,000 to the rates bill[173] while the following year he urged the voluntary hospitals to act quickly on developing a radium centre as a voluntary activity before the council attempted to take it over as a municipal idea.[174]

In Sheffield William Asbury also began to lead a changed attitude on the council to relationships with the voluntary hospital. In addition to the end to subsidies for voluntary hospital waiting list patients treated in the City General he led Labour opposition to the voluntary hospitals' key hospital plans. When the Advisory Council considered the proposals in July 1938 Sir Ronald Matthews assumed they 'would meet with general approval'. In particular, he hoped that the local authorities would contribute generously to the scheme and said they 'were looking to the Sheffield City Council to set a good example' to the adjoining county councils. Matthews also hoped the council would continue to maintain their current number of beds and that 'there would be close co-operation between the Voluntary and Municipal Hospitals'. However, Councillor Asbury was far from welcoming in his response, condemning the adjoining counties and their inhabitants for not meeting 'their responsibilities to the Sheffield Voluntary Hospitals' and stating that:

> the information given by the several documents was inadequate. In his view it was not possible to gather from them the number of beds which would be provided and the purpose for which they were to be used and the total estimated cost of the several proposals. Without more definite information he could not take the responsibility of making any recommendation upon the Voluntary Hospitals proposals.[175]

Indeed a few months later in a paper to the Royal Sanitary Institute – subsequently published in their journal – he launched a thinly veiled attack on the clear lack of consultation which had taken place in the development of the voluntary hospital scheme, stating:

> I am aware that under the Local Government Act, 1929, local authorities were compelled to consult with voluntary hospitals in their respective areas with regard to future extensions and development.
> **I do not remember any obligation being imposed on the voluntary hospitals to consult with the local authorities, and this seems to me a one-sided arrangement.**
> In any case, I doubt whether any real measure of co-ordination has been achieved. The approach to the problem must, of necessity be entirely different.[176]

Asbury, as has been noted, also abandoned the Joint Advisory Committee, refusing to call a meeting during 1939 and although he attended the two wartime meetings, the Labour members made no obvious contribution. As a result, by the time of the Ministry of Health survey of 1945 it was clear that relations between the two sectors at an official level were strained although Asbury, as with Martin, could take significant credit for developing a highly integrated hospital system for the city.

Conclusion

Politics and ideology were essential to the shaping of hospital services between the wars. But their greatest impact was on questions of ownership and control rather than specific policies, specialisms or forms of provision. That was largely determined by networks of individuals who represented a range of interests based on class, gender and professional identity. Certainly it would appear that leadership of institutions and even sectors was porous and flexible, with a diffuse form of governance characterizing most parts of both sectors. Boards of management and council committees had to share power with medical staff, co-optees, advisory committees, the contributory schemes and the medical schools. These varied interests helped to smooth service development, at a practical level at least, and to counter some of the effects of ideological battles on the council and the hustings. Conversely, medical officers of health, chairmen of management committees or advisory councils could have very limited power and autonomy as new structures and actors emerged – like the medical faculty, the medical superintendent or the contributory scheme – to offer alternative spaces for policy development and change.

This chapter has also suggested that class and gender and the local socio-economic structures which shaped them were essential in the formation of the policy battle lines. In Leeds, class was divisive, splitting the working class and uniting the middle class around a strong Conservative party. Conversely, gender proved to be a unifying factor, leading to prominent roles for women in all parts of the hospital management structure and feeding into policy around services for women such as maternity provision, general beds for women and gynaecology facilities brought together under the leadership of the LGI. The effects of gender in Sheffield were to underline the dominance of the working-class male and produce hospital services which were shaped by and for men. Yet the desire to ensure these outcomes meant that for much of the period the two sectors worked in harmony to support actions that delivered a fair deal for the working man.

As this suggests, operational experiences in Leeds and Sheffield challenge established historiographical perceptions regarding the rigid distinctions within and between sectors. How they cooperated and the extent to which they remained in competition will be the subject of the following chapter.

7 CO-OPERATION, COMPETITION AND THE DEVELOPMENT OF HOSPITAL SYSTEMS

By 1929, hospital providers in Leeds and Sheffield had assembled the buildings, the doctors and specialties, the finance and the political structures to deliver a modern hospital service to their cities. However, this process took place without any overarching control, with each hospital or authority free to inaugurate any service they wished or could afford (with some limits on the guardians and the municipality). As we have seen, finance and political will would place limits on development but the existence of a service or specialty in one institution did not preclude it being taken up by another hospital. As a result duplication was common and its potential to multiply was embedded in the 1929 Local Government Act which had encouraged the municipal authorities to take on the delivery of general hospital provision. Yet it is evident that a free-for-all was avoided and the 1930s and 1940s saw the development of integrated services in Leeds and Sheffield. This process saw the large number of independent institutions in the voluntary, poor law and municipal sectors begin to collaborate, merge and reorientate to create increasingly efficient and democratic regional services. The form this co-operation took and the speed and scale were shaped by local economic, social and political cultures and structures responding to internal imperatives and external stimulus from government, national bodies and major crises like the two world wars and the economic depression.

Yet historians have been broadly united in the view that it was a 'chaotic and highly inefficient situation'.[1] Drawing heavily on the PEP report of 1937 which

> complained about lack of unity in the two hospital systems; the 1,000 voluntary hospitals were 'self-governing institutions, jealous of their independence and only loosely associated with each other,' while the 3,000 public hospitals were distributed between hundreds of separate local authorities only remotely regulated by the health department.[2]

Supported by a highly selective reading of the Ministry of Health surveyors of 1945, a consensus has grown up summarized most effectively by Charles Webster who claimed:

The worst disjunction within the system was between the municipal and voluntary hospital sectors. From the time of the Cave Committee (1921) pressure built up for closer coordination between the two systems ... In the event it was only in isolated instances such as Liverpool, Manchester or Oxford that extensive co-operation took place. On the whole, local authorities expanded their hospital services without reference to their voluntary neighbours, or even in a spirit of competition or emulation.[3]

Abel-Smith, using the voluntary hospitals' own Sankey Report, was a little more optimistic – but not much. After describing the committees and outcomes in Liverpool, Birmingham, Sheffield and Manchester in positive terms, he concluded:

These were the main attempts to encourage co-operation, but they covered only a small part of the country. Where there was no co-ordinating body, the voluntary hospitals worked in rivalry with one another ... Over the majority of the country there was no co-ordination whatsoever.[4]

In particular, four tropes have emerged from the historiography: enduring competition within the voluntary sector; inadequate development of the services of the municipal sector; the failure of the voluntary and municipal systems to work together; and minimal progress in creating regional mechanisms for delivery.[5]

Yet these views may be rather pessimistic. Certainly evidence from Middlesbrough and the work of Levene et al. have pointed to a growing willingness on both sides to minimize competition and duplication and work towards a more efficient and effective service – for example in Barnsley.[6] Moreover, it wasn't just the bigger cities like Liverpool and Manchester where co-operation thrived, but also Bristol and Oxford, Norwich to a limited extent, and in the north-east there were developments in Newcastle, if not Sunderland.[7] There were even schemes in rural areas such as Gloucestershire and some integration for contributory scheme members in Norfolk though efforts at co-ordination in Cornwall would seem to have failed.[8] Often these developments were driven by users and by the medical staff and part of the problem historians have faced is their desire to see co-operation in formal structures emerging out of the Local Government Act, such as consultative committees. Yet, as a Ministry of Health official observed in 1933, 'in some areas where real co-operation is closest it is most difficult to find evidence',[9] as was the case in Leeds at the time. Moreover, the push for co-operation was often strongest where local pressures came to bear, for example the amalgamations of the general hospitals in Bristol, Birmingham and Sheffield were driven by a combination of major philanthropists and the medical schools while co-ordination between the voluntary and municipal sectors was pioneered in many cases by the contributors' associations.[10] Certainly there was significant duplication of services, especially core specialities like ENT, which were covered by most voluntary general hospitals and began to appear in some municipal institutions. However, in the case of the voluntary hospitals in cities with medical schools this was regarded as essential for teaching purposes while even the most advanced municipal hospitals limited their specialist outpatient facilities to their own follow-up cases.[11]

Thus, in this final chapter we will consider how such systems developed in Sheffield and Leeds. In the case of the former the high level of co-operation is well known – in part the product of their submission to the Sankey Commission.[12] However, the situation in Leeds has not attracted any attention and yet its experience is probably more representative of the gradual changes which were occurring across the hospital sector in the ten years following the 1929 Act. In the aftermath of the First World War hospital services in both cities were fragmented and in severe financial difficulty. The crisis, especially in the voluntary sector, prompted a number of responses including the establishment of the Sheffield Joint Hospital Council and the Leeds Employers' Fund which both laid the groundwork for collaboration amongst the voluntary hospitals.[13] Links to the municipal and poor law sector were also emerging, though these remained small-scale and largely commercial. However, the Local Government Act provided a stimulus which brought the municipal and poor law provision together, encouraged the municipalities to consult with the voluntary sector on their plans and even stimulated the voluntary hospitals to shake off their insularity and work together in the face of potential local government competition. In both cities high levels of co-operation emerged within and between sectors during the 1930s, with Sheffield quickly creating a highly integrated system while developments were slower but no less far-reaching in Leeds. Both cities saw the reallocation of services and joint appointments both within and between the sectors while in Sheffield there was even amalgamation and a citywide joint appeal for a new institution. But what drove these changes and what were the barriers to effective joint working?

Integration in the Voluntary Sector

Integration within the voluntary hospital sector took place at formal and informal levels and was stimulated by local and external influences and actors. Although much of the initial impetus for joint working appeared to come from the post-war financial crisis and subsequent state involvement[14] as in Bristol, Birmingham and Manchester, sustained change was often driven by the interests of the medical profession and their colleagues in the medical schools.[15] Thus in Leeds a proposal to unify the four voluntary hospitals originating from Dr Jamieson of the University Medical School was presented to the LGI Faculty and Board in 1924. Although the board – led by the surgeon Sir Berkley Moynihan – blocked the idea, it demonstrated the interest of the university in rationalizing hospital provision, an interest which returned with more effect in the 1930s when the medical faculties of both Leeds and Sheffield were instrumental in pushing reorganization and even amalgamation. Indeed, in Sheffield most of the priorities underpinning the Million Pound Appeal derived from the Medical Staff Club who produced two key memoranda for the Joint Advisory Committee.[16] Drawing on the findings of the recently published Sankey Commission,[17] the medical staff advocated the creation of a new key hospital of 750 beds adjacent to the university which would allow the SRI and the SRH to 'accomplish together what neither could separately'. The Sheffield Staff Club saw their key priorities as:

> An urgent demand for:–
>   A re-organisation of the Medical Services.
>   Maternity Beds (The Staffs are glad these are being provided)
>   A Radium Centre – The Staffs think this will soon be provided.
>   Beds for Paying Patients. The Staffs note that those at the Royal Hospital will soon be available, and note that some are included in the Jessop extensions. They trust, however, that a special block will be included in the new Key Hospital.[18]

They also advocated closer working with the Edgar Allen Institute and the amalgamation of the staff of all the hospitals in 'a single Unit Hospital built on modern lines'. To achieve this they approved the Glossop Road site as 'its proximity to the Jessop Hospital and the Children's Hospital will establish a Hospital Centre close to the University' while it would also be conveniently located as 'Practically all of the consultants live in the area between the Group of Hospitals and Fulwood, and they will be able to make more frequent visits than they would have been able to at Norton'. In addition, the teaching of students would retain a high level of efficiency while outpatients would have more convenient access to the hospital.[19]

Organizations for Co-ordination

Formal structures for co-ordination in the voluntary sector emerged from the financial crisis and particularly the state response which saw the Cave Committee secure a one-off grant to ease the pressure. But to access this support, hospitals had to form local committees to allocate the grant and explore ways in which the voluntaries could act together to eradicate duplication and increase efficiency.[20] The Sheffield Joint Hospitals Council had been initiated prior to Cave in response to medical staff concerns that current fundraising was both inefficient and unlikely to meet the need for significantly increased bed provision. A consultative committee was convened by the four hospitals in the city and its 1920 report addressed concerns over beds, nursing provision, finance and hospital locations prompting the formation of the Hospitals Council and the Penny in the Pound scheme.[21] The Sheffield Joint Hospitals Council was representative of the whole community, its sixty-two members including the Lord Mayor, Master Cutler, councillors and aldermen and appointees from the university, voluntary hospitals, contributors, the Trades and Labour Council, the Press and general practice.[22] Its main aim was to co-ordinate fundraising, and particularly the contributory scheme, and to act as a focus for donations, legacies and other joint contributions to the hospitals such as the Sunday Fund and the student Rag. But the body also took on some responsibility for co-ordinating services, in particular a citywide ambulance corps and convalescent care for contributors. Moreover, Penny in the Pound contributors were allowed emergency admittance to poor law hospitals when no bed was available in a voluntary hospital – a privilege which normally took some years to arrange in other towns; in Middlesbrough, for example, it was not arranged until 1937.[23] In response to Cave the Hospitals Council initiated a Hospitals Committee to collect information, develop co-operation on patients, finance and processes and act to protect the voluntary system. This was clearly a civic body with voluntary hospital interests balanced by those of the council and it became a 'valuable and inseparable feature of the constructive work of the Joint Hospitals' Council'.[24] Within a year the council were claiming 'co-operation by the Hospitals has indeed proved effective',[25] and certainly this was evident in the success of the Penny in the Pound scheme and in large-scale initiatives like the purchase of Norton Hall with the aim of building a new single site hospital. On the other hand, there was no attempt to limit duplication of services, with new specialities like mental health OP departments appearing at both general hospitals in the 1920s.

The situation in Leeds was less impressive. Initial joint working by the voluntary hospitals was seen in the formation of the 'Employers' Contribution Fund' in 1920, which was a 'Scheme for collecting contributions from the Employers of Labour in Leeds for the combined use' of the four institutions.[26] However, in response to Cave, the LGI decided to join with the East and West Riding Voluntary Hospitals Committee which arranged the payments to the Yorkshire hospitals, except Sheffield.[27] Much like similar bodies in other areas, this organization was short-lived. The employers' fund seems to have taken on the role of voluntary hospitals committee and continued to function as both during the 1920s, mainly concerning itself with the distribution of income collected centrally through employers and self employed schemes, the Lord Mayor's appeal of 1924 and street collections. More significantly they promoted the idea of converting the LWHF to a contributory scheme in 1928–9, with some success.[28] Many places experienced such limited progress in the 1920s; Bristol, for example, saw a number of initiatives to promote closer working sponsored by the university and leading philanthropists rebuffed by the general hospitals.[29] In Birmingham, similar pressure did produce a merger and a united hospital on a greenfield site next to the university.[30]

It was in the 1930s, however, that schemes for co-ordination developed fully, although both the LPD and Sheffield Children's Hospital were reluctant to merge their identities with the other institutions. Preparations for the introduction of the 1929 Act saw the voluntary hospitals of Leeds form a co-ordination scheme subcommittee which drew its membership from the boards of the four hospitals along with representation from the university and the faculty. Drawing on the experience of the Leeds Voluntary Hospitals Fund Committee it focused attention on the limited co-ordination between the voluntary hospitals, initially seeking to revive a 1924 plan to unify the hospitals that 'had done a great deal towards preparing the way for an amalgamation scheme'.[31] But the need to work incrementally was recognized and a subcommittee was appointed to consider four initial aims – 'to obtain co-ordination in working, (b) to have one Faculty common to the Joint Institutions (c) to represent the Voluntary Institutions as one body to the outside world (d) to facilitate the training of Students and Nurses'. In addition they were to explore the operation of a single board 'to co-ordinate the work of the Institutions in the light of their combined knowledge and experience', though beyond this the institutions were to retain local management and financial control.[32] These were radical proposals, pointing to the more efficient distribution of staff, patients and students, if not yet money and buildings.

But the plans were quickly watered down to proposals for a joint hospitals committee and a joint faculty to bring together the LGI, LMH and LHW – though even this was quite far-reaching for the time.[33] Negotiations proved slow and torturous as the committee attempted to combine the creation of a hospitals' council with the merger of the medical faculty. In effect, membership of the council would include accepting unified qualifications for staff, a joint appointments panel and the means to allocate patients across institutions. The process revealed both the increased integration of the LGI, LHW and LMH around the teaching of medical students and the autonomy of the LPD, whose chairman reported that 'The Scheme had been before his Board several times and that they had decided to remain a friendly and helpful but independent body'.[34] But following a final series of amendments, mainly around the election of medical and surgical staff and the relationship between the Maternity and Women's Hospitals, the Voluntary Hospitals Council came into being at the end of 1933. By 1939 all of the voluntary hospitals had joined the Voluntary Hospital Council but, in order to secure the co-operation of the LPD, it was decided that the joint faculty committee was no longer an essential criteria for membership.[35]

As has been seen, appeals were also significant evidence of joint working, as institutions attempted first to stagger their requests to the public and then to unite as in Sheffield's joint Million Pound Appeal of 1938. Its rational and scientific basis would allow the voluntary hospitals to build a 'great new Centre of Healing which ... will ultimately fulfil all the functions of the ideal "Key" Hospital group':

> The *medical* function is to treat the sick and injured; the *teaching* function to train the doctors and nurses; the *research* function to investigate the causes and cure of disease and, lastly, the *social* function is to raise the standard of health of the community to prevent disease.[36]

Planning like this could ensure more effective capital expansion as the financial climate became more propitious for raising large sums of money. Drawing on the experience of Birmingham, the smaller hospitals agreed to sink their individual interests. The board of the Jessop put it as follows:

> the other Sheffield Voluntary Hospitals in an exhaustive review and discussion of future hospital policy generally ... [which] With the amalgamation of the two General Hospitals and adoption of the principle of providing a new General Hospital on a new site at a future date, the extension and modernising of this Hospital on this its own site, and the development of the Children's Hospital also in its existing position, [has assured] co-ordinated service ...[37]

Even the Children's Hospital was being brought into the more central hospital work of the city, noting of their plan to build an extra storey for babies that 'the provision of these additional beds has the approval of the Boards of Management and the Honorary Medical Staffs of the other three Sheffield Voluntary Hospitals'.[38]

Challenging Duplication

Thus, formal co-ordination in committee was well advanced in both Leeds and Sheffield by the early 1930s and this provided the environment in which to challenge another criticism – duplication of delivery – as over the following fifteen years they facilitated major developments, including the reallocation of patients and the amalgamation of the two general hospitals in Sheffield. The first attempts at amalgamation had come in 1924 when Sheffield Hospitals Council co-ordinated the purchase of Norton Hall with the intention that

> each of the Hospitals, in turn, will remove all their In-Patients to this suburban site, in order to harness up the curative value of sunshine, clean air and quiet in a more generous measure to the healing work of our skilled Physicians and Surgeons.[39]

Although this scheme collapsed, the mid-1930s saw a movement to unite the city's voluntary hospitals and create a hospital centre with a new key hospital next to the university. As noted, the honorary medical staff initiated the idea, proposing 'a complete amalgamation of the Honorary Staffs which they felt should be accompanied by corresponding action in the matter of lay control'. Talks between the hospitals and the university centred on

> such recommendations as will strengthen to the utmost the position of the voluntary hospitals in the future, secure for the patients the maximum amount of efficiency in every branch of the hospital services, and maintain and extend the harmonious relationships existing between the Municipal and Voluntary Hospital Authorities.[40]

Following a resolution in July 1936 supporting amalgamation in principle, by December the two general hospitals were in discussions to acquire land for a new hospital near the university and it was 'confidently hoped that ultimately amalgamation will embrace all four Institutions'.[41] Yet, while a United Board would be formed, local management, the election of consultants and decisions on any major extensions remained with the existing committees. When formal amalgamation took place on 1 January 1939 the board of the SRI felt that although 'a certain amount of grief should be felt at parting from the old identity ... the step being taken in conjunction with the Royal Hospital is undoubtedly in the best interests of all concerned'.[42] The SRH were more prosaic, asserting that 'the primary reason for amalgamation was to join forces to provide, at the earliest possible moment, urgently needed extensions on a site near the University'.[43] Yet, there was only a limited coming together of departments at the time, and even in 1945 it was noted that the amalgamation had not gone very far towards reducing duplication. Within a year of the end of the Second World War, however, it was apparent that much more was being done to restructure the work of the two institutions.[44]

Without a doubt barriers to joint working could be acute within the voluntary sector. The LPD continued to remain outside Leeds Voluntary Hospitals' Council as long as it insisted upon minimum qualifications and joint appointments. In 1939 it was necessary to change the constitution and drop the minimum qualifications rule to secure the Dispensary's membership of the committee.[45] There were similar tensions in Sheffield when during the amalgamation discussions of the late 1930s the Edgar Allen Institute proved circumspect in its welcome to joint working, the Board of Management stating that it backed 'close co-operation' between the Voluntary Hospitals and the Institute especially in the key area of 'Orthopaedic work', reiterating that:

> it would not be in accordance with the aims and objects of the Institute if the experience of the Staff, its buildings and equipment were not available to the Orthopaedic Departments of the Royal Infirmary and Royal Hospital for the after-treatment of traumatic and orthopaedic cases.

But the council went on to assert that:

> Members of the Institute may rest assured that every care will be taken to preserve the identity of the Institute as one of the foremost centres in the country for treatment of this kind, and that the objects set out in the Memorandum of Association will not be lost sight of in considering the ultimate application of the endowments and fund.[46]

This statement did not force the Edgar Allen Institute to remain independent, and in 1947 it merged with the United Hospital to form the semi-autonomous Edgar Allen Physical Treatment Centre.[47]

These barriers notwithstanding, co-ordination between the various voluntary hospitals went from strength to strength in the 1940s, especially in Leeds, where the Ministry of Health surveyors commended the Hospitals Council and noted the very close links between the LGI and the LHW. Although the situation was less advanced in Sheffield, the merging of certain departments was commended.[48] Moreover, when the Sheffield Appeal Committee applied to the Ministry of Health to retain the money collected as part of the Million Pound Appeal after the transfer to the NHS, the level of trust and joint working in the city was met with surprise by the civil servants. As the secretary of the Jessop Hospital reported:

> We explained ... how the Appeal had originated – instead of being separate appeals on behalf of individual hospitals it was a joint appeal covering the needs of all four hospitals, administered by a joint Committee of these hospitals (plus other representatives) instead of – as normally would be the case – a committee of the individual hospitals making the appeal.

> The Officers [of the Ministry] seemed to be impressed (and a little surprised) at this evidence of the happy relationship of the Sheffield Voluntary Hospitals – joined together in common action without legal bonds.

As this suggests, by the 1940s the Ministry of Health had developed very negative views of the ability of voluntary hospitals to co-operate.[49] Yet in Leeds and Sheffield, though there were exceptions, highly sophisticated joint working had emerged.

General Services of the Local Authority

A similar pattern of co-operation was apparent within and between the elements of the local state services with early and extensive integration in Sheffield and slow but steady developments in Leeds. As has been seen, the 1920s saw the first steps come with the unification of the Boards of Guardians which led to a redistribution of responsibilities and patients between the various institutions in both cities aided by the appointment of a new medical superintendent at St James's.[50] As a result of these changes, Fir Vale in Sheffield and St James's in Leeds began to focus increasingly on general hospital work while the other institutions came to concentrate on chronic, maternity and tubercular patients. In Sheffield the first steps towards the integration of the poor law and municipal services accompanied these developments as the socialist council worked with the guardians to open Nether Edge Maternity Hospital in early 1927. As the MOH noted:

> In the past expense has probably been the prime factor preventing women from obtaining ante-natal attention, but now that we are able to offer those patients, found at the clinics to require it, the necessary hospital treatment as in-patients of Nether Edge Maternity Hospital, many of the complications of pregnancy may be lessened or averted.

Accompanying these moves, overlap between the municipality and poor law was prevented by 'close co-operation' to ensure 'certain patients are granted extra relief by the Guardians on the representation of the Tuberculosis Medical Officer'.[51] As in Sheffield, some rationalization had occurred in Leeds within the four institutions brought together by the unification of the city poor law in 1927. In particular, St Mary's became a focus for maternity while chronic and some specialist cases were moved to St George's and Holbeck.

With such extensive groundwork already laid the process of appropriation in Sheffield, along with the unification of the work of the different elements of the medical services of the city, was quickly accomplished in 1929–30. In his 1930 report the medical superintendent of Sheffield City Hospitals was able to report that Fir Vale and Nether Edge, 'which had been for years maintained as hospitals separate from the General Institution', were appropriated to the Public Health Committee as general hospitals. This process was eased by the presence of 'completely separate staffs' and 'no change was necessary in staff or buildings in order to carry this out'. Moreover, the hospitals had a staff of full-time medical officers, visiting physicians, surgeons, obstetricians and were equipped with X-ray apparatus as well as laboratory facilities and 'had all the amenities of a general hospital'.[52] The trend to specialize in chronic, TB and children at Nether Edge (which allowed the more effective development of Fir Vale as a general hospital)[53] was continued while the council aimed to reduce the proportion of their accommodation remaining in the hands of the PAC by further appropriations. As a result by the time of the Ministry of Health inspector's visit in 1933 Sheffield was commended as a fine example of the aims of the 1929 Act with unified services under the clear leadership of the MOH, medical superintendent and the Health Committee.[54]

This contrasted markedly with the situation in Leeds where the council had withdrawn a Ministry of Health approved application to appropriate three PLIs in 1930. Here the surveyors found services were split between the Health, Public Assistance, Mental Deficiency and School Medical departments, while the MOH was not the school medical officer and took 'no part in the work of the School Medical service, the Mental Deficiency service or the Public Assistance medical service'. 'Such an arrangement', the inspector noted, ran counter to the general trend which saw effective co-ordination of local authority services resting in the hands of the MOH as 'the Council's chief medical adviser' who was in a position 'to advise the Council on any matter of medical policy which may arise, under whatever statutory powers the medical services in question are administered and whatever classes of patients are concerned'. Nor were they content with assurances that the various officers co-operated urging the 'more definite and formal co-ordination of the health services' that would come from the MOH being brought into 'effective contact with the whole of the medical services'. The Minister requested clarification of how they would facilitate change and in particular drew 'special attention to the position of the Public Assistance medical service, the existing separation of which from the other medical services of the Council raises an important issue of policy under the Local Government Act, 1929'.

Indeed, the council were reminded that the Act intended local authorities to treat their sick under the Public Health Act and that as the transferred PLIs 'contain the main provision of the Council for the treatment of the sick' their appropriation as Health Committee hospitals was 'a necessary step if the policy of the Act is to be carried out'. Moreover, the Ministry confirmed their previously stated belief that 'the appropriation of some of these institutions is both desirable and practicable' and hoped 'that the Council will be in a position to formulate proposals to this end at an early date'. In an aside, the letter obliquely reassured the medical superintendent that the suggested 're-organisation and transfer of services ... would in no way affect the responsibility for the clinical care of patients which would continue to rest with the medical officers in whose charge they are placed'.[55]

In Leeds the original appropriation scheme of 1930 had assumed turning St James's into a general and acute hospital along with all of the maternity beds. St Mary's would be appropriated to take infirm cases along with Rothwell (St George's), while Holbeck would remain under the PAC to take 'institution' cases. The Ministry attempted to persuade the council to change their minds, pointing out 'the special advantage that it would facilitate for the free use of the hospitals for Maternity and Tuberculosis'.[56] However, the council stuck to their decision and the institutions passed to the PAC yet it is apparent that despite the failure to appropriate progress towards integration did occur. Thus, the shortage of accommodation at St James for the acute sick caused by the large number of infirm cases was partly addressed by using beds in Beckett Street and Holbeck to allow 'a re-distribution of the cases, with the result that the number of beds available for medical and surgical cases has been increased'.[57] By 1934 the Ministry of Health surveyor was able to comment that 'the cooperation that has been developed is creditable'.[58] He recommended that Rothwell should be taken over by the Health Committee to treat the sick and infirm while Holbeck should be left 'entirely for the non-sick', ensuring all of the sick would be 'in Public Health Act Hospitals while all the Institution inmates would be in Beckett Street and Holbeck'. This approach was adopted by the council when the hospitals were finally taken under Health Committee control by which time:

> St. James's Hospital and St. Mary's and Rothwell Infirmaries are under common medical supervision; the administration has been greatly simplified and the transfer of cases from one institution to another can be effected without unnecessary friction or delay.[59]

Yet despite further reorganization which saw a rationalization of patient types, St James's was still obliged to retain almost 150 beds for the infirm sick, while 20 special male patients remained in Rothwell.[60]

Thus by 1935 the former poor law institutions had been assimilated into the work of the Health Committees and significant reallocation of patients within and between institutions had been affected to ensure more efficient use of the resources. The Medical Officer of Health was in overall control of all hospital beds and sick patients while the institutions were run by the medical superintendents who both displayed considerable medical and managerial skill. This completion of the integration of local state provision opened the way for the development of collaboration with the voluntary sector and the first tentative steps towards a hospital system for Leeds and Sheffield.

Voluntary and Municipal Co-ordination

Despite clear evidence of local integration amongst both the voluntary and municipal providers, contemporaries and historians have focused on the absence of co-operation and the prevalence of duplication between the sectors in the interwar period. For example, Lord Dawson claimed in 1937 that the two 'rival' hospital systems were 'duplicating and even conflicting, without machinery in existence for co-ordinating their activities', while rarely is any mention made of effective systems or when they are noted they are stated to be exceptional or utilized to expose the general absence of joint working.[61] Yet it is clear that in Leeds and Sheffield there was extensive formal and informal co-operation between the two systems dating from the early 1920s. As with the developments within the voluntary sector, it was finance, especially the presence of local or national state funding and pressure from the workers' contributory schemes, which pushed early efforts at collaboration.

Thus in Sheffield, the Hospital Council quickly established good relations with the Board of Guardians and their institutions which 'heartily co-operated' with 'readiness, kindliness and absence of red tape' to take emergency cases for up to seven days.[62] These close connections with the Board of Guardians and the council paved the way for the rapid appropriation of the hospitals in 1930 which all of the partners welcomed. In Leeds, however, relations with the local authority in the 1920s were predominantly commercial. Local Boards of Guardians paid a subscription intended to cover the cost of any patients they may have to send but the councils were less forthcoming, with Sir Charles Wilson, Conservative leader of Leeds Council, seeming 'to take strong views against' the council joining the Employers Contribution Fund.[63] However, LGI did negotiate joint schemes with the local authority for the treatment of venereal disease and childhood orthopaedics – as was the case in a number of cities, including Leicester.[64] In 1924 the hospital responded positively to a scheme proposed by the MOH to unify the management of VD treatment under the LGI's VD Officer, Dr Bibby. The scheme aimed to minimize 'overlapping and confusion' with Bibby overseeing the main clinic in the Infirmary as well as treating patients at the Maternity Hospital and attending as a consultant at the council's Infant Welfare Clinics and the PLIs, where 'there is always a considerable amount of infected material, which, because of its floating character constitutes a real danger to the community'.[65] Significantly, the VD team would be 'under the administrative control of the Medical Officer of Health',[66] demonstrating both the acute awareness local hospital providers had of the complex distribution of disease cases and, more significantly, the willingness of voluntary hospital staff to serve under the MOH in appropriate circumstances.

Commercial relations were developed further when the LGI board attempted to formalize payment for schoolchildren treated through the Education Department at the voluntary hospitals.[67] The plan was initially blocked by the medical faculty who would permit a grant 'in support of the purely charitable work done by the Infirmary and other allied charities' but flatly opposed a capitation fee[68] and it was only at the third time of asking, bolstered by the prospect of other hospitals entering the field, that the staff agreed to a capitation fee to underpin the grant.[69] At the same time a scheme for severely disabled children to be treated for a fixed tariff by the orthopaedics team was mooted, in part to prevent the Education Department from setting up one of their own. Again the medical faculty initially opposed the proposals but following discussions with the Education Committee[70] a compromise emerged which aided the developing work of the Orthopaedic Surgeon, Mr Daw, and brought additional income to the hospital.[71]

Most significant, however, in facilitating the movement of patients between the different hospitals and the different sectors, were the contributory schemes. The Leeds scheme had allowed any contributor to make use of the services of any of the city voluntary hospitals from the late nineteenth century.[72] In Sheffield the establishment of the Penny in the Pound scheme in 1922 had the same effect, shifting the contributors' entitlement from a single hospital to all four institutions. Moreover, the demands of contributors for free treatment led to agreement between the Sheffield Hospitals Council and the Sheffield Board of Guardians as early as 1923 that emergency patients brought to the PLIs in the event of no bed being available in the voluntary hospitals would receive free treatment for up to a week. A similar arrangement was instituted in Leeds in 1930 between the LWHF and the Public Assistance Committee. The initial deal saw 350 patients treated by the city while fears that the agreement might lead to chronic patients languishing in the PAC institutions at the expense of the LWHF were alleviated by a clause that excluded 'Tuberculosis, Mental and Chronic Care cases'.[73] By 1938, around 5,000 LWHF members were being treated in the municipal hospitals – with St James's treating as many LWHF patients as the LGI – while in Sheffield the figure was approximately 4,000.

However, it was the 1929 Act which provided the greatest impetus to collaboration between the two sectors. The Act required municipal authorities to consult with the voluntary hospitals on their plans for service provision providing a basis for rationalization and integration – though in many case, such as Middlesbrough, this was ignored.[74] Indeed, in Leeds the voluntary hospitals were reluctant to meet officially although the council's decision to abandon appropriation took the urgency out of the situation. Conversely, co-operation got off to a flying start in Sheffield based on 'The happy relations which have always existed between the Voluntary Hospitals and the City Authorities'.[75] As early as June 1929 representatives of the voluntary hospitals and the council met to form a Joint Advisory Committee which considered the provision of inpatient, outpatient and casualty facilities, new beds, equipment and buildings:

> Financial adjustments as between the Voluntary and Municipal Hospitals for services undertaken.
> The co-ordination of Nursing Services.
> The election of visiting staffs.
> The relationship of the Sheffield Hospitals with Hospitals situate in the areas of the adjacent County Boroughs and County Councils.

This proved successful and by 1934 this 'very close co-operation' had resulted in 'several adjustments [being] made in the direction of delimiting the spheres of action of the voluntary and municipal organizations'.[76]

Formal discussions between the two sectors in Leeds began in 1936, though once again progress was incredibly slow. The key areas for negotiation were outpatients, equitable distribution of caseloads and payment for transferred cases. On the former there was fairly ready agreement that there would be one outpatient receiving department at LGI, although St James's would be allowed a 'Follow-on Department' so patients could 'be seen by the physician or surgeon who treated them when they were resident in the hospital'.[77] Such arrangements were seen elsewhere, including Liverpool, and outside of London full outpatient work was rare.[78] The joint advisory committee finally began meeting in 1937 – the same year as Bristol and Middlesbrough – with representatives from the five hospitals, the medical staff, the university and the Health Committee, with the chair alternating between the Health Committee and the Voluntary Hospitals Council.[79] Though more cautious than Sheffield, Dr Dick saw its work as 'of the highest importance, and its capacity to view the hospital problems of the city as a whole is leading to most interesting and valuable developments'. It was, he noted, 'but a short time since the revolution initiated by the Local Government Act' which had accelerated developments in municipal hospital work prompting a 'growing appreciation of the possibilities of a co-ordinated hospital service. The closer the co-operation and the more numerous the points of contact between the various hospitals in the city, the more efficient will be the service provided'.[80]

Central to the work of the advisory committees in cities like Leeds, Sheffield and Manchester was the establishment of formal spheres of influence and agreements on patient allocations, capital projects and long-term developments. Thus, in Sheffield, among the initial recommendations of the Health Committee was the extension of the City General at a total cost of around £57,000 to include a new outpatient department, operating theatre and maternity block, along with an addition to the nurses' home, and the centralization of all ambulances – municipal and voluntary – under the control of the Joint Hospital Council.[81] But central to the policy was the decision to initiate patient transfers. Based on a survey which showed the voluntary hospitals had over 2,000 names on waiting lists for their 1,000 beds while the appropriated general hospitals had 1,500 beds and no waiting lists,

> An arrangement was made by which the City General Hospital undertook to relieve the voluntary hospitals of patients on their waiting lists up to 500 in number in each year at an inclusive charge to the voluntary hospital concerned of 25/– per case.

Moreover, the service was in effect free as the corporation – utilizing an obscure clause in the 1925 Public Health Act – gave a donation to the Joint Hospitals Council of £625, distributed according to the number of patients taken – thus balancing the payments made and satisfying the Ministry of Health's insistence that all general hospital patients paid for their treatment. The scheme was policed by a subcommittee of the medical superintendent, steward and resident surgical officer of the City General along with the secretary of the two voluntary hospitals to determine who should be transferred with a stipulation that 'no person is to be admitted to the Sheffield City General Hospital unless the

Medical Superintendent has first approved, and also that Section 16 of the Local Government Act is not to be applied to any such person'. The initial two-year deal saw waiting lists at the SRH and SRI fall from 2,446 in 1930 to 1,648 by the end of 1933 while at the Jessop it had come down to 439 from 504 over the same period. The arrangement was continued until 1937 when the council pulled out; by that time it had relieved the lists by a total of 3,240 patients – 2,632 from the SRI and 608 from the SRH.[82]

In Leeds there was no such formal agreement, and some confusion existed over who would meet the cost of transferred patients, the MOH cautioning that direct transfer from the Infirmary OP Department would be possible 'provided that satisfactory arrangements could be made for this'.[83] However, although Martin had tried to avoid financial responsibility for transferred patients, Johnstone Jervis had to admit that 'where cases were admitted to the Infirmary for special treatment not available at the local authority's hospital it would be possible to reimburse the Infirmary the cost of such treatment'.[84] Patient transfers were also extensive in Manchester by the later 1930s and beginning, slowly, in Middlesbrough. In Bristol an agreement on case distribution was signed in 1938 aiming to minimize waiting times while allocating 'cases requiring more prolonged treatment' to the municipal general.[85]

Positive views of municipal voluntary relations were promoted into the second half of the decade. In response to the Sankey Commission's questionnaire, the Sheffield Hospitals Council noted the existence of very good relations with the City of Sheffield though they were critical of the surrounding county councils for not setting up joint committees or making particular progress with the development of their own services. They noted their support for the principles of co-operation and complementarity expressed in the 1929 Act, commented favourably on the waiting list scheme and drew attention to the Joint Committee, 'to which are referred all questions of common interest'.[86] However, following the launch of the key hospital programme in 1936–7, relations between the two sides cooled and the Joint Committee effectively ceased to operate by 1940.

In Leeds the initial agreements of 1936–7 focused on formalizing the discussions of the previous three years to confirm that there would be no OP Department at St James's, but there would be a follow-up unit for returning inpatients. There was also an agreement to establish facilities for the interchange of inpatients and outpatients between LGI and St James's which would be governed by the availability of beds, with the exception of certain classes of patients: those requiring special treatment only available at LGI such as deep X-ray, and particular cases required for teaching (agreed to by both sides). Patients transferred to St James's also had to be Leeds residents. In the years up to the outbreak of war the Joint Committee considered various approaches to the reduction or diminution of duplication in service delivery.[87]

While committees and agreements emerged to formalize arrangements between the two sectors in the 1930s, informal understandings, especially at the level of key individuals such as the medical superintendent, municipal hospital consultant or twin-tracking board members like George Martin, were crucial to the transformation of relations. Thus, although no formal arrangements existed in Leeds until the later 1930s, unofficial joint working had been underway for some time through a variety of channels. For example, in 1934 the voluntary hospital working group agreed to allow the Labour chair of the PAC access to the joint faculty scheme, while the PAC had three co-opted members from the voluntary hospitals. Progress was such that the city was one of those places where collaboration was strongest where it was least obvious, the Ministry of Health surveyor commenting that, 'Leeds seems to be a good example of the achievement of very satisfactory co-operation without formal consultation'.[88]

In the main this was due to close links at the level of individual medical and administrative personnel and especially the medical superintendent who was able to negotiate a range of informal processes for the effective distribution of patients between the different sectors. Admittedly these could be a source of tension. Like all municipal doctors, Dr Dick was concerned that the LGI might try to use St James's as a 'dumping ground' for their unwanted cases.[89] In response to an accusation that St James's had refused to accept cases from the LGI, he explained that 'they did not refuse to accept cases referred direct from the Receiving Room but that difficulties were experienced regarding the dumping of cases which have been treated in the Infirmary and then sent to St James's'.[90] Similarly, he assured the MOH inspector that he was happy to take patients 'who seemed to be more suitable for a public assistance hospital' but expected the voluntary hospital to ask if St James's would accept the patient and justify the transfer. Among the type of case he would reject were appendicitis patients a few days after their operation, or 'troublesome and noisy cases which the voluntary hospital doctor was not prepared to label as requiring to be admitted for observation to a mental ward'. Moreover, he claimed the voluntary hospitals were increasingly willing to accept his position – an assertion confirmed to the inspector by the voluntary hospitals.[91]

The fair allocation of cases remained a concern for the municipality in the 1936 negotiations with the voluntary hospitals. Although a generally fair system of transfer was 'extensively practised now, both from the casualty and receiving departments', Johnson Jervis felt 'there should be no bias towards either institution but that the reference of cases should be governed by the available accommodation and not merely by the desire to retain a particularly interesting type of case'.[92] The LGI were conciliatory, the Chairman A. P. Nicholson promising receiving officers would get 'definite instructions not to send "star" cases to one particular hospital', while chief physician Dr Watson urged trust, for 'unless the two bodies trusted each other no good could come of co-ordination'.[93]

Mirroring developments in Manchester, Bristol, Middlesbrough, Leicester and even Newcastle,[94] by the mid-1930s arrangements were in place in both cities to exchange patients and to co-ordinate and even develop joint services. However, integration proved easier in some areas than in others. In particular, orthopaedics, maternity and cancer saw the closest working, as these were the areas where expertise was limited, demand was high, state support was available or patients required both acute *and* long-term treatment. Certainly both sides sought to avoid a hierarchical approach, and while the municipal hospitals continued to take most chronic cases it was agreed in Leeds that 'Special departments should not be wholly centralised at the General Infirmary, but that certain departments should be provided at other institutions with the proviso that there should not be unnecessary duplication of staff and equipment'.[95] For example, in 1939, a neurosurgeon was appointed in a consultant role at St James's and plans were tabled to reorganize the work to avoid expensive duplication.

Similarly, joint working was seen as essential to the effective operation of fracture and orthopaedic services. In Sheffield the medical staff club recognized that, to set up an adequate fracture and orthopaedic service for the city and surrounding area, co-operation between sectors and with other agencies was vital,

> both on account of the large number of accident cases, and on account of the provision of long stay beds for the Orthopaedic cases. Such co-operation will provide a really efficient and complete service. Already a start has been made with the help of the South Yorkshire Miners' Welfare Committee for their injuries.[96]

A similar scheme was discussed in Leeds, although by 1939 Dr Dick was of the opinion that a joint fracture service 'could not proceed to a satisfactory conclusion until the Government had definitely indicated the extent to which it would provide financial assistance'.[97] Yet as we have seen, fracture clinics were operating in both sectors by the outbreak of the Second World War, culminating in the major unit opened in Sheffield in 1946.

The treatment of cancer was another suitable field for a unified approach. As an emergent speciality with a very broad patient base requiring both intensive radium treatment and long-term chronic care, it was an obvious area for collaboration. Although surgery remained the primary treatment for cancer throughout the first half of the twentieth century, by the First World War some doctors were promoting the potential of radium to treat certain types of patient.[98] Following a public appeal in 1914, Sheffield established a radium centre controlled by a committee representing the voluntary hospitals, the university and the city council,[99] while ten years later the loan of a substantial quantity of the element by the Yorkshire Council of the British Empire Cancer Campaign (BECC) allowed the establishment of a Radium Department at the LGI managed by a medical officer, A. A. Diges La Touche FRCS.[100] With the establishment of the National Radium Commission to allocate national stocks of radium and limit the number of centres engaging in radium therapy, both Sheffield and Leeds were recognized as national radium centres in 1930. These recognized centres were all linked to university medical schools and physics departments to ensure safety, encourage research and permit the use of the larger radium 'bombs' based on substantial loans of the element from the NRC and BECC.[101]

Following some teething problems,[102] the Sheffield centre was established in 1931 with Frank Ellis as director (until 1943), assisted by a physicist and costs being met by all four voluntary hospitals. Ellis was a Sheffield man and graduate of the university who pioneered a number of techniques and practices, including the development of wooden wedge-shaped filters 'to deflect a radiation beam to avoid sensitive organs such as the eye'.[103] Once established these centres proved effective and the number of patients grew, with Leeds treating 685 people with a mixture of radium and X-ray by 1938, while over a thousand were attending the Sheffield centre by the early 1940s.[104] This compared favourably with the problems at Bristol where inexperience and competition between the two hospitals held up the effective development of the city's radium centre.[105]

Co-operation was essential, as cancer patients were spread across all of the voluntary hospitals and the public sector institutions. Both the Jessop and the LHW undertook some cancer treatment by radium while patients from the municipal sector were also included. In 1934 Sheffield City Council joined the Radium Institute and contributed to the core funding, while the Sheffield MOH noted that 540 voluntary hospital, 53 municipal hospital and 56 private patients received radium treatment in 1937. Moreover, the medical staff of the centre worked in the 'closest co-operation with the four principal Voluntary Hospitals and the Municipal General Hospital. The Radium Treatment is administered in these hospitals and is in all cases given under the supervision of the Medical Director of the Radium Centre.'[106] Similarly, in Leeds from the early 1930s St James's was involved in the interchange of patients on a regular basis, for example deep X-ray and radium patients were sent from St James's to the LGI via an arrangement formalized in 1936, when it was agreed all deep X-ray patients would be treated in the LGI. Joint working developed further in the later 1930s as both WRCC and Leeds Corporation agreed to pay capitation fees of ¹²/₆ d or twelve shillings and six pence per patient treated at the radium centre while St James's made 6–8 beds available for recovering patients from Leeds and the West Riding to be treated by the medical director who would be given status of visiting physician in relation to these patients.

As has been seen, a particular concern for the voluntary hospitals was the pressure created on beds by the growing number of motor vehicle accidents. At the heart of the 1930 arrangements in Sheffield was the development of a casualty block with two new operating theatres at the City General mainly to take traffic accidents from the northern side of the city.[107] By 1934 the casualty block was operational and arrangements were made with the police to ensure that casualties were assigned to the appropriate institution. Although this took fewer patients annually than the city centre casualty departments, it went a long way to relieving the pressure on the accident and emergency facilities.[108] Developments in Leeds were less successful. Although informal discussions over the allocation of road accident casualties had taken place in the early 1930s, as in Manchester little progress was made. Dr Dick reported in 1937 that 'The question of the Casualty Department has not yet received more than preliminary thought'.[109]

A third area for joint working was children and maternity. In Leeds the new Advisory Committee agreed on the need for an institution for children to meet the needs of city and county

> though a difference of opinion exists as to whether the new hospital should take long-term cases only, acute cases continuing to be admitted to the Leeds General Infirmary and 'infectious cases' to St James's Hospital, or whether it should deal with children of all types.[110]

By the following year it had been agreed that the new hospital would be the responsibility of the local authority advised by the committee 'to ensure that in construction, equipment and staffing the new hospital shall embody all that is best in modern hospital practice'. Sheffield's reorganization placed particular emphasis on creating an integrated maternity service, including the building of a new maternity block at the municipal hospital and the creation of a central maternity clinic which allocated mothers to specific hospitals from both sectors. Although the Ministry of Health was critical of the Maternity and Child Welfare Services, which they saw as too centralized and conservative, the maternity block was commended as 'indicating the close planning being undertaken in the city to meet hospital needs and make the most efficient use of resources'.[111] But as has been noted, the dominant centralizing ideology apparent at the council and deteriorating relations with the voluntary sector meant little was done to integrate maternity provision as was to happen in Leeds.[112]

The medical staff were involved in promoting a number of cross-sector initiatives, although their role was less prominent than it had been in instigating joint action within the voluntary hospitals. Thus, in 1924, while considering the issue of waiting lists, the LGI Faculty urged the board to 'lead the way' by harnessing the 'great movement going on in the country' for closer links with the Union hospitals, enabling 'the available bed accommodation there to be utilised and at the same time suitably controlled and administered by specialists'.[113] In Sheffield ten years later the Medical Staff Club's memoranda on the development of a key hospital system made a number of references to joint working with the municipality, but these were frequently in ancillary or supplementary roles and it is clear the plans did not include a central place for the city hospitals. This reflected the less integrated nature of medical relations in the city, for while formal arrangements were strong, the consultants in the municipal hospitals were semi-detached, often only attending on request and not taking control of beds or cases. This contrasted with the case in Leeds where strong links had grown up, especially in areas like paediatrics and cancer therapy while, as in Bristol, from 1944 municipal appointments were being made through the joint panel and increasing numbers of consultants worked in the corporation institutions, often with control of their own beds.

Similar differences were apparent in the role of the medical schools in promoting inter-sector collaboration. Prior to the First World War both Leeds and Sheffield had brought clinical teaching into the medical faculty although at this time this only included the staff of the main general hospitals and a 1924 plan floated by the university to merge the staff of all three Leeds hospitals was blocked by the LGI until a 'future date'.[114] But this did not prevent some integration taking place, especially in the newer, more scientific areas such as radium therapy, rheumatism research and pathology, and unglamorous infectious disease work such as TB, VD and public health which were concentrated in the municipal hospitals for teaching and consultant posts. Moreover, the work of the university, which in Leeds privileged access to appropriate 'teaching material' over institutional labels, played a positive role in bringing the sectors together. Jervis was already a professor and teacher on the Diploma in Public Health and in 1930 he was joined by his chief TB officer who was appointed to the new post of lecturer in tuberculosis (with a £10 honorarium).[115] In Sheffield there were also moves from the medical staff to extend teaching and specialization to the council hospitals to escape the traditional areas of midwifery, TB, public health and infectious disease, the Staff Club considering it 'desirable' that teaching should be 'extended to include the available material at the City General Hospital'.[116] It is notable that this did not happen, a memo prepared for the Vice Chancellor of Sheffield University in 1939 showed no teaching was done on the general wards of municipal hospitals, while even in 1945 Fir Vale 'contributes little to the medical teaching facilities in comparison with its large share of the clinical work of this centre'.[117] This was in marked contrast to Leeds, where a professorial unit was established at St James's in 1945.[118]

Co-operation or Competition?

As this suggests, there were barriers to closer working and some of these can be attributed to areas of criticism highlighted by contemporaries and historians, including hierarchical attitudes, petty jealousies and political interference, though others arose from institutional rigidities, financial concerns and competition for lucrative patients. The key institutional rigidity was the geographical origin of patients, a problem evident in many towns and cities able to provide some specialist hospital services. For while the voluntary hospitals had a regional patient base – often drawing a third or more of their admissions from outside the city – the municipal hospitals were obliged by law to restrict themselves to those with settlement in the local authority.[119] As such, councils were restricted in which patients they could take, prompting the Sheffield and East Midlands surveyors of 1945 to complain that co-ordination was hampered:

> The worst anomalies arise from the artificial divisions of local government boundaries. The large county boroughs are natural centres within which hospital provision of various kinds could most readily be made for considerable areas around. An arbitrary line drawn on a map often determines whether a patient shall have access to a well-staffed, relatively modern hospital in a natural hospital centre or be sent some distance away to an unsatisfactory institution[120]

Thus in Leeds there was initial hostility expressed by the LGI to working with the council, as only city patients could be transferred to St James's.[121] But there was also growing resentment in Sheffield, especially due to the feeling that the council were operating to reduce waiting lists at the voluntary hospitals only for the freed places to go to external patients. This led the Sheffield Health Committee to terminate the waiting list scheme in 1937. The official reasons were pressure on Health Committee funds and that the arrangement had been a temporary expedient to 'enable the Waiting Lists to be reduced to such an extent that the Voluntary Hospitals would then be able to deal with their Waiting Lists in the ordinary way'.[122] Certainly, the growing waiting lists at the City General, noted earlier, did not justify the continuation of the arrangement but it seems likely that the decision was partly ideological, the town clerk alluding to 'certain views expressed when the question was under consideration' by the Labour Council's Finance Consultative Committee.[123] This situation was one reason why a more competitive approach emerged in the city by the later 1930s as the council looked to build a new general hospital for Sheffield citizens.

Problems over who could be admitted to which institution were exacerbated by enduring hierarchical attitudes and petty jealousies. Again, these appear to have been worse in Sheffield than in Leeds. In the 1920s traditional medical protectionism meant honorary staff aimed to resist new entrants while at the same time looking to utilize capacity in the local authority institutions for their own patients. For example, a proposal to allow Leeds Education Department medics to oversee treatment of disabled children in the LGI orthopaedic wards was deemed 'quite unsuitable for acceptance, for obvious reasons'.[124] Yet the honorary staff expected to retain control over any of 'their' patients transferred to municipal institutions under waiting list reduction schemes – a particular stumbling block to integration in Middlesbrough.[125] This did ease in the 1930s, especially in Leeds, where cancer specialists from the LGI were given some beds in St James's, and by 1945 the visiting consultants were 'specifically in clinical charge of the cases in the wards'.[126] But despite this there is evidence that some medics continued to see the municipal role as subsidiary and marginal to the work of their increasingly specialized institutions. In the planning for the new hospital centre in Sheffield the amalgamation of the voluntary hospitals around the university was at the core with no real attempt to include the municipal provision directly except within the traditional role of beds for chronic cases.

Thus, while the 'goodwill and active co-operation' of the municipal services were required, the latter's role would be supplementary to the voluntary hospitals, as they were 'the older foundation and whatever may be their shortcomings there is no doubt that the high state of efficiency in the practice of medicine in this country has developed under this system'. The 'more recent' municipal hospitals had more accommodation as they were 'compelled to provide beds for all kinds of chronic cases which may be bed-ridden for years'. Moreover, they were confined to their locality for the patients they could treat, their staff were full-time and paid and they did not provide complete outpatient services – nor was it likely they would, as these would 'require considerable additional equipment and an increase in the existing staff'. Although they paid lip-service to the requirement to work together to ensure the 'production of an efficient Hospital Service for the City'[127] and offered the municipality the possibility of providing 'a further number of beds for acute cases from within the City of Sheffield', it was the older institutions that would be responsible for developing new specialist services particular to the city, like fractures, brain damage or chest diseases. Such specialist work would be done in departments and clinics at the SRH and SRI where 'the surgeons in charge ... would have the advantage of widening their experience', while the municipal hospitals would deal with the large number of accident cases and provide the 'long stay' beds for the orthopaedic, chest and brain cases, 'such co-operation' providing 'a really efficient and complete service'.[128]

Even the medical school could prove a barrier to cross-sector integration and sometimes the best interests of the broader hospitals service. Thus, when Sheffield was planning its new hospital complex the medical staff insisted on a city centre site at Glossop Road, for while a suburban hospital may have been better for inpatients, they rightly pointed to the fact that:

> Treatment of in-patients is not the whole work of a hospital. The out-patient practice of the Voluntary Hospital is equally important. Many are unable to walk more than a few yards. They often attend at least once a week for long periods. There are also casualties to be considered.[129]

But of greater significance was the position of medical students and their clinical teaching. As the senior students had to undertake their practical work in the hospitals while still attending lectures and labs at the university, it was vital to keep the hospitals in close proximity to the school of medicine, thus minimizing travel time. Moving the key hospital to suburban Norton would make 'conditions for Students ... very difficult indeed' and could necessitate moving the medical school too.

> It may appear at first sight that this question of students and teaching is one of secondary importance in comparison with the best interests of the sick, but actually the two are so intimately interwoven that it is impossible to separate them.

This call to protect the interests of the medical students was often utilized to promote or block a particular development, Charles Lupton cited their needs in his opposition to a children's hospital in Leeds after the First World War while, as we will see, Austyn Barran claimed a single maternity unit was necessary for teaching purposes.[130]

As this suggests, the voluntary hospitals remained convinced of their superior status and totally opposed to municipal control or municipal expansion into areas they currently occupied. As Sheffield Voluntary Hospital Council told the Sankey Commission, they desired 'full and friendly relations and working arrangements between ... the voluntary hospitals and the local authorities ... to secure the most efficient and economical provision of hospital services'. However, they were 'of the opinion that the voluntary hospitals should be encouraged to continue their present services to the public' and that:

> Nothing should be encouraged to impair their efficiency or to reduce them to a position subordinate to that of local government hospitals. If and when voluntary effort fails or is unable to fulfil the legitimate claims of the public for hospital services then and only then should the local government hospital be called upon to make good the deficiency.

Somewhat cynically, however, they did not wish to 'exclude ... the giving and acceptance of financial assistance ... under Section 64 of the Local Government Act, 1925, and other assistance from public funds such as the maintenance of beds'.[131]

As this demonstrates finance could be a strong driver for collaboration but it could also prove to be an area of contention as the two sectors began to compete for lucrative patients and as the local authorities began to resent their subsidies to the voluntary hospitals. Yet how these difficulties were resolved – or not – was central to the ongoing relationship between the two sectors in Leeds and Sheffield.

The key area where competition emerged was maternity beds where both council grants and NI maternity benefit created a desire on both sides to increase provision. Although the 1920s had seen local authorities making block grants to voluntary maternity hospitals, from around 1927 poor law infirmaries opened maternity units of their own for paying patients.[132] In the case of Sheffield this policy was actively pushed by the Socialist council who subsidized the unit. In the early 1930s general agreement underpinned the extension of local authority accommodation, but in 1934 Austyn Barran, president of Leeds Maternity Hospital, made a concerted effort to nip municipal provision in the bud by making a bid to monopolize all of the institutional births in his hospital. But while the arrogance of the voluntary hospitals led to the breakdown of relations between the sectors in Sheffield, strong leadership and a voice for the municipal service within the voluntary hospital camp protected joint working at the expense of the ambitions of the LMH.

In his campaign, Barran targeted both the Ministry of Health and the Leeds Voluntary Hospital Council to secure their support for his proposal, arguing to the ministry that:

> it would be a satisfactory arrangement if maternity beds were concentrated in the maternity hospital (now 110 beds), which had a specialist staff and was available for the instruction of both medical students and pupil midwives, for whom an increased number of cases would be very valuable.[133]

Moreover, he suggested the LMH could add a further fifty beds and that 'the maternity beds now at St. James's Municipal Hospital (about 50) should be transferred to the Maternity Hospital', making more beds available at St James's for surgical and medical patients. However, the Ministry of Health refused to commit publicly, stating that 'the matter was essentially one for local discussion', although privately they concluded that 'without knowing the Council's views, I think we should be careful to avoid giving Mr Barran the impression that we are in favour of such an agreement being made'.[134] Indeed, the surveyors had already advised the council to increase and improve its maternity provision to assist the 'seriously overtaxed' LMH, while the plan for appropriation – which the Minister of Health had approved – included the retention of the maternity departments in St. James's and St. Mary's.

Barran had no more success with the Voluntary Hospitals Committee. Initially he had stressed the importance of closer co-operation with the municipality and some LMH cases had been transferred to St James's and St Mary's with the PAC receiving the payments.[135] However, in early 1935 he submitted a memorandum to the Voluntary Hospitals Committee, 'suggesting the centralization of the maternity services of the City in that Institution' along with a plan for an additional fifty-seven beds, arguing that 'the reason for submitting it was due, in large measure, to requests received from the University for better facilities at the Maternity Hospital for the training of Medical Students'. In particular, all the obstetric specialists were already at the LMH and his institution had better facilities for clerkships.

Although the committee tried to bury the idea in discussion of a 'comprehensive scheme' for co-ordination across the whole city,[136] Barran urged prompt action, fearing the 'provision of additional maternity accommodation at St. James Hospital was contemplated at an early date'.[137] His plan for concentration was 'in the interests of the mothers of the City', as the LMH honorary staff were the city's obstetric consultants; the hospital could provide continuity of care by experienced staff at all stages; and anaesthetics were always used, while the transfer of beds would permit St James's to extend its accommodation for general cases. His trump card was that 'in view of the wide interest which is being taken in Maternal Mortality throughout the Country, the merits of the foregoing scheme are strongly urged'.[138] But concentration would not only benefit medical students and midwives, it also offered a considerable financial bonus for the LMH. In particular, it saw this as a way of broadening its narrow income base by increasing the grant from the council to meet both the perceived underfunding of the council cases and the increased workload which would be part funded by the savings the Health Committee would make by winding up the St James's unit. But the Voluntary Hospitals Committee continued to resist his requests for support[139] and the scheme was finally killed off by Alderman Martin, wearing his Health Committee hat, who

> expressed the view that the proposals as attached would not meet with the approval of the Health Committee, who, for various reasons, were strongly opposed to the discontinuance of Maternity work at their Institutions. He was of [the] opinion that there was no likelihood of the proposals being accepted and that it would be unwise to put them forward at the present time.

Barran admitted defeat while the Voluntary Hospital Committee agreed to call attention to 'the difficulties which exist in giving adequate training in Maternity work' and to ask that this be considered by the Joint Municipal Voluntary Hospital Committee.[140]

From 1936 Barran took a different tack, arguing instead for a specialist centre at the LMH, which had reached its maximum size in a city where demand for institutional delivery was amongst the highest in the country. In a letter sent to the Minister of Health, MOH and the Health Committee he emphasized the importance of specialization, arguing that 'by virtue of the status of our Medical Faculty, we should be regarded as a hospital for consultation, research and training rather than a hospital for the reception of general maternity cases'. Given they already had 'clinical material which we are led to understand is equal to, if not better than, that existing in other large cities', to add more beds 'would not improve our position as a consultant hospital', as they already took nearly all of the abnormal cases from Leeds and the West Riding. Any future development would focus on improving facilities for research and teaching. The Minister of Health was largely supportive, but urged:

> I very much hope that your Board will formulate their plans for reorganisation in consultation with the City Council, so that the maternity needs of the City may be fully explored and a suitable scheme of development worked out with due regard to all the available resources.[141]

On the back of this letter Barran received approval from the Voluntary Hospital Council to open direct negotiations with the council over the allocation of cases along the lines suggested, leading the Joint Advisory Council to note

> That to meet the shortage of maternity bed accommodation resulting from the increased hospitalisation of maternity cases, a solution would need to be found either by increasing the accommodation or by a process of selection of cases for admission, or both.[142]

By 1938, a co-ordinated system of allocation was in place and this was developed further by the time of the Ministry of Health survey of 1945 when the hospital had 'had to restrict its practice to primiparae and to emergencies or difficult cases'.[143] This example shows how collaboration could be sustained where relations were good and consultation was effectively pursued. It also demonstrates the impact of twin-tracking administrators, with Martin using his role on the VHC to promote the interests of the Health Committee.

In Sheffield, arrangements had worked well for most of the 1930s, with the city co-operating with the voluntary sector to expand maternity provision. However, the limited degree of consultation around the super hospital plan angered the Labour council, prompting Councillor Asbury to comment that while the municipal authorities were obliged to consult with the voluntary sector about their plans, clearly this did not apply in reverse.[144] Thus, when the plan to extend the Jessop was first mooted, Ronald Matthews assured the Joint Committee that:

> There was no intention to ask the Corporation for any financial assistance towards the Scheme. What they desired was the good-will and co-operation of the Corporation. He, however, suggested that the Corporation might consider making some contribution to the cost of the maintenance of the proposed additional beds at the Jessop Hospital.

Although Asbury, Labour chair of the Health Committee, did note that 'the Corporation were desirous that maternity beds should be provided to meet the needs of the whole of the City' – presumably a jibe at the closed pool of potential Jessop Hospital patients – and that the council had approved plans to add thirty-two new beds at the City General, he:

promised that the question regarding the financial assistance in respect of the Jessop Hospital ... would be submitted to the Health Committee, and that so far as the members of the Council who were present at this meeting were concerned, he thought he could say that they received with every good will the proposals of the Voluntary Hospitals outlined in the Statement above referred to.[145]

However, the final decision of the Jessop to build a large extension with additional general and private maternity provision prompted the chair of the Health Committee to object both at the Joint Committee and in public. Once again, he suggested that the decision had been taken without consultation and that the new beds would not benefit Sheffield citizens, hardening the resolve of the council to build another maternity block and deepening competition between the two sectors. Moreover, it would appear that it was around this date that the council withdrew from active involvement in the Joint Advisory Council, Asbury failing to convene a meeting in 1939 and stating in 1941 'that he did not think there was any necessity to hold a further meeting'.[146] One was held in 1942 under the chairmanship of Ronald Matthews of the SRH, but it achieved little.

Regional Developments

As the preceding sections suggest, co-operation and integration was well advanced in both cities and across all sectors by the 1940s but was this the case at a regional level? Overall regional issues were emerging as a significant barrier to joint working, as institutions sought to address patient payment, regional organization and regional services and meet the constraints imposed by geography and authority boundaries. An enduring problem was payment by patients from outside the city with both sectors trying to extract payment from other areas, either through their local authorities or their contributory schemes.[147] Voluntary hospitals had always had a regional role, with around a third of all voluntary hospital patients coming from outside the cities, prompting long-running anxieties about the geographical distribution of income. Moreover, increased specialization saw their regional position expand, bringing them into conflict with both institutions and their funders in other districts[148] while – as discussed previously – legal restrictions prevented municipal provision from developing on a comparable scale. But discussion of and action on the regionalization of services was apparent from the mid-1930s. For example, it was noted that:

There is a general desire to get as complete co-ordination as possible between the Hospitals not only in the city but over a much wider area. One thing that emerges after 8 years working of the Local Government Act is the fact that Hospital areas under that Act are too small. Many hope that the efforts of the British Hospital Association will result in such modifications as will make for a re-distribution of the rural areas round the Key Hospital Centres.[149]

Sheffield Voluntary Hospital Council's evidence to the Sankey Commission gave strong backing to a regional hospital council which 'should be empowered alone to negotiate with the county councils and county boroughs on questions of general hospital policy for the area'. Moreover, these should have significant power to make deals and then convince the constituent hospitals to accept any new arrangements – though not to force compliance.[150] Such moves were aided by the merger in 1945 of LGI and the small miners' hospital in Normanton, fifteen miles to the south-west of the city, and by the strongly regional nature of the Sheffield Penny in the Pound scheme which had expanded to include local committees in towns like Barnsley and as far away as Retford.[151]

Key to these developments was the creation or expansion of regional services. During the early stages of planning for the amalgamation of the SRH and SRI it was hoped that in addition to a radium centre:

> there will be less over-lapping and duplication in the treatment of patients, but more specialisation. There will be more 'regional' surgery and medicine. Specialised treatment of fractures in accordance with the latest techniques has been decided on as a first step. It is also hoped that there may be soon a Clinic for diseases of the respiratory organs such as Asthma and Hay Fever; industrial diseases such as Silicosis, and for Anti-gas treatment.[152]

These would be supported by specialists in 'regional diseases', including diseases of the chest, brain and nervous system and orthopaedics and fractures, with some success seen in these areas when the Fracture Centre opened in 1946.[153] Leeds also saw increased regional planning in the later 1930s, including the development of a long-stay children's hospital to meet a distinct regional weakness, a fashionable joint orthopaedic and fracture service for the city and county, an orthopaedic hospital to be developed in combination with the West Riding County Council, and a radium institute. The Joint Hospital Council demonstrated a regional approach from the start, co-opting representatives from WRCC. A development committee with representatives from the Advisory Council, WRCC and the Marguerite Hepton Orthopaedic Hospital was formed to explore a county orthopaedic facility, while a similar body including representatives from city, county, the voluntary hospitals and the BECC was brought together to plan a radium institute. Indeed cancer treatment, encouraged by the NRC and the BECC, proved to be the most successful regional venture of the period.

Although surgery remained the primary treatment for cancer, specialists were demanding better facilities for the use of radium. By 1939 – prior to the Cancer Act – both cities had plans in place for major regional cancer institutes of around ninety beds based largely on the model of the Christie Hospital in Manchester, with dedicated staff, outpatient and operating facilities and all of the required technologies for deep therapy and radium treatment.[154] The priority placed on new facilities was informed by national and international developments, Ellis travelling 'all over America and Canada seeing the latest technique practised there', while the Leeds director argued that the 'Best results appear to be obtained where there are separate Institutes or Departments devoted to Radiotherapy, e.g. Stockholm Radiumhemmet and the Radium Institutes at London, Manchester and Paris'. Equally important was local competition, as the 'real need for such Departments is shown by the fact that other Centres are either planning or building such Departments, e.g. Bradford, Sheffield, Middlesex Hospital'.[155]

As this suggests, by the later 1930s regional centralization was emerging as the main response to cancer treatment by radium, based in units 'adequate for the work of treatment, research and recording' and close to key hospitals and medical schools.[156] In part this central role had been promoted by the BECC and the NRC since 1930, but it was increasingly developed as part of a hierarchical regionalism which placed Leeds and Sheffield at the centre of networks linking clinics and smaller units in neighbouring towns. Thus, in 1938 LGI's regional role was crucial as it was 'the only hospital in the District at which Radiotherapeutic facilities are provided and, therefore, patients have no alternative but to come here'.[157] Moreover, the Radium officer estimated more than a third of the patients he treated were from the West Riding, making it vital that the Leeds centre was developed in close collaboration with Leeds and West Riding councils. In Sheffield the plans received a boost with the creation of the Graves Radiotherapy Trust endowed with £100,000 in 1942, and by 1945 the 'well organised special centre' in Sheffield served around 1.5 million people through links to Doncaster and 'satellite diagnostic and follow up clinics' in Chesterfield, Rotherham and Barnsley as well as 'some cases from even further afield'.[158] Thus the history of cancer treatment provides an object lesson in high level public/ voluntary co-operation over the long term, suggesting that joint working may have been easier in new areas with few existing power bases and a patient profile which crossed traditional sectoral and specialist boundaries.

But regional working was constrained by certain factors. The geographical position of Leeds at the heart of the West Riding smoothed working with the county council who had been doing deals on various patient groups since the 1920s. However, the 1929 Act merely made Sheffield's situation more complex, as for them 'it was necessary that the position of the County Councils of the West Riding of Yorkshire, Derbyshire, Lincolnshire and Nottinghamshire should be clearly defined'.

Voluntary hospital managers were certainly keen to work with external authorities to create the most efficient services, the Sheffield Staff Club claiming that West Riding County Council's

declared policy ... is one of co-operation both in the provision of new accommodation and in future maintenance. The W.R.C.C. consider the larger Voluntary
Hospitals should undertake specialised work and that grants should be made to them
towards capital and maintenance costs in proportion to their use by residents of the
Administrative County.[159]

West Riding County Council's relations with Leeds suggest a similar preference
for subcontracting services from the voluntary hospitals on a regional basis well
into the 1930s. However, the increasingly parochial nature of Sheffield's socialist
council reflected in their opposition to regional boards in 1940 and their attack
on neighbouring authorities in 1938 proved a bigger barrier to regionalization
than the oft-cited case of voluntary hospital independence.[160]

Overall, it would seem that the excellent relations between the two sectors
which had characterized the early 1930s in Sheffield moved from co-operation
to competition, while in Leeds the opposite movement appeared to be taking
place. The Second War amplified these emergent trends. In Leeds joint working strengthened with joint faculty appointments, close working in the advisory
board, commended by the Ministry of Health surveyors and further extension of municipal involvement in teaching.[161] The surveyors were particularly
impressed by the city's Voluntary Hospitals Council and especially the Joint
Medical Faculty with its insistence on Royal College membership for all hospital
appointments, while they found the Leeds Joint Hospitals Advisory Committee
a 'useful example' of an organization to develop co-operation.[162] Indeed:

> The Public Health Authority ... impressed the Surveyors with their sincere desire
> to develop intimate relationship with the university teaching school. There already
> exist arrangements for the training of medical students in maternity work, the deputy
> medical superintendent is recognised by the University as a lecturer in obstetrics,
> and the representatives of the Health Committee expressed themselves as desirous of
> extending this into other spheres of medical education.[163]

On the other hand, although the Sheffield surveyors found some further progress in terms of joint working prompted by the needs of the university this was
limited, especially in relation to the municipal hospitals. For example, they noted
that while Lodge Moor Hospital for Infectious Diseases was used regularly for
teaching students, 'The two chronic hospitals are not associated with the teaching school at all and the City Hospital has hitherto been only casually associated
with it mostly for the partial training of medical students in midwifery'. Nor were
relations within the voluntary sector particularly strong, for while they provided
'the main basis for the consultant centre established in Sheffield ... the association between the individual hospitals is not nearly as close as it might be'.[164] Joint
working was identified amongst the newer specialists but 'the medical staffs do
not function as one' and in general the absence of 'an effective common medi-

cal staff' resulted in wasteful duplication of special departments. Furthermore, although the City General employed various part-time consultants, unlike Leeds they had no allocated beds, nor any continuing responsibility for patients. On the other hand, separation of casualties was noted as a feature of the city,[165] and this and the radium centre were the only joint ventures in the city to attract praise, the surveyors ranking the latter 'one of the foremost in the country'.[166]

Conclusion

How might we assess the development of collaboration in Leeds and Sheffield in the light of the common criticisms of contemporaries and historians of the interwar hospital system? In both cities considerable progress was made towards the integration of voluntary hospital provision with the joint faculty approach of Leeds creating distinct responsibilities in the three main institutions – gynaecology at the LHW, maternity at the LMH and all other work at the LGI. Although the LPD remained semi-detached from these developments, its role as a city centre accident and outpatient unit was complementary to rather than in competition with the LGI.[167] Although the pattern was a little different in Sheffield, the merger of the competing general hospitals held out the prospect of greater integration in the planned new hospital – as had recently happened in Birmingham – and the apparent slow progress to minimize duplication prior to 1945 owed much to the significant disruption wrought by the war.[168] Similarly, both municipal sectors expanded rapidly following appropriation. As was the case in Bristol and Middlesbrough, extensive relocation and more effective classification of patients across the whole municipal provision allowed the health departments to significantly increase their throughput of patients and especially their surgical and maternity work. Both cities benefitted from the opportunity to appropriate more than one PLI and to develop this inheritance in complementary ways, as seen by the concentration of maternity and TB provision at Nether Edge and St Mary's.[169] Some new departments were added, especially in Leeds in the 1940s, though in Sheffield there is the suggestion some of this had the potential to be competitive.

These developments were similar to trends in many towns and cities, as we now know, but what of integration between the two sectors? Again the message is largely positive, with effective advisory committees established by the second half of the 1930s which defined responsibilities, planned service developments and, like Manchester and Bristol, established protocols for the exchange of staff and patients. However, here the outcome was not linear – for in Sheffield, where joint working dated back to the 1920s, by the end of the 1930s the two sides were becoming more competitive and there seems to have been few areas of common ground after 1938. On the other hand in Leeds, where formal joint working was very slow to arrive, it seems to have flourished after 1936, operating at a regional level even before the publication of the Sankey findings. And this points to the final area of concern, namely regionalization. Certainly it would be difficult to claim that an extensive and conscious level of regional development had taken place around either city by 1946. However, there are definite signs of a positive desire to work beyond the boundaries of the city. In Leeds, especially, a number of projects were being developed with the county council while close links with satellite institutions had even resulted in a merger. In Sheffield the positive role of the Penny in the Pound scheme was creating a regional patient base and in both cities this was obviously demonstrated by the activities of their radium centres. But to a great extent the barrier to regionalization was the limitations on the county boroughs which both restricted their ambitions to operate on a regional level without the agreement of their neighbours and promoted insularity in the face of voluntary hospital expansion. It is worth remembering that the regional agenda had had very little chance to develop prior to the war and without government support would continue to be stifled by local authority limitations. Overall, therefore, we can see that collaboration, rather than competition, shaped much of the development in Leeds and Sheffield, creating a hospital system that was increasingly rationalized, integrated and regional by the middle of the 1940s.

CONCLUSION

Historians of the pre-NHS hospital system have addressed a number of themes in recent years: the scale and speed of development of both voluntary and municipal hospitals;[1] the rise of specialist services;[2] the central part played by finance in hindering or promoting change;[3] the role of politics;[4] and the extent of collaboration and co-operation within and between the sectors at an urban and regional level.[5] This book has been concerned with exploring each of these themes in two localities, providing a comparison of developments within Leeds and Sheffield and placing those trends within their wider national context. The two cities examined here provide important perspectives; by focusing on regional centres with medical schools, we have been able to assess change in the most highly developed part of the contemporary hospital system. Historians have often dismissed such places as atypical with their experiences having little to tell us about small towns, rural areas or places struggling with limited resources and the effects of depression. Yet, as Pickstone observed in relation to his study of the north-west:

> To gain a more adequate perspective we must also consider Manchester itself: not just because any hospital service planned for a nation must solve the peculiar problems of large cities but because the problems which were more evident in Manchester than elsewhere in the Region, came to dominate the planning of the NHS.[6]

Thus how Leeds and Sheffield faced their challenges in this period is essential to understanding the viability and challenges of the pre-NHS system. In particular, the extent to which their responses were shaped by their localities reveals much about the trajectory of the hospital system in the thirty years following the First World War, providing some order to the apparent chaos seen by outsiders.

The central unifying theme of this book, therefore, has been the importance of local social, economic and political cultures in the shaping of the hospital system. In the cases of Leeds and Sheffield it has demonstrated the prominence of long-term developments such as heavy, masculine industries in Sheffield and female-dominated light trades in Leeds; labour cultures shaped by the industrial wing in the former city and socialists in the latter; a narrow and divided middle class in the steel city in contrast to a deep, wide and long-established bourgeois culture in Leeds; and geo-political factors such as Sheffield's isolation on the boundary of three administrative areas in contrast to the central place advantages of Leeds. These all played their part in the general and specialist services, funding structures and extent of co-operation observed. Thus, the economic hardship of the 1920s and early 1930s limited the ability of the hospitals to build major extensions leading them to focus on increasing capacity and throughput by more efficient use of existing space, improved utilities and services like laundries, investment in laboratories for scientific testing, administrative facilities for sorting and classifying potential patients and improved amenities for staff. Although predominantly a feature of the voluntary sector, such changes were also found in the municipal hospitals where appropriation provided the stimulus to a major reorganization of the classificatory and physical arrangements of the institutions. These developments provided the space to accommodate the significant rise in inpatients and outpatients and to move towards the more systematic distribution of patients across the cities. Indeed, this study confirms the centrality of outpatient organization as a major factor in transforming medicine supporting Cooter and Sturdy's contention that it was managerial rather than scientific technologies which were at the heart of interwar hospital modernity.[7]

Moreover, who those patients were and the conditions of their admittance were equally shaped by socio-economic and political factors. The corporatist response of Sheffield workers and employers produced a funding and admissions system which privileged the needs of working-class men and industry while the more complex funding streams supporting the hospitals of Leeds reflected strong mutualist structures, the enduring commitment of the middle class and the more prominent role of women in the city and the structures of hospital governance.[8] In the latter case this was reflected in the extensive service provision for women in the city and the commensurately high rates of female admissions. But these features also shaped the pattern of specialist services. For while many of the specialities which operated in both cities were common to large hospitals across the country – ENT, dermatology, ophthalmology – the emergence of an orthopaedic specialty in Sheffield was demonstrably linked to the needs of local industry while the significant commitment to maternity services in Leeds by both the voluntary and public sector owed much to demand from the city's women and their notable political role.

Certainly Leeds and Sheffield were not unique in developing orthopaedic or maternity services – Manchester pioneered provincial fracture clinics, Liverpool could offer more maternity beds, if not a higher proportion of institutional births.[9] Nor was Sheffield alone in creating a Penny in the Pound corporate scheme – they followed in Birmingham and Liverpool[10] – while the mix of indirect and direct payment along with the healthy survival of voluntary income in Leeds was unusual but shared characteristics with Manchester, Bristol and Nottingham by the end of the 1930s.[11] However, this diversity does reflect local imperatives as much as serendipity, chaos or inequality in the shaping of services. Moreover, while we can see many characteristics which support Sturdy and Cooter's analysis of specialist development from the late nineteenth century – the wish for order, efficiency and effective patient throughput rather than scientific developments or the pressure of medical markets[12] – to this should be added a growing awareness of the role of key medical centres in providing services which met the specific as well as the general needs of their area. There are hints at this in the literature for other localities, especially the emergence of an industrial diseases centre in Birmingham and the pioneering of orthopaedics around the docks of Liverpool, but this is a theme that could be explored more fully in future research.[13]

Building on these findings, the second half of this book has been concerned with the influence of local structures and cultures on finance, control and collaboration. As we have seen, finance was pivotal to infrastructure, access and even specialist development, but it also influenced the leadership of the hospitals and the willingness of institutions to collaborate within and across sectors. Admittedly the work of Gorsky, Mohan and Willis has questioned the ability of contributory schemes and their leaderships to make much impact on collaboration outside of their catchment areas or to gain much of a foothold in hospital management.[14] But this is a little pessimistic. Certainly the evidence for a prominent role for the contributory scheme and the impact of its leadership comes mainly from Sheffield where the scheme proved effective in rationalizing services, promoting patient transfer and incorporating outlying areas. Indeed, the Penny in the Pound scheme was unperturbed by local authority boundaries, drawing its membership from the coalfield community which crossed easily into Derbyshire and Nottinghamshire as well as up through Rotherham to Barnsley.[15] The Leeds scheme was far less effective in this respect, driving the LGI to bypass the LWHF and extract payment directly from outlying collecting and contributory schemes. It is possible that this approach laid the basis for the takeover of the Normanton and Castleford Hospital by the LGI and weakened the power of the LWHF in negotiations with the senior hospital. Undoubtedly neither scheme had the access to power afforded to the hospital based schemes of the north-east, especially Middlesbrough, where contributors were the largest group on the board of the North Riding Infirmary.[16] However, they could and did exert considerable negative influence, using their financial muscle to block or change policies most notably in the stand-off over free treatment for higher paid workers which rocked Sheffield in 1938.

The effects of socio-economic structures on local labour politics also had an impact on the politics of the contributory schemes. The more ideological basis for labour politics in Leeds meant hostility towards the voluntary sector in general and an arms-length approach to the LWHF. Certainly some of the older, labourist members of the party gave support to the LPD and the LWHF, but it remained a separate mutualist body with few links to the socialist Labour party or even the unions. As a result, it could do little to act as a bridge between a Labour-controlled council and the voluntary sector. In Sheffield, however, labour politics was dominated, for much of the period, by trade unionists whose key aim was to secure good services and a 'fair deal' for working people, especially working men. A number of leading Labour party figures held roles on the executive of the contributors associations and secured seats on the hospital boards. Thus, as in Barnsley, Preston and to a lesser extent Middlesbrough, interactions between the two sectors were underpinned by interlinking memberships and cross-sector understanding.[17]

Nor were these links limited to the contributory schemes. A range of interests including voluntary hospital consultants, medical superintendents – a much under-rated group – medical schools and external agencies like the National Radium Commission and the BECC promoted city- and regional-level collaboration. Contemporary commentators and historians have tended to focus on the activity or inactivity of official committees, recognizing the existence of a few 'pioneers' while contending most areas lacked co-ordination within, let alone between, sectors.[18] In Leeds and Sheffield local political cultures did produce diverse outcomes. Within the voluntary sectors the depression and the influence of the medical staff and medical school forced the main general hospitals of Sheffield to seek amalgamation, as in Birmingham, as a preliminary to the building of a new hospital.[19] In Leeds the merging of the faculties, also at the suggestion of the medical school, had been achieved by 1933 in the case of the LGI, LHW and LMH, securing the rational allocation of patients and the avoidance of duplication.[20] Admittedly the smaller institutions in both cities were reluctant to get too closely involved with the big general hospitals, but even here duplication was minimized. Similarly, Sheffield's interlinked voluntary and municipal leadership quickly agreed to joint action between the two sectors in the 1930s, although political hostility in Leeds held off official agreement for a number of years. Yet below this level local networks were operating to ensure collaboration and the reduction of duplication. Thus the medical superintendent worked closely with the receiving room at the LGI and with the raft of consultants working at St James's and St Mary's by the mid-1930s, to smooth the transfer of patients and maximize the use of the available resources – evidenced by the thousands of contributory scheme members in both cities admitted to the municipal hospitals by 1939. The role of the medical staff, especially the medical superintendents and the municipal hospital consultants, warrants further study. There were undoubtedly some consultants who were only occasional visitors but many were active on the wards and some had their own patients and beds. Similarly, the medical superintendents – who have invariably been overlooked in favour of consideration of the role of the Medical Officers of Health – were an integral part of their medical communities, playing a pivotal role in managing relations between the two sectors.

Local structures and cultures could also shape regional developments. Clearly the voluntary hospitals of Leeds and Sheffield operated on a regional basis, drawing around one-third of their patients from outside the administrative boundaries of their cities.[21] However, while local industrial cultures may have facilitated the extension of the Penny in the Pound scheme to a regional level, Sheffield's position at the intersection of four counties limited its ability to make arrangements with neighbouring authorities, unlike Leeds which developed close links with West Riding County Council and was proposing joint ventures by the later 1930s. Moreover, the increasingly parochial approach of Sheffield Council challenged the voluntary hospitals' regional role. Yet regional services were being promoted successfully by external agencies like the BECC which supported the development of radium institutes, with the centre in Leeds attracting strong support from WRCC. So while regional hospital councils on the Oxford model may have been slow to emerge,[22] organic interactions were increasing and paving the way for patient exchange and rational organization.

These findings restore some agency to individuals and groups in the creation of local hospital systems and in particular they challenge images of sharply divided institutions and sectors rarely 'organically linked with their neighbours'.[23] Associational links and structures were obviously important manifestations of developing co-operation both within the voluntary sector and between voluntary and local authority hospitals. Yet, as the Leeds case very clearly shows, personal connections and inter-institutional working at an operational level could be equally or even more effective than formal joint advisory boards. Equally, individuals like Sir George Martin, William Asbury, Moses Humberstone and Charles Lupton criss-crossed the sectors and determined the extent and form of competition and co-operation. As with the relations between the doctors, so these 'amphibious' elites did much to unify their own sectors and facilitate the creation of a 'real service' with increasingly unified aims, objectives and even personnel. These figures, unlike the national leaders of political parties, the Royal Colleges and the BMA had to balance the interests of their institutions with those of their wider communities and in particular the need to provide the most comprehensive, effective and efficient service for their citizens. Indeed, their role highlights the much overlooked fact that interwar hospital systems were entirely the responsibility of localities whose concerns and interests were in stark contrast to those of metropolitan elites. This study has focused on the part played by the labour movement in shaping hospital politics but there is a need for more studies of non-socialist authorities. For while some, like West Hartlepool, can be characterized as penny-pinching, many of the most prominent municipal services were instigated by Conservative authorities and a greater understanding of their relationships with the voluntary sector and neighbouring authorities will enhance our appreciation of service development in the years leading up to the NHS.

Yet we should not be either overly determinist or unduly parochial, for hospital providers in both cities had to deal with a wide range of general issues and modern problems. In addition to satisfying the rapid growth in demand for basic medical treatment, they also had to address the challenges posed by road accidents, cancer, fractures and maternity and the extent to which these problems were tackled across both sectors has received very little attention within the broad framework of hospital services. Glimpses are available in the local studies referenced throughout this study, most of which show progress in some, if not all of these areas, but they are too few to challenge pessimistic accounts. Thus, in characteristic fashion Webster claimed theirs was a 'lack of co-ordinated services for cancer, orthopaedics, gynaecology, etc'.[24] but from these case studies it is apparent that hospital managers were aware of the issues and were acting, often on a regional and cross sector basis, to tackle them. Especially in the case of cancer and orthopaedics they were actively pursuing improvements which suggest that, contrary to pessimistic accounts, they were meeting these big challenges. Furthermore, they were meeting these challenges on a regional basis, which made the replication of services in every town unnecessary as suggested here and to some extent by Cherry.[25] It could rightly be argued that these are not representative places – but then very few places are. Yet we need to consider how much we can learn from a study of just two cities, especially two very large university towns? Certainly, as Mohan has pointed out, co-ordination was easier when there was something to co-ordinate.[26] Moreover, the impetus to co-operation would appear to be strongest in cities with medical schools. These provided a neutral space for negotiation and generally had a set of interests which favoured concentration rather than dispersal and the pursuit of 'material' over the interests of particular institutions.[27] Very few places had these advantages. Nor did most have the benefit of more than one ex-poor law institution or of clearly defined specialist institutions dealing with specific demographic groups.[28] Yet the extent to which medium sized towns linked up their own services and plugged them into regional developments has received very little attention.

Moreover, as regional centres Leeds and Sheffield offer a much wider perspective than might be the case for 'normal' towns. Although in addressing the differences inherent in regional centres we need to view them in relation to the other towns and services in the region. This has not been possible here but there are suggestive glimpses of a wider remit, like the take over of Normanton, or the spread of the Penny and the Pound scheme into Barnsley or the reach of the Radium Institutes by 1945. Taking a regional approach that drills down to explore the relationships between institutions in satellite towns and main centres will help to clarify the extent to which specialist services – like those for cancer or fractures – were deficient or regional networks were emerging. Similarly many more comparative studies – especially of the midlands, east and south of England – are required which address the transformation of services within particular places holistically, and that draw on locally generated records rather than external surveys, to consider why superficially similar towns produced very different hospital services. Furthermore, we would benefit from studies which examined the relationship between the hospital services of major cities and their hinterlands and other health services, including the school medical service, general practice, mental health and mental deficiency services, private midwives and municipal and voluntary services in other towns and surrounding counties.[29] To date little use has been made of the Ministry of Health surveys of county council services in the early 1930s yet a full understanding of urban provision relies on a greater awareness of developments in surrounding localities and wider health care infrastructure.

Overall the aim of this book has been to provide a richly textured comparison between two large but quite different cities to explore the impact of social, economic and political cultures on the development of hospital systems in the dynamic interwar period. It has shown that choices were determined and shaped by these local elements within the context of generally growing numbers of beds, staff, specialists and income and expenditure. Co-ordination and co-operation were evident in both cities from before the 1929 Act while the interchange of personnel at all levels, medical and lay, ensured that these were not closed or selfish institutions. The holistic approach has sought to view the work of the two sectors together as a de facto, if not a de jure, system. In doing so it has emphasized the similarities of approach and the broad acceptance of hierarchical realities rather than the normal emphasis on difference, competition and defensiveness. Moreover, it seeks to encourage historians to look at the distance travelled by local hospital systems between 1918 and 1948, at the huge gains made across provision in both sectors and the enormous improvements which benefitted over 100,000 people a year in each city. These successes have been too readily dismissed by historians eager to highlight the perceived failures of small towns and poor authorities. Yet such an approach does a considerable disservice to the huge effort of both voluntary and municipal workers who oversaw the growth and democratization of these institutions. This democratization – greater possibly in the voluntary than in the municipal sector – meant these were already the people's hospitals shaped, funded and run by citizens and meeting the challenges of modern medicine in a highly effective manner.

NOTES

Introduction

1. Sheffield Hospital Contributors Association, 'Annual Report of the Executive Committee for the Year Ended 31st December, 1946', in *Annual Report, 1946*, pp. 25–32, on p. 27.

2. The key text on the long-term development of hospitals is B. Abel-Smith, *The Hospitals, 1800–1948: A Study in Social Administration in England and Wales* (London: Heinemann, 1964), though see also S. Cherry, *Medical Services and the Hospitals in Britain, 1860–1939* (Cambridge: Cambridge University Press, 1996). The initial statistical material presented by R. Pinker, *English Hospital Statistics, 1861–1938* (London: Heineman, 1966) has been significantly enhanced by the outputs of the Hospitals Database, at http://www.hospitalsdatabase.lshtm.ac.uk/the-voluntary-hospitals-database-project.php [accessed 9 September 2010], which draws on the *Hospitals Yearbook*. These include M. Gorsky, J. Mohan and M. Powell, 'British Voluntary Hospitals, 1871–1938: The Geography of Provision and Utilization', *Journal of Historical Geography*, 25 (1999), pp. 463–82; M. Gorsky, J. Mohan and M. Powell, 'The Financial Health of Voluntary Hospitals in Interwar Britain', *Economic History Review*, 55:3 (2002), pp. 533–57. Understanding of municipal provision has been enhanced significantly by the team of Martin Powell, John Stewart, Alysa Levene and Becky Taylor, especially M. Powell, 'An Expanding Service: Municipal Acute Medicine in the 1930s', *Twentieth Century British History*, 8 (1997), pp. 334–57; A. Levene, M. Powell and J. Stewart, 'Patterns of Municipal Health Expenditure in Interwar England and Wales', *Bulletin of the History of Medicine*, 78 (2004), pp. 635–69; A. Levene, M. Powell and J. Stewart, 'The Development of Municipal Hospital Care in English County Boroughs in the 1930s', *Medical History*, 50:1 (2006), pp. 3–28; and A. Levene, M. Powell, J. Stewart and B. Taylor, *Cradle to Grave: Municipal Medicine in Interwar England and Wales* (Bern: Peter Lang, 2011). No work has emerged to challenge Rivett on London, but see J. Stewart, '"The Finest Municipal Hospital Service in the World"? Contemporary Perceptions of the London County Council's Hospital Provision, 1929–1939', *Urban History*, 32:2 (2005), pp. 327–44.

3. J. Mohan, *Planning, Markets and Hospitals* (London: Routledge, 2002); J. V. Pickstone, *Medicine and Industrial Society: A History of Hospital Development in Manchester and its Region* (Manchester: Manchester University Press, 1985); G. Rivett, *The Development of the London Hospital System, 1823–1982* (London: King Edward's Hospital Fund, 1986).

4. There are some excellent urban studies, including M. Gorsky, '"For the Treatment of Sick Persons of All Classes": The Transformation of Bristol's Hospital Service, 1918–39', in

P. Wardley (ed.), *Bristol Historical Resource CD-ROM* (Bristol: University of the West of England, 2000) [hereafter Gorsky, 'Bristol']; J. Reinarz, *Healthcare in Birmingham: A History of the Birmingham Teaching Hospitals, 1779–1939* (Woodbridge: Boydell and Brewer, 2009), J. Welshman, *Municipal Medicine: Public Health in Twentieth-Century Britain* (Oxford and New York: Peter Lang, 2000); and especially Pickstone, *Medicine and Industrial Society*.

5.   M. Powell, 'Did Politics Matter? Municipal Public Health Expenditure in the 1930s', *Urban History*, 22:3 (1995), pp. 360–79.

6.   M. Gorsky, J. Mohan and T. Willis, *Mutualism and Health Care: British Hospital Contributory Schemes in the Twentieth Century* (Manchester: Manchester University Press, 2006); C. Webster, *The Health Services since the War: Problems of Health Care. The National Health Service before 1957* (London: HMSO, 1988); C. Webster, 'Conflict and Consensus: Explaining the British Health Service', *Twentieth Century British History*, 1:2 (1990), pp. 115–51.

7.   R. Earwicker, 'The Labour Movement and the Creation of the National Health Service 1906–1948' (PhD thesis, University of Birmingham, 1982); B. M. Doyle, 'Labour and Hospitals in Three Yorkshire Towns: Middlesbrough, Leeds, Sheffield, 1919–1938', *Social History of Medicine*, 23:2 (2010), pp. 374–92; J. Stewart, '"For a Healthy London": The Socialist Medical Association and the London County Council in the 1930s', *Medical History*, 41:4 (1997), pp. 417–36; T. Willis, 'Politics, Ideology and the Governance of Health Care in Sheffield before the NHS', in R. J. Morris and R. H. Trainor (eds), *Urban Governance: Britain and Beyond since 1750* (Aldershot: Ashgate, 2000), pp. 218–49.

8.   Earwicker, 'Labour Movement'; J. Stewart, *'The Battle for Health': A Political History of the Socialist Medical Association, 1930–51* (Aldershot: Ashgate, 1999).

9.   The key texts here from an array of recent works include S. Cherry, 'Before the National Health Service: Financing the Voluntary Hospitals, 1900–1939', *Economic History Review*, 50 (1997), pp. 309–27; Gorsky, Mohan and Powell, 'Financial Health'; Gorsky, Mohan and Willis, *Mutualism and Health Care*.

10. Levene et al., *Cradle to Grave*; A. Levene, 'Between Less Eligibility and the NHS: The Changing Place of Poor Law Hospitals in England and Wales, 1929–1939', *Twentieth Century British History*, 20:3 (2009), pp. 322–45; Powell, 'An Expanding Service'.

11. This has received little attention but see M. Gorsky, '"Threshold of a New Era": The Development of an Integrated Hospital System in North-East Scotland, 1900–39', *Social History of Medicine*, 17:2 (2004), pp. 247–67; Mohan, *Planning*; Pickstone, *Medicine and Industrial Society*.

12. Each of these areas remains curiously under-researched from the perspective of their effect on hospital services. The bald facts of road accidents have recently been reviewed in M. J. Law, 'Speed and Blood on the Bypass: The New Automobilities of Inter-War London', *Urban History*, 39:3 (2012), pp. 490–509; cancer in J. Melling and P. Dale, 'Britain's Medical Officers of Health, Gender and the Provision of Cancer Services by Local and National Government, c. 1900–1940', *Medical History*, 53:4 (2009), pp. 537–60; while institutional births feature in A. Nuttall, 'Maternity Charities, the Edinburgh Maternity Scheme and the Medicalisation of Childbirth, 1900–1925', *Social History of Medicine*, 24:2 (2011), pp. 370–88.

13. These concerns inform the works of Pickstone, *Medicine and Industrial Society*; Welshman, *Municipal Medicine* and Doyle, 'Labour and Hospitals'. Levene et al., *Cradle to Grave* includes four case studies but the 'urban ecology' of the towns is not a central concern.

14. Webster, *Health Services since the War*, p. 1.
15. For popular views see N. Timmins, *The Five Giants: A Biography of the Welfare State* (London: Fontana, 1995), p. 104; and the BBC4 *Timeshift* programme 'Health before the NHS: A Medical Revolution', first broadcast 1 October 2012.
16. In addition to the works cited in p. 211, n. 2, above, see B. Taylor, J. Stewart and M. Powell, 'The Development of Central-Local Relations in the 1930s', *English Historical Review*, 122:496 (2007), pp. 397–426; S. Cherry, 'Accountability, Entitlement and Control Issues and Voluntary Hospital Funding, c. 1860–1939', *Social History of Medicine*, 9:2 (1996), pp. 215–33; M. Gorsky, M. Powell and J. Mohan, 'British Voluntary Hospitals and the Public Sphere: Contribution and Participation before the National Health Service', in S. Sturdy (ed.), *Medicine, Health and the Public Sphere in Britain, 1600–2000* (Abingdon and New York: Routledge, 2002), pp. 123–44; M. Powell, 'Hospital Provision before the NHS: Territorial Justice or Inverse Care Law', *Journal of Social Policy*, 21:2 (1992), pp. 145–63.
17. Pickstone, *Medicine and Industrial Society*, p. 266.
18. Ibid.
19. Abel-Smith, *The Hospitals*; Cherry, *Medical Services*; C. Webster (ed.), *Caring for Health: History and Diversity*, 2nd edn (Buckingham: Open University Press, 1993).
20. Some attention is paid to co-operation in Pickstone, *Medicine and Industrial Society*, pp. 272–96; Welshman, *Municipal Medicine*, pp. 264–71; Levene et al., *Cradle to Grave* in each of the case studies, chs 4–7; B. M. Doyle, 'Competition and Cooperation in Hospital Provision in Middlesbrough, 1918–48', *Medical History*, 51:3 (2007), pp. 337–56, and in a very pessimistic assessment in Mohan, *Planning*, pp. 55–9.
21. S. Cherry, 'Beyond National Health Insurance: The Voluntary Hospitals and Hospital Contributory Schemes: A Regional Study', *Social History of Medicine*, 5:3 (1992), pp. 455–82; S. Cherry, 'Medical Care since 1750', in C. Rawcliffe and R. Wilson (eds), *Norwich since 1550* (London: Hambledon and London, 2004), pp. 271–94; B. M. Doyle, *A History of Hospitals in Middlesbrough* (Middlesbrough: South Tees Hospitals NHS Trust, 2002); N. Hayes, '"Our Hospitals"? Voluntary Provision, Community and Civic Consciousness in Nottingham before the NHS', *Midland History*, 37 (2012), pp. 84–105; B. M. Doyle, 'Power and Accountability in the Voluntary Hospitals of Middlesbrough, 1900–1948', in A. Borsay and P. Shapley (eds), *Medicine, Charity and Mutual Aid: The Consumption of Health and Welfare, c. 1550–1950* (Aldershot: Ashgate, 2007), pp. 207–24.
22. Pickstone, *Medicine and Industrial Society*; Mohan, *Planning*; Levene et al., *Cradle to Grave*; Welshman, *Municipal Medicine*; Reinarz, *Birmingham*; Gorsky, 'Bristol'.
23. Abel-Smith, *The Hospitals*; R. Cooter, 'The Meaning of Fractures: Orthopaedics and the Reform of British Hospitals in the Inter-War Period', *Medical History*, 31:3 (1987), pp. 306–32; S. Sturdy and R. Cooter, 'Science, Scientific Management, and the Transformation of Medicine in Britain, c. 1870–1950', *History of Science*, 36 (1998), pp. 1–47; J. V. Pickstone, 'Contested Cumulations: Configurations of Cancer Treatments through the Twentieth Century', *Bulletin of the History of Medicine*, 81:1 (2007), pp. 164–96; Pinker, *Hospital Statistics*.
24. Pickstone, *Medicine and Industrial Society*, p. 266.
25. L. Granshaw, 'Introduction', in L. Granshaw and R. Porter (eds), *The Hospital in History* (London: Routledge, 1989); M. Powell, 'Hospital Provision before the NHS: A Geographic Study of the 1945 Hospital Survey', *Social History of Medicine*, 5:3 (1992), pp. 483–504; Powell, 'Did Politics Matter?'.

26. R. Ellis, 'The Asylum, the Poor Law and the Growth of County Asylums in Nineteenth-Century Yorkshire', *Northern History*, 45:2 (2008), pp. 279–93.

27. Sturdy and Cooter, 'Scientific Management'.

28. Cherry, 'Before the National Health Service'; M. Daunton, 'Payment and Participation: Welfare and State-Formation in Britain 1900–1951', *Past and Present*, 150:1 (1996), pp. 169–216; B. M. Doyle, 'The Economics, Culture and Politics of Hospital Contributory Schemes: The Case of Inter War Leeds', *Labour History Review*, 77:3 (2012), pp. 289–315; G. C. Gosling, '"Open the Other Eye": Payment, Civic Duty and Hospital Contributory Schemes in Bristol, *c.* 1927–1948', *Medical History*, 54:4 (2010), pp. 475–94; Gorsky, Mohan and Powell, 'British Voluntary Hospitals'; N. Hayes and B. M. Doyle, 'Eggs, Rags and Whist Drives: Popular Munificence and the Development of Provincial Medical Voluntarism between the Wars', *Historical Research*, 86:234 (November 2013), pp. 712–40; Reinarz, *Birmingham*; and the articles in M. Gorsky and S. Sheard (eds), *Financing Medicine: The British Experience since 1750* (London: Routledge, 2006).

29. S. Cherry, 'Hospital Saturday, Workplace Collections and Issues in Late Nineteenth-Century Hospital Funding', *Medical History*, 44:4 (2000), pp. 461–88; Gorsky, Mohan and Willis, *Mutualism and Health Care*.

30. Cherry, 'Accountability, Entitlement and Control'; Daunton, 'Payment and Participation', p. 195; Doyle, 'Hospital Contributory Schemes'; Gorsky, Mohan and Powell, 'Financial Health'.

31. Levene et al., *Cradle to Grave*, pp. 75–86; Pickstone, *Medicine and Industrial Society*; Powell, 'An Expanding Service'; Willis, 'Health Care in Sheffield'.

32. B. M. Doyle, 'The Changing Functions of Urban Government: Councillors, Officials and Pressure Groups', in M. Daunton (ed.), *The Cambridge Urban History of Britain: Volume 3, 1830–1950* (Cambridge: Cambridge University Press, 2001), pp. 287–313; Doyle, 'Competition and Cooperation'.

33. Hayes and Doyle, 'Eggs, Rags and Whist Drives'.

34. Levene, Powell and Stewart, 'Municipal Hospital Care'; Powell, 'Did Politics Matter?'; Welshman, *Municipal Medicine*.

35. Stewart, 'Healthy London'; Stewart, *Battle for Health*; Stewart, 'Finest Municipal Hospital Service'; Taylor, Stewart and Powell, 'Central-Local Relations'; Willis, 'Health Care in Sheffield'; T. Willis, 'The Bradford Municipal Hospital Experiment of 1920: The Emergence of the Mixed Economy in Hospital Provision in Inter-War Britain', in Gorsky and Sheard (eds), *Financing Medicine*, pp. 130–41; T. Willis, 'The Politics and Ideology of Local Authority Health Care in Sheffield, 1918–1948' (PhD thesis, Sheffield Hallam University, 2009).

36. Pickstone, *Medicine and Industrial Society*, pp. 278–93; Gorsky, 'Bristol', secs 5.3, 6 which also discusses Birmingham; G. C. Gosling, 'Charity and Change in the Mixed Economy of Healthcare in Bristol, 1918–1948' (PhD thesis, Oxford Brookes University, 2012), pp. 141–60, which also discusses Oxford.

37. Mohan, *Planning*, ch. 3; Levene et al., *Cradle to Grave*, pp. 215–21; Doyle, 'Competition and Cooperation', pp. 352–3; Welshman, *Municipal Medicine*, pp. 267–70.

38. Gorsky, 'Bristol', sec. 5.3; Gorsky, 'Threshold of a New Era'; Pickstone, *Medicine and Industrial Society*, p. 279 for medical schools; pp. 253–4 for managers in Preston and pp. 285–92 for the role of consultants in shaping a joint system after 1935, including a joint faculty.

39. Ibid., p. 2.

40. Gorsky, 'Bristol'; Mohan, *Planning*; Cherry, 'Medical Care'.

41. For a preliminary assessment see Doyle, 'Labour and Hospitals'.
42. S. Cherry, 'Regional Comparators in the Funding and Organisation of the Voluntary Hospital System, *c.* 1860–1939', in Gorsky and Sheard (eds), *Financing Medicine*, pp. 59–76; Willis, 'Health Care in Sheffield'.
43. W. S. Porter, *The Royal Infirmary, Sheffield: An Epitome* (Oldham: Allan Hanson, 1921); C. Shaw, 'Aspects of Public Health', in C. Binfield, R. Childs, R. Harper, D. Hey, D. Martin and G. Tweedale (eds), *The History of the City of Sheffield 1843–1993*, 3 vols (Sheffield: Sheffield Academic Press, 1993) vol. 2, pp. 110–17; E. F. Skinner, *A Short History of the Sheffield Royal Hospital: 1832–1932* (Sheffield: Printed by Greenup & Thompson, Limited, 1932); S. Sturdy, 'The Political Economy of Scientific Medicine: Science, Education and the Transformation of Medical Practice in Sheffield, 1890–1922', *Medical History*, 36:2 (1992), pp. 125–59; H. Swan, 'Medical Education', in Binfield et al. (eds), *The History of the City of Sheffield*, vol. 2, pp. 130–41.
44. S. T. Anning, *The General Infirmary at Leeds: Volume II the Second Hundred Years, 1869–1965* (Edinburgh: Livingstone, 1966); S. T. Anning, 'The History of Medicine in Leeds', *Proceedings of the Leeds Philosophical and Literary Society: Literary and Historical Section*, 16 (1978), pp. 207–46.
45. M. Meadowcroft, 'The Years of Political Transition', in D. Fraser (ed.), *A History of Modern Leeds* (Manchester: Manchester University Press, 1980), pp. 410–36; A. Thorpe, 'The Consolidation of a Labour Stronghold 1926–1951', in Binfield et al. (eds), *The History of the City of Sheffield*, vol. 1, pp. 85–118.
46. Pickstone, *Medicine and Industrial Society*, p. 266.

1 Leeds and Sheffield: Economic, Social and Political Change

1. Abel-Smith, *The Hospitals*; Webster, *Health Services since the War*; Mohan, *Planning*; Levene et al., *Cradle to Grave*.
2. Pickstone, *Medicine and Industrial Society*, p. 2.
3. For the idea of urban ecology see ibid., p. 2.
4. C. J. Morgan, 'Demographic Change, 1771–1911', in Fraser (ed.), *A History of Modern Leeds*, pp. 46–71, on p. 48; A. D. H. Crook, 'Appendix: Population and Boundary Changes, 1801–1981', in Binfield et al. (eds), *The History of the City of Sheffield*, vol. 2, pp. 482–5.
5. Morgan, 'Demographic Change', pp. 52–7.
6. A. M. Craven, 'Housing before the First World War', in Binfield et al. (eds), *The History of the City of Sheffield*, vol. 2, pp. 65–75.
7. A. D. H. Crook, 'Needs, Standards and Affordability: Housing Policy after 1914', in Binfield et al. (eds), *The History of the City of Sheffield*, vol. 2, pp. 76–99, on pp. 92–6.
8. 'Leeds', in *Survey Reports, County Boroughs: Hastings to Leicester*, The National Archives [hereafter TNA] Ministry of Health [MH] 66/1072 [hereafter Leeds Survey Report, TNA MH66/1072], p. 3.
9. 'Sheffield', in *Survey Reports, County Boroughs: Rotherham to Southampton*, [hereafter Sheffield Survey Report, TNA MH66/1076], p. 4.
10. J. J. Jervis, 'Foreword: A Review of the Public Health Services of the City during the Thirty-One Years 1916–1948', in Medical Officer of Health for the City of Leeds, *Report on the Health and Sanitary Administration of the City* (Leeds: Leeds Corporation) [hereafter MOH Leeds, *Annual Report*], 1946, pp. 1–19.

11. T. McIntosh, '"A Price Must be Paid for Motherhood": The Experience of Maternity in Sheffield, 1879–1939' (PhD thesis, University of Sheffield, 1997), pp. 46–55 [hereafter 'Maternity in Sheffield'].

12. S. Taylor, 'The Industrial Structure of the Sheffield Cutlery Trades, 1870–1914', in Binfield et al. (eds), *The History of the City of Sheffield*, vol. 2, pp. 194–210, on pp. 206–7.

13. Ibid.; G. Tweedale, 'The Business and Technology of Sheffield Steelmaking', in Binfield et al. (eds), *The History of the City of Sheffield*, vol. 2, pp. 142–93.

14. Ibid., pp. 167–8.

15. G. Tweedale, *Steel City: Entrepreneurship, Strategy, and Technology in Sheffield 1743–1993* (Oxford: Clarendon, 1995), part 2.

16. S. Pollard, 'Labour', in Binfield et al. (eds), *The History of the City of Sheffield*, vol. 2, pp. 260–78.

17. Tweedale, 'Sheffield Steelmaking', pp. 166–76; Pollard, 'Labour', pp. 272–3;

18. Ibid., p. 272; B. J. Elliott, 'The Last Five Years of the Sheffield Guardians', *Transactions of the Hunter Archaeological Society* (1977), pp. 132–7.

19. Pollard, 'Labour', pp. 272–3.

20. For a list of major conditions affecting Middlesbrough iron workers see Doyle, 'Competition and Cooperation', pp. 342–3; and V. Brown, 'Public Health Issues and General Practice in the Area of Middlesbrough, 1880–1980' (PhD thesis, University of Durham, 2012).

21. Similar concerns with the dangers of the steel industry in Middlesbrough are examined in Doyle, 'Competition and Cooperation', pp. 342–3. The wider risks associated with heavy industry, especially mining, are covered by A. McIvor and R. Johnson, *Miners' Lung: A History of Dust Disease in British Coal Mining* (Aldershot: Ashgate, 2007); A. McIvor, 'Germs at Work: Establishing Tuberculosis as an Occupational Disease in Britain, c. 1900–1951', *Social History of Medicine*, 25:4 (2012), pp. 812–29; M. W. Bufton and J. Melling, 'Coming Up for Air: Experts, Employers and Workers in Campaigns to Compensate Silicosis Sufferers in Britain, 1918–1939', *Social History of Medicine*, 18:1 (2005), pp. 63–86.

22. B. M. Doyle, 'Managing and Contesting Industrial Pollution in Middlesbrough, 1880–1940', *Northern History*, 47:1 (2010), pp. 135–54; Brown, 'Public Health Issues'.

23. C. Webster 'Healthy or Hungry Thirties?', *History Workshop*, 13 (1982), pp. 110–29; M. Mitchell, 'The Effects of Unemployment on the Social Condition of Women and Children in the 1930s', *History Workshop Journal*, 19 (1985), pp. 105–27; K. Laybourn, *Britain on the Breadline: A Social and Political History of Britain, 1918–1939* (Stroud: Sutton, 1998); J. Winter, 'Unemployment, Nutrition and Infant Mortality in Britain, 1920–1950, in J. M. Winter (ed.), *The Working Class in Modern British History* (Cambridge: Cambridge University Press, 1983), pp. 232–56; McIntosh, 'Maternity in Sheffield'.

24. D. Hey, 'Continuities and Perceptions', in Binfield et al. (eds), *The History of the City of Sheffield*, vol. 2, pp. 7–16.

25. Taylor, 'Cutlery Trades'; C. Binfield and D. Hey (eds), *Mesters to Masters: A History of the Company of Cutlers in Hallamshire* (Oxford: Oxford University Press, 1997).

26. Tweedale, *Steel City*, pp. 133–6.

27. G. Tweedale, 'Steelmakers as Masters Cutler: A Look at a Sheffield Industrial Elite', in Binfield and Hey (eds), *Mesters to Masters*, pp. 63–84; C. Stevens, 'The Conservative Club Movement in the Industrial West Riding, 1880–1914', *Northern History*, 38:1 (2001), pp. 121–43.

28. H. Scurfield, Medical Officer of Health, *City of Sheffield Health Statistics*, 1918 (Sheffield: Sheffield Corporation, 1919). The average birthrate for 1907–16 was 28.4 per 1,000. McIntosh, 'Maternity in Sheffield', p. 49. For a similar pattern in Middlesbrough, F. Bell, *At the Works: A Study of a Manufacturing Town with a new introduction by Jim Turner* (Middlesbrough: University of Teesside, 1st edn 1907; repub. 1997).

29. GB Historical GIS/University of Portsmouth, Sheffield MB/CB through time/Industry Statistics/Persons of Working Age by Sex & 1921 Occupational Order, *A Vision of Britain through Time*, at http://www.visionofbritain.org.uk/unit/10152513/cube/OCC_ORD1921; GB Historical GIS/University of Portsmouth, Sheffield MB/CB through time/Industry Statistics/Persons of Working Age by Sex & 1931 Occupational Order, *A Vision of Britain through Time*, at http://www.visionofbritain.org.uk/unit/10152513/cube/OCC_ORD1931 [26 September 2013].

30. Pollard, 'Labour', p. 270.

31. H. E. Mathers, 'Sheffield Municipal Politics, 1893–1926: Parties, Personalities and the Rise of Labour' (PhD thesis, University of Sheffield, 1979).

32. Willis, 'Health Care in Sheffield', p. 133; Sheffield Hospitals Council Incorporated, *Sheffield 1d in the £ Scheme: 1919–1948* (Sheffield: Sheffield Hospitals Council, 1949) [hereafter SHC].

33. Webster, 'Healthy or Hungry'; Mitchell, 'Effects of Unemployment'; but for a contrary view see Winter, 'Unemployment'. McIntosh, 'Maternity in Sheffield' drew a similar conclusion to the one presented here.

34. See Willis, 'Local Authority Health Care'.

35. Medical Officer of Health, *Annual Report on the Health of the City of Sheffield for the Year*, 1928 (Sheffield: Sheffield Corporation, 1929), p. 7 [hereafter MOH Sheffield, *Annual Report*, followed by year].

36. McIntosh, 'Maternity in Sheffield', p. 126.

37. Sheffield Survey Report, TNA MH66/1076, pp. 183–4.

38. T. McIntosh, '"An Abortionist City": Maternal Mortality, Abortion and Birth Control in Sheffield, 1920–1940', *Medical History*, 44:1 (2000), pp. 75–96.

39. A. Digby, 'Poverty, Health, and the Politics of Gender in Britain 1870–1948', in A. Digby and J. Stewart (eds), *Gender, Health and Welfare* (London: Routledge, 1996), pp. 67–90.

40. McIntosh, 'Maternity in Sheffield', pp. 102–5.

41. Doyle, 'Pollution in Middlesbrough', p. 144; Brown, 'Public Health Issues', p. 61.

42. MOH Sheffield, *Annual Report*, 1927, p. 12.

43. Ibid., p. 13.

44. MOH Sheffield, *Annual Report*, 1938, pp. 16–20.

45. Bell, *At the Works*, pp. 90–1.

46. The Royal Infirmary, Sheffield, *One Hundred and Thirty-Ninth Annual Report for the Year ended 31st December 1936*, p. 6 [hereafter SRI, *Annual Report* followed by year].

47. See ch. 4.

48. MOH Sheffield, *Annual Report*, 1928, p. 7.

49. Swan, 'Medical Education', pp. 137–9; Sturdy, 'Political Economy', pp. 140–3.

50. For similar merger campaigns led by medical schools in Bristol and Birmingham see Reinarz, *Birmingham*, pp. 213–14, 235–8; Gorsky, 'Bristol', sec. 5.3.

51. L. G. Parsons, S. Clayton Fryers and G. E. Godber, *Hospital Survey: The Hospital Services of the Sheffield and East Midlands Area* (London: HMSO, 1945) [hereafter Parsons, *Hospital Survey: Sheffield*].

52. Doyle, 'Changing Functions of Urban Government'.
53. For a discussion of the possible impact of ideology on service provision in health care see Levene et al., *Cradle to Grave*, pp. 86–98. For a general discussion, Doyle, 'Changing Functions of Urban Government', p. 309.
54. Elliott, 'Sheffield Guardians', p. 132.
55. Levene, Powell and Stewart, 'Municipal Hospital Care', p. 4.
56. R. Lloyd-Jones and M. J. Lewis, 'Business Structure and Political Economy in Sheffield: The Metal Trades, 1880–1920' and H. Mathers, 'The City of Sheffield, 1893–1926', in Binfield et al. (eds), *The History of the City of Sheffield*, vol. 2, pp. 211–33 and vol. 1, pp. 53–84; Stevens, 'The Conservative Club Movement'.
57. This was a relatively common experience after 1908. T. Adams, 'Labour and the First World War: Economy, Politics and the Erosion of Local Peculiarity?', *Journal of Regional and Local Studies*, 10 (1990), pp. 23–47.
58. Mathers, 'Politics, 1893–1926', pp. 75–7; Thorpe, 'Labour Stronghold', pp. 97–9.
59. Thorpe, 'Labour Stronghold', pp. 86–9; Sheffield City Council Labour Group, *Six Years of Labour Rule in Sheffield, 1926–32* (Sheffield: E. G. Rowlinson, 1932), p. 8; Crook, 'Housing Policy after 1914', pp. 78–80.
60. S. Davies and B. Morley, 'The Reactions of Municipal Voters in Yorkshire to the Second Labour Government, 1929–32', in M. Worley (ed.), *Labour's Grass Roots: Essays on the Activities of Local Labour Parties and Members, 1918–45* (Aldershot: Ashgate, 2005), pp. 124–46.
61. Thorpe, 'Labour Stronghold', pp. 98–9; Davies and Morley, 'Voters in Yorkshire', p. 141. For the national politics of the period and controversies around the means test and the collapse of the Macdonald government see Laybourn, *Britain on the Breadline*; and J. Shepherd, J. Davis and C. Wrigley (eds), *The Second Labour Government: A Reappraisal* (Manchester: Manchester University Press, 2011).
62. For a general discussion of municipal hospital politics and policy see Levene et al., *Cradle to Grave*.
63. Crook, 'Housing Policy after 1914', p. 79.
64. Sheffield Labour Party, *Labour Accomplishes: What Has Been Done – What Will Be Done* (Sheffield, 1945).
65. E. J. Connell and M. Ward, 'Industrial Development, 1780–1914', in Fraser (ed.), *A History of Modern Leeds*, pp. 142–76, on p. 143 quoting an 'observer' from 1858.
66. Ibid., K. Grady, 'Commercial, Marketing and Retailing Amenities, 1700–1914', in Fraser (ed.), *A History of Modern Leeds*, pp. 177–99, M. W. Beresford, 'Prosperity Street and Others: An Essay in Visible Urban History', in M. W. Beresford and G. R. J. Jones (eds), *Leeds and its Region* (Leeds: For the British Association for the Advancement of Science, 1967), pp. 186–99.
67. Connell and Ward, 'Industrial Development', pp. 162–4; Morgan, 'Demographic Change', pp. 46–71.
68. Connell and Ward, 'Industrial Development', p. 164.
69. K. Honeyman, *Well Suited: A History of the Leeds Clothing Industry, 1850–1990* (Oxford and New York: Pasold Research Fund: Oxford University Press, 2000).
70. K. Honeyman, 'Montague Burton Ltd.: The Creators of Well-dressed Men', in J. Chartres and K. Honeyman (eds), *Leeds City Business, 1893–1993: Essays Marking the Centenary of the Incorporation* (Leeds: Leeds University Press, 1993), pp. 186–216.

71. Honeyman, *Well Suited*, pp. 55–7; 86–7; A. J. Kershen, *Uniting the Tailors: Trade Unionism Amongst the Tailors of London and Leeds, 1870–1939* (Ilford: Frank Cass, 1995), pp. 48–9.

72. G. F. Rainnie and R. K. Williamson, 'The Economic Structure', in Beresford and Jones (eds), *Leeds and its Region*, pp. 215–39, on p. 229.

73. J. Benson, *The Rise of Consumer Society in Britain, 1880–1980* (London: Longman, 1994); Connell and Ward, 'Industrial Development'; Honeyman, *Well Suited*; J. Buckman, 'Later Phases of Industrialisation, to 1918', in Beresford and Jones (eds), *Leeds and its Region*, pp. 156–66.

74. J. Chartres, 'Joshua Tetley and Son, 1890s to 1990s: A Century in the Tied Trade', in Chartres and Honeyman (eds), *Leeds City Business*, pp. 112–44.

75. J. Chartres, 'John Waddington PLC, 1890s to 1990s: A Strategy of Quality and Innovation' and K. Honeyman, '"Soapy Joes": The History of Joseph Watson and Sons Ltd., 1893–1993', in Chartres and Honeyman (eds), *Leeds City Business*, pp. 145–85; 217–43.

76. P. Wainwright, 'Chas. F. Thackray Ltd.: Suppliers to the Surgeons', in Chartres and Honeyman (eds), *Leeds City Business*, pp. 244–69.

77. Grady, 'Commercial, Marketing and Retailing', pp. 186–90; M. Collins, 'The History of Leeds Permanent Building Society, 1893–1993', in Chartres and Honeyman (eds), *Leeds City Business*, pp. 57–79.

78. R. J. Morris, *Men, Women and Property in England, 1780–1870* (Cambridge: Cambridge University Press, 2005).

79. B. J. Barber, 'Aspects of Municipal Government, 1835–1914', in Fraser (ed.), *A History of Modern Leeds*, pp. 301–26.

80. Meadowcroft, 'Years of Political Transition', pp. 430–1.

81. Honeyman, *Well Suited*, pp. 56; 87–90.

82. P. Atkinson, 'Cultural Causes of the Nineteenth-Century Fertility Decline: A Study of Three Yorkshire Towns' (PhD thesis, University of Leeds, 2010).

83. Calculations based on *Vision of Britain through Time*, Leeds, at http://www.visionofbritain.org.uk/unit/10108809/cube/OCC_ORD1921 and http://www.visionofbritain.org.uk/unit/10108809/cube/OCC_ORD1931 [accessed 21 November 2013].

84. Honeyman, *Well Suited*, pp. 181–90; Honeyman, 'Montague Burton Ltd', pp. 200–4.

85. G. Cookson, 'Kitson, James, first Baron Airedale (1835–1911)', *ODNB*.

86. T. Woodhouse, 'The Working Class', in Fraser (ed.), *A History of Modern Leeds*, pp. 327–52, on p. 379.

87. T. Woodhouse, *Nourishing the Liberty Tree: Liberals and Labour in Leeds, 1880–1914* (Keele: Keele University Press, 1996), pp. 37–41.

88. Morgan, 'Demographic Change', p. 62; Kershen, *Uniting the Tailors*, pp. 25–59.

89. Honeyman, *Well Suited*, pp. 86–7.

90. Doyle, 'Hospital Contributory Schemes'; Woodhouse, *Liberty Tree*.

91. Morris, *Men, Women and Property*; R. J. Morris, *Class, Sect and Party: The Making of the British Middle Class, Leeds 1820–1850* (Manchester: Manchester University Press, 1990); S. Gunn, *The Public Culture of the Victorian Middle Class: Ritual and Authority in the English Industrial City 1840–1914* (Manchester: Manchester University Press, 2000).

92. Ibid.; R. J. Morris, 'Middle-Class Culture, 1700–1914', in Fraser (ed.), *A History of Modern Leeds*, pp. 200–22.

93. For commentary on the city's death rate see MOH Leeds, *Annual Report*.

94. MOH Leeds, *Annual Report*, 1918, p. 5.

95. MOH Leeds, *Annual Report*, 1946, p. 14.
96. MOH Leeds, *Annual Report*, 1939, p. 69.
97. MOH Leeds, *Annual Report*, 1946, p. 8.
98. Ibid., p. 3.
99. Ibid.
100. C. Murphy, 'A History of Radiotherapy to 1950: Cancer and Radiotherapy in Britain, 1850–1950' (PhD thesis, University of Manchester, 1986) and this volume, ch. 7.
101. Barber, 'Muncipal Government'; R. J. Marshall, 'Town Planning in Sheffield', in Binfield et al. (eds), *The History of the City of Sheffield*, vol. 2, pp. 17–32; Shaw, 'Aspects of Public Health', pp. 110–14.
102. Leeds Survey Report, TNA MH66/1072, p. 2; MOH Leeds, *Annual Report*, 1946, p. 13.
103. 'Report on Maternity and Child Welfare Services of Leeds', TNA MH66/1072. See ch. 4.
104. See ch. 3.
105. Meadowcroft, 'Political Transition'; F. J. Fowler, 'Urban Renewal, 1918–1966', in Beresford and Jones, ed., *Leeds and its Region*, pp. 175–85.
106. MOH Leeds, *Annual Report*, 1946, pp. 15–16.
107. S. Mosley, *The Chimney of the World: A History of Smoke Pollution in Victorian and Edwardian Manchester* (London: White Horse, pb edn, 2008); MOH Leeds, *Annual Report*, 1939, p. 101; W. Asbury, 'Presidential Address on "Smoke Abatement"', *Journal of the Royal Sanitary Institute*, 50 (1929–30), pp. 389–93.
108. See ch. 7.
109. MOH Leeds, *Annual Report*, 1946, p. 6.
110. Pickstone, *Medicine and Industrial Society*, p. 246; Gosling, 'Charity and Change'.
111. M. Hogarth, 'Campbell, Dame Janet Mary (1877–1954)', *ODNB*.
112. 'Report on Maternity and Child Welfare Services of Leeds', Leeds Survey Report, TNA MH66/1072, p. 27.
113. MOH Leeds, *Annual Report*, 1946, p. 11.
114. S. T. Anning and W. K. J. Walls, *A History of the Leeds School of Medicine: One and a Half Centuries, 1831–1981* (Leeds, 1981), p. 103.
115. Pickstone, *Medicine and Industrial Society*; Gorsky, 'Bristol', sec. 5.3; and Reinarz, *Birmingham* which is largely concerned with the role of the Medical School.
116. H. Eason, R. Veitch Clark and W. H. Harper, *Hospital Survey: The Hospital Services of the Yorkshire Area* (London: HMSO, 1945), pp. 31–3 [hereafter Eason, *Hospital Survey: Yorkshire*].
117. Barber, 'Muncipal Government', pp. 316–23.
118. P. M. Pennock, 'The Evolution of St James's, 1845–94: Leeds Moral and Industrial Training School, Leeds Union Workhouse and Leeds Union Infirmary', *Publications of the Thoresby Society*, 59 (1984), pp. 129–76.
119. P. Proctor, 'St. James's Hospital Leeds: 1900 to 1970, A Study of its Development, from Poor Law Infirmary to the Largest General Hospital in this Country' (Unpublished typescript, Leeds, 1970); Leeds Board of Guardians, *Yearbook, 1925–26* (Leeds, 1926), p. 21; *1929–30* (Leeds, 1930), p. 27.
120. D. Fraser, *Urban Politics in Victorian England: The Structure of Politics in Victorian Cities* (Leicester: Leicester University Press, 1976); W. R. Meyer, 'Charles Henry Wilson: The Man Who was Leeds', *Publications of the Thoresby Society*, second series, 8 (1998), pp. 78–96, on pp. 80–1. Thanks to Steve Burt for this reference.

121. Woodhouse, *Liberty Tree*, pp. 116–17; Woodhouse, 'Working Class', pp. 360–3.
122. Meyer, 'Wilson', pp. 84–5.
123. Woodhouse, *Liberty Tree*, pp. 122–33.
124. Meadowcroft, 'Political Transition', pp. 424–5.
125. For the context of Yorkshire Labour politics see J. Reynolds and K. Laybourn, *Labour Heartland* (Bradford: Bradford University Press, 1986).
126. Ibid.; Meyer, 'Wilson'.
127. Levene et al., *Cradle to Grave*, pp. 86–98; Doyle, 'Changing Functions of Urban Government'.
128. Barber, 'Muncipal Government'; Meadowcroft, 'Political Transition'; A. Ravetz, *Model Estate: Planned Housing at Quarry Hill* (London: Croom Helm in association with Joseph Rowntree Memorial Trust, 1974).
129. MOH Leeds, *Annual Report*, 1939, p. 107.
130. For the politics of slum clearance in Leeds and the development of Quarry Hill see Ravetz, *Model Estate*.
131. *Leeds Mercury*, various dates 1931.
132. *Leeds Citizen*, various dates 1935.
133. See ch. 6, p. 166.
134. Mohan, *Planning*; Gosling, 'Charity and Change'; Pickstone, *Medicine and Industrial Society*; Reinarz, *Birmingham*.

2 Hospital Provision: Voluntary and Municipal

1. Pinker, *Hospital Statistics*; Cherry, *Medical Services*, p. 46.
2. Levene, Powell and Stewart, 'Municipal Hospital Care'.
3. Abel-Smith, *The Hospitals*, p. 404.
4. C. Webster, *The National Health Service: A Political History*, 2nd edn (Oxford: Oxford University Press, 2002), p. 5.
5. H. Marland, *Medicine and Society in Wakefield and Huddersfield, 1780–1870* (Cambridge: Cambridge University Press, 1987), p. 382.
6. Pickstone, *Medicine and Industrial Society*; Gorsky, 'Bristol'; Gorsky, 'Threshold of a New Era'; Cherry, 'Medical Care'; Doyle, 'Labour and Hospitals'.
7. Sturdy and Cooter, 'Scientific Management'.
8. Ellis, 'Growth of County Asylums' and A. Brumby, 'From "Pauper Lunatics" to "Rate-Aided Patients": Dismantling the Poor Law of Lunacy in Mental Health Care: 1888–1930' (PhD in progress, University of Huddersfield).
9. Abel-Smith, *The Hospitals*, ch. 1, though this largely concentrates on London; M. Gorsky, *Patterns of Philanthropy: Charity and Society in Nineteenth-Century Bristol* (Woodbridge: Boydell and Brewer, 1999); Pickstone, *Medicine and Industrial Society*, ch. 1; J. Taylor, *The Rebirth of the Norfolk and Norwich Hospital, 1874–1883: An Architectural Exploration* (Norwich: Wellcome Unit for the History of Medicine, 2000).
10. The General Infirmary at Leeds was the official title of the hospital as used in its annual reports and the official history. The hospital was generally known as Leeds General Infirmary, and the abbreviation LGI used here and throughout this volume reflects this general term.
11. S. T. Anning, *The General Infirmary at Leeds: The First Hundred Years, 1767–1869* (Edinburgh: Livingstone, 1963); Anning, 'Medicine in Leeds', p. 208.
12. Porter, *Royal Infirmary*, pp. 29, 41.

13. Anning, 'Medicine in Leeds', p. 220.
14. Skinner, *Royal Hospital*; *The Annual Report of the Board of the Leeds Public Dispensary and Hospital* 1932–3 (Leeds, 1933), p. 7 [hereafter LPD, *Annual Report* followed by date (mid-year to mid-year until 1936)].
15. Skinner, *Royal Hospital*, pp. 2–3.
16. Ibid., pp. 31–5.
17. Gorsky, *Patterns of Philanthropy*; Doyle, *Hospitals in Middlesbrough*.
18. Cherry, *Medical Services*, pp. 45–8.
19. S. Clayton Fryers, 'The General Infirmary at Leeds: A Short History', *University of Leeds Review*, 3 (1952–3), pp. 341–9.
20. Porter, *Royal Infirmary*; Skinner, *Royal Hospital*.
21. Anning, 'Medicine in Leeds', p. 221.
22. See p. 57.
23. Granshaw, 'Introduction'.
24. Reinarz, *Birmingham*, p. 38.
25. Anning, 'Medicine in Leeds', pp. 221–2.
26. Pickstone, *Medicine and Industrial Society*, pp. 114–16; Reinarz, *Birmingham*, p. 82.
27. A. M. Claye, *A Short History of the Hospital for Women at Leeds, 1853–1953* (Leeds: Walter Gardham Ltd., 1953), p. 7.
28. Reinarz, *Birmingham*, p. 82.
29. *Manchester Guardian*, 5 October 1875.
30. The Jessop Hospital for Women, Sheffield, *Sixty-Fourth Annual Report* (Sheffield, 1927), p. 11 [hereafter Jessop, *Annual Report* and year].
31. For similar involvement at an earlier date in Manchester see Pickstone, *Medicine and Industrial Society*, pp. 115–16.
32. Claye, *Hospital for Women*; Leeds Maternity Hospital, *Third Annual Report for the Year 1907–08* (Leeds, 1908) [hereafter LMH, *Annual Report*, and year]; LMH, *Annual Report*, 1947, p. 16.
33. Reinarz, *Birmingham*, p. 74.
34. P. Harvey, *Up the Hill to Western Bank: A History of the Children's Hospital, Sheffield, 1876–1976* (Sheffield: The Centenary Committee, Children's Hospital, 1976).
35. Pickstone, *Medicine and Industrial Society*, ch. 9.
36. Doyle, 'Changing Functions of Urban Government'.
37. Levene et al., *Cradle to Grave*; and Welshman, *Municipal Medicine*, who concentrates on tuberculosis treatment only.
38. R. G. Hodgkinson, *The Origins of the National Health Service: The Medical Services of the New Poor Law, 1834–1871* (London: The Wellcome Historical Medical Library, 1967).
39. Pennock, 'Evolution of St James's', p. 167.
40. J. Flett, *The Story of the Workhouse and the Hospital at Nether Edge* (Sheffield: n.p., [1984]).
41. P. Speck et al., *The Institution and Hospital at Fir Vale, Sheffield: A Centenary History of the Northern General Hospital* (Sheffield: Nothern General Hospital, 1978).
42. Doyle, *Hospitals in Middlesbrough*; Pickstone, *Medicine and Industrial Society*, p. 216.
43. Cherry, 'Medical Care', p. 291.
44. For the financial climate for local authorities at the time see F. Bell and R. Millward, 'Public Health Expenditure and Mortality in England and Wales, 1870–1914', *Continuity and Change*, 13:2 (1998), pp. 221–49; Doyle, 'Changing Functions of Urban Government'.

45. Proctor, 'St. James's Hospital', unpaginated but information from ch. 1.
46. Flett, *Nether Edge*, pp. 16–18.
47. Speck, *Fir Vale*, pp. 26–32.
48. Ibid., p. 22.
49. Doyle, 'Competition and Cooperation'; Gorsky, 'Bristol', sec. 2.3.
50. Abel-Smith, *The Hospitals*, pp. 127–30.
51. Pickstone, *Medicine and Industrial Society*, ch. 8; J. Gray, *Edinburgh City Hospital* (East Linton: Tuckwell, 1999).
52. Pickstone, *Medicine and Industrial Society*, p. 181.
53. Anning, 'Medicine in Leeds', pp. 210–13.
54. Leeds Corporation Sanitary Committee, *Leeds City Hospitals: Seacroft and Killingbeck. Opened by the Right Nonourable, the Lord Mayor and Lady Mayoress, September 29th 1904* (Leeds: Leeds Corporation, 1904).
55. Ibid.; Leeds Hospital Management Committee B Group, *50th Anniversary of the Opening of Seacroft and Killingbeck Hospitals* (Leeds: Leeds HMC, 1954).
56. Pickstone, *Medicine and Industrial Society*, ch. 8, on infectious diseases.
57. For a detailed study of a local tuberculosis policy see Welshman, *Municipal Medicine*, ch. 3.
58. Leeds HMC, *Seacroft*; Pickstone, *Medicine and Industrial Society*, pp. 229–35; Doyle, 'Competition and Cooperation', p. 347.
59. MOH Leeds, *Annual Report*, p. 36.
60. MOH Leeds, *Annual Report*, 1919, p. 40. See also the discussion of an extension to Thorp Arch in 1938 in ch. 7.
61. Levene et al., *Cradle to Grave*; Doyle, 'Competition and Cooperation'.
62. For the financial implications of new building see ch. 5, and Hayes and Doyle, 'Eggs, Rags and Whist Drives'.
63. Both of the Sheffield hospitals had annexes for preoperative and aftercare cases.
64. Hayes, 'Our Hospitals'; Hayes and Doyle, 'Eggs, Rags and Whist Drives'.
65. The General Infirmary at Leeds, *One Hundred and Fifty-Sixth Annual Report*, 1923 (Leeds, 1924) [hereafter LGI, *Annual Report*, followed by year].
66. Jessop, *Annual Report*, 1927, p. 7. See also ch. 7.
67. Leeds Survey Report, Letter from P. Austyn Barran to Minister of Health, 17 January 1936, MH66/1072. Eason, *Hospital Survey: Yorkshire*, pp. 32–3; *Seventy-Sixth Annual Report of the Hospital for Women and Children, Coventry Place Leeds*, 1928, p. 20; 1933, p. 21; 1937, p. 30; 1939, p. 6 [hereafter LHW, *Annual Report*, followed by year].
68. Pickstone, *Medicine and Industrial Society*, p. 265; Reinarz, *Birmingham*, pp. 212, 243.
69. Gosling, 'Charity and Change', ch. 5.
70. Ibid., pp. 254–5.
71. See the evidence from Middlesbrough presented by R. Lewis, R. Nixon and B. Doyle, 'Health Services in Middlesbrough: North Ormesby Hospital 1900–1948' (Unpublished AHRC Final Report, Middlesbrough, 1999), and p. 79.
72. Claye, *Hospital for Women*, p. 18.
73. LMH, *Annual Report*, 1933, p. 8.
74. 'The New Jessop Hospital Maternity and Pay Bed Block', in Jessop, *Annual Report*, 1937. LGI, *Annual Report*, 1940, pp. 12–13; Anning, *General Infirmary: Vol. II*, pp. 45–6.
75. Reinarz does catalogue these developments in the various Birmingham hospitals but does not tie them to efforts to organize patients and increase efficiency. See for example Reinarz, *Birmingham*, pp. 185–6 on the city's Ear Hospital.

76. Jessop, *Annual Report*, 1937, p. 15.
77. 'The Nurses Home', Sheffield Royal Hospital, *The One Hundred and Third Annual Report of the Sheffield Royal Hospital to 31st December, 1935* (Sheffield, 1935) adjoining p. 48 [hereafter SRH, *Annual Report* followed by year].
78. SRH, *Annual Report*, 1935, p. 12.
79. Claye, *Hospital for Women*, p. 19; The United Leeds Hospitals, *First Report Covering the Period 5th July 1948 to 31st March 1950* (Leeds: Kelly & Barratt, 1950) [hereafter, United Leeds Hospitals, *First Report*], pp. 35–7; LGI, *Annual Report*, 1940, p. 12.
80. Study and Cooter, 'Scientific Management', p. 9. In Bristol, outpatients grew substantially at the General Hospital but very little at the Royal where bed numbers increased by around a quarter. Gorsky, 'Bristol', table 2.
81. Claye, *Hospital for Women*, p. 19.
82. SRI, *Annual Report*, 1935.
83. SRH, *Annual Report*, 1927, p. 8. See also ch. 3 for a discussion of the impact of road accidents.
84. See ch. 7.
85. Sturdy and Cooter, 'Scientific Management'.
86. Reinarz notes existing or new pathology labs in the Ear, Eye, Children's and Women's hospitals of Birmingham and more sophisticated bacteriology and biochemical facilities at the Queen's and General hospitals, the latter undertaking all of the biochemical work for the Maternity Hospital. Reinarz, *Birmingham*, ch. 9.
87. Jessop, *Annual Report*, 1927, pp. 7–8; LMH, *Annual Report*, 1934, p. 30; 1936, p. 30.
88. Jessop, *Annual Report*, 1929, p. 9; 1938, p. 21.
89. United Leeds Hospitals, *First Report*, p. 37.
90. Ibid., p. 36.
91. Skinner, *Royal Hospital*, p. 62; Sturdy, ' Political Economy'.
92. Parsons, *Hospital Survey: Sheffield*.
93. Ibid., p. 28; Doyle, *Hospitals in Middlesbrough*, p. 93.
94. For a discussion of the development of UV treatment in Birmingham see Reinarz, *Birmingham*, pp. 191–2; Preston Infirmary acquired electro-massage and UV therapy equipment in the 1920s and radium in 1933, Pickstone, *Medicine and Industrial Society*, p. 255; developments were even more extensive in Bristol, Gorsky, 'Bristol', sec. 3.1.
95. SRH, *Annual Report*, 1937, p. 11.
96. SRI, *Annual Report*, 1941, back page.
97. Harvey, *History of the Children's Hospital, Sheffield*, pp. 37–9.
98. Gorsky, 'Bristol', sec. 3.1.
99. LGI, *Annual Report*, for example 1922, p. 14.
100. Cooter, 'Meaning of Fractures'; and R. Cooter, *Surgery and Society in Peace and War: Orthopaedics and the Organization of Modern Medicine, 1880–1948* (Basingstoke: Macmillan in Association with the Centre for the History of Science, Technology and Medicine, University of Manchester, 1993).
101. See ch. 7.
102. Gorsky gives a brief mention to 'technology which increased efficiency: electric lifts, up to date equipment for the laundries and kitchens, hospital wireless, electric clocks, telephone systems and so on'. Gorsky, 'Bristol', sec. 3.1.
103. LGI, *Annual Report*, 1927, p. 16; LMH, *Annual Report*, 1933, p. 6; SRI, *Annual Report*, 1940, p. 14.

104. LMH, *Annual Report*, 1933, p. 6; Harvey, *History of the Children's Hospital, Sheffield*, p. 38.

105. See ch. 5.

106. For discussion of the priorities of four specific towns – Barnsley, Eastbourne, Newport and West Hartlepool - see Levene et al., *Cradle to Grave*; and for services in Manchester and some other Lancashire towns see Pickstone, *Medicine and Industrial Society*, pp. 256–64.

107. For descriptions of the hospitals see Leeds Survey, Appendices TNA MH66/711; Sheffield Survey Appendices O–Z, TNA MH66/873; and Eason, *Hospital Survey: Yorkshire* and Parsons, *Hospital Survey: Sheffield*.

108. Flett, *Nether Edge*, p. 18; Speck, *Fir Vale*, p. 33; Leeds Board of Guardians, *Yearbook, 1929–30*, p. 27; J. J. Jervis, *Scheme for the Utilization of Poor Law Institutions under the Local Government Act, 1929* (Leeds: Leeds Corporation, 1934).

109. For an upbeat assessment of post appropriation improvements see Powell, 'An Expanding Service', pp. 343–9.

110. Leeds Survey Report, TNA MH66/1072, p. 65 and Sheffield Survey Report, TNA MH66/1076, p. 143.

111. Powell, 'An Expanding Service'. See also Levene et al., *Cradle to Grave*, ch. 3.

112. Mohan, *Planning*; Stewart, 'Finest Municipal Hospital Service'; Pickstone, *Medicine and Industrial Society*; Doyle, 'Competition and Cooperation'; and Gorsky, 'Bristol'.

113. Ibid., sec. 4.3; Pickstone, *Medicine and Industrial Society*, pp. 256–64; Cherry, 'Medical Care', p. 291.

114. MOH Sheffield, *Annual Report*, 1930, pp. 57–8.

115. Sheffield Survey Report, TNA MH66/1076, pp. 164–77 and Sheffield Survey Appendices O19–O21, TNA MH66/873.

116. See chs 6, 7.

117. MOH Sheffield, *Annual Report*, 1934, p. 86.

118. Speck, *Fir Vale*, pp. 39–40.

119. Jervis, *Utilization of Poor Law*.

120. Leeds Survey Report, TNA MH66/1072, pp. 48–9.

121. Jervis, *Utilization of Poor Law*, pp. 8–9 and appendix.

122. City of Leeds, *Opening of the New Extensions at St. James's Hospital by the Minister of Health ... September 30th 1940* (Leeds: Leeds Corporation, 1940), p. 5.

123. Leeds (Group A) Hospital Management Committee, *Report for the Period, 5th July 1948 to 31st December 1949* (Leeds: Leeds HMC, 1950), pp. 15–16 [hereafter Leeds A, *Annual Report* followed by year].

124. City of Leeds, *Opening of the New Extensions at St. James's Hospital*, p. 9.

125. Cherry, 'Medical Care', p. 291.

126. Levene, Powell and Stewart, 'Municipal Hospital Care', p. 13; Eason, *Hospital Survey: Yorkshire*, pp. 62–5.

127. City of Leeds, *Opening of the New Wards for Women at Killingbeck Sanatorium by the Minister of Health ... July 9th 1936* (Leeds: Leeds Corporation, 1936).

128. MOH Sheffield, *Annual Report*, 1935, p. 61.

129. Cherry, 'Medical Care', p. 289; Gorsky, 'Bristol', sec. 4.3; Doyle, 'Competition and Cooperation', p. 347.

130. For the basis of the EHS see Webster, *Health Services Since the War*, pp. 20–4. There are very few local studies of the operation of the EMS but see Rivett, *London Hospital System*, pp. 239–43.

131. LGI, *Annual Report*, 1941, p. 12; 'Jessop Hospital for Women Newscuttings Book vol. 6, 1938–48', Sheffield City Archives [hereafter SCA] NHS12/1/7/1/6.
132. J. J. Jervis, *The Health Services of the City after the War* (Leeds: City of Leeds, 1945), pp. 5, 11, 17.
133. Sheffield Labour Party, *Labour Accomplishes*, pp. 5–6.
134. LMH, *Annual Report*, 1939, p. 6; A. J. Ward and T. Ashton, (eds), *Cookridge Hospital, 1867–1972* (Leeds: Cookridge Hospital, 1997).
135. SRI, *Annual Report*, 1943, p. 5.
136. Royal Sheffield Infirmary and Hospital, *Annual Report for the Year Ended 1948*, p. 25 [hereafter SUH, *Annual Report*, followed by the year].
137. LHW, *Annual Report*, 1941; LGI, *Annual Report*, 1940. For the decline in pay beds nationally see Gosling, 'Charity and Change', p. 251.
138. MOH Leeds, *Annual Report*, 1940, pp. 23, 30–5.
139. Flett, *Nether Edge*, p. 24; Speck, *Fir Vale*, p. 44.
140. Flett, *Nether Edge*, p. 24; Harvey, *History of the Children's Hospital, Sheffield*, pp. 40–2; SUH, *Annual Report*, 1941, p. 3; 'Jessop Newscuttings, vol. 6', SCA NHS12/1/7/1/6.
141. Jervis, *Health Services*. See also Eason, *Hospital Survey: Yorkshire*; Parsons, *Hospital Survey: Sheffield*.
142. Eason, *Hospital Survey: Yorkshire*, pp. 31–3.
143. Parsons, *Hospital Survey: Sheffield*, pp. 18–23.
144. Eason, *Hospital Survey: Yorkshire*, p. 31.
145. Ibid., p. 33.
146. Ibid., p. 74.
147. Ibid., p. 32.
148. Ibid., p. 32.
149. Parsons, *Hospital Survey: Sheffield*, p. 18.
150. Ibid., p. 19.
151. Ibid., p. 20.
152. Ibid., p. 20.
153. Ibid., p. 21.
154. SUH, *Annual Report*, 1947, p. 11.
155. SUH, *Annual Report*, 1945, p. 7; 1946, p. 8.
156. Flett, *Nether Edge*, p. 24; Speck, *Fir Vale*, p. 46.
157. LGI, *Annual Report*, 1945, p. 20.
158. Leeds A, *Annual Report*, 1948–9, p. 62. The Ministry of Health surveyors had recommended the closure of this unit once the war was over. Eason, *Hospital Survey: Yorkshire*, pp. 32–3.
159. Ibid., p. 33.
160. Leeds (Group B) Hospital Management Committee No. 22, *First Annual Report for the Period Ended 31st March 1949 with Statistical Tables for the Year Ended 31st December 1948* (Leeds: Leeds HMC, 1949), p. 6 [hereafter Leeds B, *Annual Report* followed by year].

3 Patients and Access

1. There are no figures for patients treated in this period. Pinker does provide information on average patient numbers but the increase in bed occupancy and the decrease in length of stay of patients provide a sense of the growth in the numbers treated nationally. Pinker, *Hospital Statistics*, chs 12–15.

2. For a general discussion see A. Hardy, *Health and Medicine in Britain since 1860* (Basingstoke: Palgrave, 2001), p. 91. For an extensive consideration of changing demographic and epidemiological profiles see D. Coleman and J. Salt, *The British Population: Patterns, Trends and Processes* (Oxford: Oxford University Press, 1992).

3. Abel-Smith, *The Hospitals*, pp. 4–7; Cherry, *Medical Services*; K. Waddington, *Charity and the London Hospitals, 1850–1898* (Woodbridge: Boydell and Brewer, 2000).

4. Cherry, 'Before the National Health Service'; Gorsky, Mohan and Willis, *Mutualism and Health Care*.

5. National hospital politics are covered in Abel-Smith, *The Hospitals*; Webster, 'Conflict and Consensus'; M. Gorsky, J. Mohan and T. Willis, 'Hospital Contributory Schemes and the NHS Debate 1937–1946: The Rejection of Social Insurance in the British Welfare State?', *Twentieth Century British History*, 16 (2005), pp. 170–92; and from a local perspective critical of much national history, Pickstone, *Medicine and Industrial Society*. Other key local studies include, Mohan, *Planning*; Gorsky, 'Bristol'; Reinarz, *Birmingham*; Hayes, 'Our Hospitals'; Doyle, 'Competition and Cooperation'.

6. Abel-Smith, *The Hospitals*, pp. 119–32; Levene, 'Less Eligibility'; Levene et al., *Cradle to Grave*.

7. Levene et al., *Cradle to Grave*, pp. 9–12 and case studies; Powell, 'An Expanding Service'; Stewart, 'Finest Municipal Hospital Service'; Doyle, 'Competition and Cooperation'.

8. Cherry, 'Medical Care', p. 275.

9. E. A. Heaman, *St Mary's: The History of a London Teaching Hospital* (Montreal and Liverpool: McGill-Queen's University Press, 2003), p. 24; North Riding Infirmary, *Annual Report for the Year Ending 31st December 1933* (Middlesbrough: Appleyard, 1934), p. 54.

10. 'Extracts from the Rules and Bye-Laws', LGI, *Annual Report*, 1920, p. 140.

11. Sheffield Royal Hospital, *Rules of Sheffield Royal Hospital* (Sheffield: n. p., 1911), p. 1.

12. SRI, *Annual Report*, 1919, front cover.

13. SRI, *Annual Report*, 1929, p. 27.

14. LPD, *Annual Report*, 1919–20, p. 35.

15. *Fifty-Seventh Annual Report of the Children's Hospital, Sheffield for the Year Ended 31st December, 1932* (Sheffield: The Children's Hospital, 1933) [hereafter Children's Hospital, *Annual Report*, followed by year], p. 46.

16. LMH, *Annual Report*, 1913, p. 36. Emphasis in original.

17. See ch. 5, pp. 133–4.

18. See p. 55. For examples elsewhere see Welshman, *Municipal Medicine*, p. 147.

19. Pickstone, *Medicine and Industrial Society*, pp. 258–9; Doyle, *Hospitals in Middlesbrough*, p. 72; Gorsky, 'Bristol', sec. 4.3.

20. Leeds Survey Report, TNA MH66/1072, p. 152.

21. Gorsky, Mohan and Willis, *Mutualism and Health Care*, p. 82.

22. LGI, *Annual Report,* 1932, p. 15. For national utilization rates see J. Mohan, 'Voluntarism, Municipalism and Welfare: The Geography of Hospital Utilization in England

in 1938', *Transactions of the Institute of British Geographers*, new series, 28 (2003), pp. 56–74.

23. Pickstone, *Medicine and Industrial Society*, p. 265; In Birmingham this was most obvious at the Orthopaedic Hospital, Reinarz, *Birmingham*, p. 202; Cherry, 'Beyond National Health Insurance', pp. 466–9.

24. Reinarz, *Birmingham*, p. 82; Mohan, *Planning*, p. 58.

25. LHW, *Annual Report*, 1920, pp. 45–8.

26. An 'ingenuous' system designed by the medical superintendent to admit non-Sheffield patients is described in Sheffield Survey Report, TNA MH66/1076, pp. 134–5.

27. For the development of regional services see ch. 7.

28. B. M. Doyle and R. Nixon, 'Voluntary Hospital Finance in North-East England: The Case of North Ormesby Hospital, Middlesbrough, 1900–1947', *Cleveland History*, 80 (2001), pp. 5–19; Gorsky, Mohan and Powell, 'British Voluntary Hospitals', p. 476; Gorsky, 'Bristol', sec. 3.3.

29. SRI, *Annual Report*, 1911, p. 24.

30. SRH, *Annual Report*, 1913, p. 99.

31. Gosling, 'Charity and Change', p. 187; Reinarz, *Birmingham*, p. 195.

32. From 1930 there were also private wards. LHW, *Annual Report*, 1920, pp. 45–8; 1935, pp. 63–7.

33. Pickstone, *Medicine and Industrial Society*, pp. 117, 265; Gorsky, 'Bristol', sec. 3.3; Hayes, 'Our Hospitals', p. 97.

34. SRH, *Annual Report*, 1922, p. 18. Emphasis in the original.

35. LMH, *Annual Report*, 1913, p. 36.

36. LMH, *Annual Report*, 1933, pp. 35–6. See also Reinarz, *Birmingham*, pp. 196–8.

37. Jessop, *Annual Report*, 1935, p. 33.

38. Abel-Smith, *The Hospitals*, p. 128. There is no direct reference to this in Levene et al., *Cradle to Grave*, but the high cost and under-utilization of the borough's infectious disease provision is discussed on pp. 152–3.

39. Sheffield Survey Report, TNA MH66/1076, pp. 210–1.

40. A note headed 'Public Assistance Administration: Voluntary Institutions', Leeds Survey Report, TNA MH66/1072.

41. Minutes of 'Members of the Health Committee Meeting with Representatives of the Voluntary Hospitals Committee to Discuss Co-ordination of Hospital Services', 19 October 1936, Leeds Central Library, Local Studies Department [hereafter 'Co-ordination of Hospital Services']. Martin was also Chairman of the Public Health Committee of Leeds City Council from 1936.

42. Eason, *Hospital Survey: Yorkshire*, p. 32.

43. Cherry, 'Hospital Saturday'.

44. Doyle, 'Hospital Contributory Schemes'.

45. Gorsky, Mohan and Willis, *Mutualism and Health Care*, pp. 32–7.

46. Ibid., p. 1; Gosling, 'Charity and Change', ch. 4.

47. Gorsky, Mohan and Willis, *Mutualism and Health Care*; Cherry, 'Accountability, Entitlement and Control'; Gosling, 'Open the Other Eye'.

48. Pickstone, *Medicine and Industrial Society*, pp. 272–3, 263; Cherry, 'Beyond National Health Insurance', pp. 473–4.

49. Sheffield Joint Hospitals' Council, *A Record of 1923* (Sheffield: Sheffield Hospitals Council, 1923), p. 22.

50. Doyle, 'Hospital Contributory Schemes'; Pickstone, *Medicine and Industrial Society*, p. 263 for the arrangements in Salford.
51. Doyle, 'Hospital Contributory Schemes'; *Sheffield Independent*, 7 September 1938. For a wider discussion of this issue, see Gorsky, Mohan and Willis, *Mutualism and Health Care*, pp. 46–8; Abel-Smith, *The Hospitals*, pp. 323–37.
52. Gorsky, Mohan and Willis, *Mutualism and Health Care*, p. 47.
53. For Sheffield see ch. 5 and for provident schemes see Gosling, 'Charity and Change'.
54. Ibid., pp. 190–1.
55. See ch. 5.
56. Timmins, *The Five Giants*, p. 104; H. Jones, *Health and Society in Twentieth Century Britain* (Harlow: Longman, 1994), p. 21.
57. Gosling, 'Charity and Change'.
58. Anning, *General Infirmary: Vol. II*, pp. 96–7.
59. LMH, *Annual Report*, 1928, p. 12; LGI, *Annual Report*, 1932, pp. 15–16.
60. LGI, *Annual Report*, 1935, p. 21.
61. *Sheffield Telegraph*, 18 May 1938.
62. LHW, *Annual Report*, 1936, p. 4.
63. SRI, *Annual Report*, 1938, pp. 44–7.
64. SRI, *Annual Report*, 1930, inside front cover.
65. *The Shape of Things to Come: The Sheffield Voluntary Hospitals' Million Pound Appeal* (Sheffield: Appeal Committee, 1938), pp. 3, 12 [hereafter *Shape of Things*].
66. Liverpool Hospitals Commission [Chair Lord Cozens-Hardy], *Report on the Voluntary Hospitals of Liverpool* (Liverpool: Liverpool University Press, 1935) [hereafter, LHC, *Hospitals of Liverpool*], pp. 38–41.
67. Gosling, 'Charity and Change'. On changing social relations see Hayes, 'Our Hospitals'. On the needs of medical schools and the rise of the observation case see LHC, *Hospitals of Liverpool*, p. 41.
68. Gorsky, 'Bristol', table 2. See also Hayes, 'Our Hospitals', p. 101; Reinarz, *Birmingham*, pp. 206–7.
69. Only two copies of the annual report for the Children's Hospital were found. Figures for the 1930s are based on those contained in the Sheffield Hospital Council *Annual Reports*. There were also no extant annual reports for LMH before 1928 or LPD after 1944.
70. Ibid., pp. 196–9.
71. Gosling, 'Charity and Change', p. 75. Births at the Birmingham Maternity hospital also doubled in the decade to 1938. Reinarz, *Birmingham*, p. 199.
72. Powell, 'An Expanding Service', p. 344.
73. Gorsky, 'Bristol', sec. 4.3; Pickstone, *Medicine and Industrial Society*, pp. 272–3.
74. Powell, 'An Expanding Service', p. 345.
75. Waddington, *London Hospitals*, pp. 87–95.
76. Sturdy and Cooter, 'Scientific Management', p. 9.
77. Gorsky, 'Bristol', sec. 3.1 enumerates the new equipment and the volume of work undertaken with new technologies such as X-ray and UV lamps. Reinarz, *Birmingham*, ch. 10 relates the growth of a range of outpatient departments and their specialties between the wars, many building on pre-war developments.
78. Gorsky, 'Bristol', sec. 3.1; Reinarz, *Birmingham*; LHC, *Hospitals of Liverpool*, p. 5; Cherry, 'Medical Care', p. 277; Hayes, 'Our Hospitals'.

79. A similar pattern was observed in Bristol where the Infirmary experienced significant inpatient and minimal outpatient growth while the General saw more modest inpatients but a marked rise in outpatients. Gorsky, 'Bristol', table 2.
80. Harvey, *History of the Children's Hospital, Sheffield*, p. 38.
81. LHC, *Hospitals of Liverpool*, pp. 6–7.
82. See pp. 182–3.
83. MOH Leeds, *Annual Report*, 1938, pp. 94–5, 100–1; MOH Sheffield, *Annual Report*, 1938, pp. 79–83, 87, 113–43, 172–90.
84. Gorsky, 'Bristol', sec. 4.3; Webster, *Health Services since the War*, p. 8.
85. Hardy, *Health and Medicine*, pp. 87, 83–4.
86. A. Digby and J. Stewart, 'Welfare in Context', in A. Digby and J. Stewart (eds), *Gender, Health and Welfare* (London: Routledge, 1996), pp. 1–30; V. Berridge, 'Health and Medicine', in F. M. L. Thompson (ed.), *The Cambridge Social History of Britain, 1750–1950: Volume 3 Social Agencies and Institutions* (Cambridge: Cambridge University Press, 1990), pp. 171–242; Webster, 'Healthy or Hungry', pp. 122–3.
87. Evidence from Middlesbrough does suggest that women were more likely to remain on waiting lists for longer than men. Lewis, Nixon and Doyle, 'Health Services in Middlesbrough', pp. 32–41.
88. Sheffield Survey Report, TNA MH66/1076, p. 190 and discussion of cases, pp. 191–4.
89. Most children's hospitals were operating a free service by the later nineteenth century, including Bristol and Birmingham. E. Lomax, 'Small and Special: The Development of Hospitals for Children in Victorian Britain', *Medical History Supplement*, 16 (1996), pp. 50–2. Gosling, 'Charity and Change', p. 187; Reinarz, *Birmingham*, p. 78. For Sheffield see Children's Hospital, *Annual Reports*.
90. The LGI, *Annual Report* listed the number of children treated each year, e.g. 1922 p. 9; 1930, p. 12; 1938, p. 18; 1946, p. 15.
91. LPD, *Annual Report*, 1924, p. 13; 1935, p. 15. For Barnsley, see Levene et al., *Cradle to Grave*, pp. 129–30.
92. Leeds Survey Report, TNA MH66/1072, pp. 20–1.
93. MOH Sheffield, *Annual Report*, 1927, p. 83. For similar observations of the reducing burden of lumbar TB see Doyle, *Hospitals in Middlesbrough*, p. 34.
94. Leeds Joint Hospitals Advisory Committee, *First Annual Report* (1936–7) (Leeds, 1937), pp. 6–7 [hereafter LJHAC]; Eason, *Hospital Survey: Yorkshire*, pp. 26–7, 33.
95. For the changing profile of patients in Barnsley, Levene et al., *Cradle to Grave*, p. 133; Bristol, Gorsky, 'Bristol', sec. 4.3; Doyle, *Hospitals in Middlesbrough*, pp. 67–73.
96. Gorsky, 'Bristol', sec. 4.3.
97. For a discussion of the politics of these differences see ch. 7.
98. LJHAC, *First Annual Report*, p. 2.
99. This was the case in Barnsley but less so in Middlesbrough. Levene et al., *Cradle to Grave*, p. 133; Doyle, *Hospitals in Middlesbrough*, p. 71.
100. Sheffield Survey Report, TNA MH66/1076, p. 163.
101. Doyle, *Hospitals in Middlesbrough*, p. 72.
102. *Sheffield Independent*, 7 September 1938.
103. Gorsky, Mohan and Willis, *Mutualism and Health Care*, pp. 46–7; Cherry, 'Beyond National Health Insurance', p. 472; Hayes, 'Our Hospitals', pp. 97–102; Gosling, 'Open the Other Eye'.
104. See pp.47–8.

105. For a full discussion of these aspects see Gosling, 'Charity and Change', ch. 5 and this volume, ch. 5.
106. Jessop, *Annual Report*, 1937, p. 12.
107. Hayes, 'Our Hospitals'; Reinarz, *Birmingham*; Gosling, 'Charity and Change'; Lewis, Nixon and Doyle, 'Health Services in Middlesbrough'.
108. Ibid.
109. There have been relatively few discussions of accidents by historians and seemingly even fewer about how they were treated. B. Luckin and R. Cooter (eds), *Accidents in History: Injuries, Fatalities and Social Relations* (Amsterdam: Rodopi, 1997); B. Luckin, 'Accidents, Disasters and Cities', *Urban History*, 20:2 (1993), pp. 177–90.
110. Gorsky, 'Bristol', sec. 3.2.
111. For example Hardy, *Health and Medicine*, p. 84, although see claims by Moses Humberstone that panel doctors were sending patients to casualty who they should have treated. *Sheffield Independent*, 9 June 1932.
112. See below, pp. 82–4, n. 131 for further discussion of road accidents.
113. Explicit discussion of the growth in casualty numbers is rare in the secondary literature, though Cherry, 'Medical Care', does allude to concerns about outpatient 'abuse' (p. 277).
114. Sturdy and Cooter, 'Scientific Management', p. 9.
115. LGI, *Annual Report*, 1925, p. 15. For St Thomas' see Abel-Smith, *The Hospitals*, p. 334.
116. SRI, *Annual Report*, 1930, pp. 5–6. See also Sturdy and Cooter, 'Scientific Management', p. 5 and Gorsky, 'Bristol', sec. 3.2 for discussion of these trends elsewhere.
117. Even in the 1950s problems remained with the recording of outpatients and casualty patients as shown by the survey in Middlesbrough. A. D. Airth and D. J. Newell, *The Demand for Hospital Beds: Results of an Enquiry on Tees-side* (Newcastle: King's College, Newcastle, 1962), pp. 62–70.
118. SRI, *Annual Report*, 1933, p. 10.
119. Sturdy and Cooter, 'Scientific Management'. The Infirmary owned a copy of American College of Surgeons, *Hospital Standardization Report* of 1927, SCA NHS17/1/9/4/9. For the registration block see above, p. 49.
120. MOH Sheffield, *Annual Report*, 1930, p. 57.
121. Sheffield Survey Report, TNA MH66/1076, pp. 181–2.
122. Pickstone, *Medicine and Industrial Society*, p. 273.
123. *Sheffield Independent*, 25 April 1935; MOH Sheffield, *Annual Report*, 1934, p. 86.
124. Figures from Parsons, *Hospital Survey: Sheffield*. A similar plan in Manchester was slow to develop. Pickstone, *Medicine and Industrial Society*, p. 273.
125. Parsons, *Hospital Survey: Sheffield*, p. 19.
126. LJHAC, *First Annual Report*, p. 6. See also ch. 4, p. 97.
127. Dr Dick Medical Superintendent, 'Leeds City General Hospitals', MOH Leeds, *Annual Report*, 1937, p. 98.
128. MOH Leeds, *Annual Report*, 1938, pp. 94–5.
129. C. Pooley and J. Turnbull, 'Commuting, Transport and Urban Form: Manchester and Glasgow in the Mid-Twentieth Century', *Urban History*, 27:3 (2000), pp. 360–83, Law, 'Speed and Blood'.
130. S. O'Connell, *The Car and British Society: Class, Gender and Motoring, 1896–1939* (Manchester: Manchester University Press, 1998). For an international perspective see I. Borowy, 'Road Traffic Injuries: Social Change and Development', *Medical History*, 57:1 (2013), pp. 108–38. For the return of high mortality in the early years of the Second World War see B. Luckin, 'War on the Roads: Traffic, Accidents and Social Tension in

Britain, 1939–45', in Luckin and Cooter (eds), *Accidents*, pp. 234–54; and B. Luckin and D. Sheen, 'Defining Early Modern Automobility: The Road Traffic Accident Crisis in Manchester, 1939–45', *Cultural and Social History*, 6:2 (2009), pp. 211–30.

131. For example *Sheffield Star*, 27 November 1926. National road accident statistics for this period are discussed in Law, 'Speed and Blood', p. 499.
132. SRH, *Annual Report*, 1928, p. 11.
133. The figures in Leeds were generally well above average for large English cities, Luckin, 'War on the Roads', p. 238.
134. Pickstone, *Medicine and Industrial Society*, p. 273. For other cities Reinarz, *Birmingham*, p. 211 and Gorsky, 'Bristol', sec. 3.2.
135. LGI, *Annual Report*, AGM 1926, p. 25. This concern was still being expressed ten years later, LGI, *Annual Report*, 1935, p. 20.
136. SRI, *Annual Report*, 1933, p. 12.
137. LPD, *Annual Report*, 1927–8, p. 13.
138. LGI, *Annual Report*, AGM 1927, pp. 25–6.
139. SRI, *Annual Report*, 1926, p. 4.
140. Ibid.
141. LPD, *Annual Report*, 1927–8, p. 13.
142. LGI, *Annual Report*, AGM 1927, pp. 25–6.
143. SRH, *Annual Report*, 1929, p. 12.
144. Abel-Smith, *The Hospitals*, p. 325; SRH, *Annual Report*, 1931, p. 13.
145. SRI, *Annual Report*, 1931, pp. 10–1.
146. Pickstone, *Medicine and Industrial Society*, p. 273.
147. LGI, *Annual Report*, 1932, p. 15.
148. LGI, *Annual Report*, 1934, p. 16.
149. J. Moran, 'Crossing the Road in Britain', *Historical Journal*, 49:2 (2006), pp. 477–96; M. Gorsky, 'Public Health in Interwar England and Wales: Did It Fail?', *Dynamis*, 28 (2008), pp. 175–98; Luckin, 'War on the Roads', p. 247.
150. SRH, *Annual Report*, 1934, p. 10.
151. SRH, *Annual Report*, 1935, pp. 11–2.
152. For the situation in Manchester see Luckin and Sheen, 'Early Modern Automobility'.
153. For the problems in Hull see Levene, Powell and Stewart, 'Municipal Hospital Care', p. 13, and Eason, *Hospital Survey: Yorkshire*, pp. 62–5.

4 Specialization and the Challenges of Modern Medicine

1. G. Rosen, *Specialization in Medicine* (New York: Froben Press, 1944); R. Stevens, *Medical Practice in Modern England: The Impact of Specialization and State Medicine* (New Haven, CT: Yale University Press, 1966).
2. A. Digby, *Making a Medical Living: Doctors and Patients in the English Market for Medicine, 1720–1911* (Cambridge: Cambridge University Press, 1994).
3. L. Granshaw, '"Fame and Fortune by Means of Bricks and Mortar": The Medical Profession and Specialist Hospitals in Britain, 1800–1948', in Granshaw and Porter (eds), *The Hospital in History*, pp. 199–220; L. Granshaw, 'The Hospital', in W. F. Bynum and R. Porter (eds), *Companion Encyclopedia of the History of Medicine*, 2 vols (London: Routledge, 1993), vol. 2, pp. 1180–203.

4. Granshaw, 'Fame and Fortune', p. 206; LHC, *Hospitals of Liverpool*, pp. 5, 14; Reinarz, *Birmingham*, chs 2, 4 for eye and ear hospitals; Pickstone, *Medicine and Industrial Society*, chs 3, 6; Anning, 'Medicine in Leeds', pp. 221–3.

5. Heaman, *St Mary's*, pp. 106–9; Sturdy and Cooter, 'Scientific Management', p. 5.

6. C. Murphy, 'From Friedenheim to Hospice: A Century of Cancer Hospitals', in Granshaw and Porter (eds), *The Hospital in History*, pp. 221–41.

7. R. Dingwall, A. M. Rafferty and C. Webster, *An Introduction to the Social History of Nursing* (London: Routledge, 1988); Doyle, *Hospitals in Middlesbrough*, p. 49 for work of nurses in the eye department of the North Riding Infirmary.

8. LHC, *Hospitals of Liverpool*, p. 5; Reinarz, *Birmingham*; Pickstone, *Medicine and Industrial Society*.

9. Anning, *General Infirmary, Vol. II*; Anning, 'Medicine in Leeds', p. 222.

10. See ch. 3.

11. Harvey, *History of the Children's Hospital, Sheffield*.

12. Reinarz, *Birmingham*, pp. 207–14; Gorsky, 'Bristol', sec. 5.1; Doyle, 'Competition and Cooperation', pp. 351–4.

13. For a discussion of the introduction of the Finsen Lamp in Bradford Infirmary see A. Jamieson, 'More Than Meets the Eye: Revealing the Therapeutic Potential of 'Light', 1896–1910', *Social History of Medicine*, 26:4 (2013), pp. 715–37.

14. L. A. Hall, 'Venereal Diseases and Society in Britain from the Contagious Diseases Act to the National Health Service', in R. Davidson and L. A. Hall (eds), *Sex, Sin and Suffering: Venereal Disease and European Society since 1870* (London: Routledge, 2001), pp. 120–36.

15. Reinarz, *Birmingham*, pp. 115–16, 154–5. For developments elsewhere see Gorsky, 'Bristol', sec. 2.2.

16. Sturdy and Cooter, 'Scientific Management', pp. 6–8; LGI, *Annual Report*, 1936, pp. 38–9.

17. Sturdy and Cooter, 'Scientific Management', p. 13; A. Digby, *The Evolution of British General Practice, 1850–1948* (Oxford: Oxford University Press, 1999).

18. See pp. 186–7.

19. SRH, *Annual Report*, 1925, p. 9; Swan, 'Medical Education', pp. 139–40; Sturdy, 'Political Economy'.

20. LHW, *Annual Report*, 1932, p. 5.

21. Anning, *General Infirmary: Vol. II*.

22. Cherry, 'Medical Care', p. 279; Reinarz, *Birmingham*, p. 186.

23. MOH Leeds, *Annual Report*, 1918, pp. 49–50.

24. LGI, *Annual Report*, 1919, pp. 21–2.

25. See ch. 7.

26. Leeds B, *Annual Report*, 1948, p. 6.

27. Sheffield Survey Report, TNA MH66/1076, pp. 93–4.

28. Reinarz, *Birmingham*, p. 207; Gorsky, 'Bristol', sec. 3.1, Pickstone, *Medicine and Industrial Society*, p. 254.

29. Birmingham introduced a similar clinic around the same time. For a description of the techniques involved see Reinarz, *Birmingham*, pp. 192–3.

30. SRI, *Annual Report*, 1934, p. 10.

31. Pickstone, *Medicine and Industrial Society*, pp. 288–9.

32. SUH, *Annual Report*, 1944, p. 6.

33. MOH Leeds, *Annual Report*, 1944, p. 32; SUH, *Annual Report*, 1945, p. 5.

34. For the development of West Yorkshire mental health services see Ellis, 'Growth of County Asylums'.
35. Brumby, 'Dismantling the Poor Law of Lunacy'.
36. Reinarz, *Birmingham*, p. 206.
37. SRH, *Annual Report*, 1927, p. 9.
38. SRH, *Annual Report*, 1928, p. 11.
39. SRI, *Annual Report*, 1932, p. 7.
40. Brumby, 'Dismantling the Poor Law of Lunacy'.
41. LGI, *Annual Report*, 1934, p. 23.
42. Sheffield Survey Report, TNA MH66/1076, pp. 163–4; Pickstone, *Medicine and Industrial Society*, pp. 256–7; Gorsky, 'Bristol', sec. 4.3. For the experience of a range of appropriated hospitals see Powell, 'An Expanding Service'; and Levene, Powell and Stewart, 'Municipal Hospital Care'.
43. Leeds Survey Report, TNA MH66/711, Appendix O 1A.
44. Gorsky, 'Bristol', sec. 4.3. See also Pinker, *Hospital Statistics*, p. 77.
45. Pickstone, *Medicine and Industrial Society*, p. 273.
46. LJHAC, *First Annual Report*, p. 5–6.
47. MOH Sheffield, *Annual Report*, 1935, p. 89.
48. Sheffield Survey Report, TNA MH66/1076, p. 171.
49. MOH Sheffield, *Annual Report*, 1935, p. 88.
50. MOH Sheffield, *Annual Report*, 1935, p. 82.
51. *Sheffield Independent*, 5 September 1938.
52. For a similar situation in the south-west of England see M. Gorsky, 'Local Government Health Services in Interwar England: Problems of Quantification and Interpretation', *Bulletin of the History of Medicine*, 85:3 (2011), pp. 384–412, on pp. 399–400.
53. Cooter, 'Meaning of Fractures'. For the broader issues involved see Cooter, *Surgery and Society*, especially ch. 3.
54. Ibid., chs 3, 6, 10.
55. Ibid., ch. 10.
56. For example *Final Report of the Inter-departmental Committee on the Rehabilitation of Persons Injured by Accidents* (London: HMSO, 1939) [Chairman, Malcolm Delevingne]. For an example of the development of rehabilitation services in the coalfields of Wales, see A. Borsay, '"Fit to Work": Representing Rehabilitation on the South Wales Coalfield during the Second World War', in A. Borsay (ed.), *Medicine in Wales c. 1800–2000: Public Service or Private Commodity?* (Cardiff: University of Wales Press, 2003), pp. 128–53.
57. A. Borsay, 'Disciplining Disabled Bodies: The Development of Orthopaedic Medicine in Britain, c. 1800–1939', in D. M. Turner and K. Stagg (eds), *Social Histories of Disability and Deformity: Bodies, Images and Experiences* (London: Routledge, 2006), pp. 97–116.
58. Reinarz, *Birmingham*, p. 114.
59. Borsay, 'Disciplining Disabled Bodies', p. 103; R. Cooter, 'Jones, Sir Robert, first baronet (1857–1933)', *ODNB*.
60. Cooter, *ODNB*; Reinarz, *Birmingham*, p. 201.
61. Cooter, *ODNB*.
62. In particular Jones's team at the Southern Hospital in Liverpool and one or two other younger surgeons influenced by Jones and Americans like the Mayo brothers, Cooter, *Surgery and Society*, ch. 3.

63. Cooter, *ODNB*; Cooter, 'Meaning of Fractures', p. 307, n. 7.
64. Cooter, *ODNB*; M. Harrison, *The Medical War: British Military Medicine in the First World War* (Oxford: Oxford University Press, 2010).
65. Cooter, 'Meaning of Fractures', pp. 308–9.
66. Pickstone, *Medicine and Industrial Society*, pp. 286–7; Cooter, 'Meaning of Fractures', pp. 310–2.
67. Reinarz, *Birmingham*, pp. 206, 215. See also p. 203 for number of orthopaedic hospitals and clinics operating by 1938.
68. MOH Sheffield, *Annual Report*, 1927, pp. 83–4, which showed a halving of the length of stay at King Edward VII's and a doubling of the number of admissions between 1920 and 1927. Indeed, the hospital was admitting patients from outside Sheffield by this time.
69. The Edgar Allen Institute, Report and Statement of Accounts, *c.* 1934 (Sheffield, 1934) [hereafter Edgar Allen Institute, *Annual Report* followed by year].
70. For Edwardian discussion of rehabilitation of injured workers see Cooter, *Surgery and Society*, p. 201.
71. Edgar Allen Institute, *Annual Report*, 1933, pp. 6–7.
72. Pickstone, *Medicine and Industrial Society*, pp. 286–9; Reinarz, *Birmingham*, pp. 206, 215.
73. He served in the RAMC throughout the First World War and spent some time in a specialist unit concerned with 'penetrating wounds of the chest'. See his obituary in *British Medical Journal* [hereafter *BMJ*] (10 June 1961), p. 1690. For his work on scoliosis see R. G. Abercrombie, 'The Pathology of Adolescent Scoliosis', *BMJ* (27 January 1938), pp. 215–17.
74. 'Obituary: J. B. Ferguson Wilson, M.S. F.R.C.S.', *BMJ* (24 October 1959), p. 829.
75. 'Obituary Notices: Sir Frank Holdsworth, M.A., M.Chir, F.R.C.S.', *BMJ* (27 December 1969), p. 812.
76. SRH, *Annual Report*, 1938, p. 10. For the development of X-rays at the Sheffield hospitals see W. H. J. Coombs, *The History of Radiology and Radiography in the United Sheffield Hospitals* (Sheffield: Privately printed, 1981).
77. SRI, *Annual Report*, 1935, p. 12.
78. SRI, *Annual Report*, 1936, p. 11.
79. SRI, *Annual Report*, 1937, p. 14.
80. Ibid., pp. 14–15.
81. Cooter, *Surgery and Society*, pp. 199–217.
82. 'Obituary Notices: Sir Frank Holdsworth', p. 812.
83. Similar relationships between the Miners' Welfare and hospitals were not a feature of mining areas in Scotland, Wales or the north-east of England, according to the Wellcome Trust project on mining and disability led by Anne Borsay, Vicky Long and Arthur McIvor, *Disability and Industrial Society: A Comparative Cultural History of British Coalfields, 1780–1948*, at http://www.dis-ind-soc.org.uk/en/index.htm [accessed 12 December 2013].
84. SRH, *Annual Report*, 1932, p. 18.
85. See pp. 50–1.
86. SRI, *Annual Report*, 1939, pp. 10–1; Cooter, *Surgery and Society*.
87. SRI, *Annual Report*, 1937, p. 15.
88. SRI, *Annual Report*, 1937, pp. 14–15.
89. SRH, *Annual Report*, 1937, p. 12.
90. 'Obituary Notices: Sir Frank Holdsworth', p. 812.

91. 'Rehabilitation of Injured Miners', *BMJ* (24 June 1944), p. 851.
92. SUH, *Annual Report*, 1945, p. 7.
93. Cooter, 'Meaning of Fractures'.
94. SUH, *Annual Report*, 1945, p. 7.
95. SUH, *Annual Report*, 1944, pp. 5–6.
96. LPD, *Annual Report*, 1937, p. 9.
97. LPD, *Annual Report*, 1936, p. 9.
98. LPD, *Annual Report*, 1935, p. 10.
99. LGI, *Annual Report*, 1922, p. 14.
100. 'Daw, Samuel Wilfrid (1875–1944)', *Plarr's Lives of the Fellows Online* http://liveson-line.rcseng.ac.uk/biogs/E003948b.htm [accessed 20 November 2013].
101. LGI Faculty Minutes, 1913–29, 12 September 1924, West Yorkshire Archives Leeds [hereafter WYL] 2295/5/3. Also see ch. 7.
102. *BMJ* (14 April 1984), p. 1170.
103. LGI, *Annual Report*, 1936, p. 29.
104. *Final Report of the Inter-departmental Committee on the Rehabilitation of Persons Injured by Accidents*.
105. LJHAC, *First Annual Report*, pp. 6–7; *Second Annual Report*, p. 6.
106. LJHAC, *First Annual Report*, pp. 6–7; *Second Annual Report*, p. 6.
107. LGI, *Annual Report*, 1938, p. 46.
108. LGI, *Annual Report*, 1932, p. 32.
109. 'New Hope for Foot Sufferers', *Sheffield Independent*, 23 June 1938. This suggests that the layman did not see a particular separation between bedside and bench, a view recently put forward by S. Sturdy, 'Looking for Trouble: Medical Science and Clinical Practice in the Historiography of Modern Medicine', *Social History of Medicine*, 24:3 (2011), pp. 739–57.
110. LGI, *Annual Report*, 1937, p. 26.
111. Edgar Allen Institute, *Annual Report*, 1936, p. 4.
112. See ch. 3.
113. Hardy, *Health and Medicine*, p. 105. Webster gives a figure of 35 per cent of notified births in hospital but no reference to a source, Webster, *Health Services since the War*, p. 7. They had reached around 80 per cent in London according to Cherry, *Medical Services*, p. 59, while in Lancashire the figures, including Manchester, were not as high as Leeds. Pickstone, *Medicine and Industrial Society*, pp. 241–7.
114. Parsons, *Hospital Survey: Sheffield*, pp. 15–16.
115. Nuttall, 'Maternity Charities'.
116. Gorsky, 'Bristol', sec. 4.3; Pickstone, *Medicine and Industrial Society*, pp. 275–6.
117. Nuttall, 'Maternity Charities', pp. 371–4; joint working was particularly evident in Bristol in the 1920s, Gorsky, 'Bristol' and Gosling, 'Charity and Change', pp. 73–5.
118. MOH Leeds, *Annual Report*, 1946, p. 8.
119. Beds in Maternity Hospitals increased from 3,000 to 10,000 between 1921 and 1938. Pinker, *Hospital Statistics*, pp. 73, 77.
120. MOH Leeds, *Annual Report*, 1946, p. 8.
121. This is also the conclusion of Nuttall from her work on Edinburgh. For a survey of the literature critical of the medicalizing effects of the Act, see Nuttall, 'Medical Charities', pp. 371–5.
122. See ch. 7.
123. MOH Leeds, *Annual Report*, 1918, p. 45.

124. MOH Leeds, *Annual Report*, 1919, p. 49.

125. MOH Leeds, *Annual Report*, 1920 p. 87.

126. MOH Leeds, *Annual Report*, 1923, p. 122. For the pessimistic case see Webster, 'Healthy or Hungry'. Gorsky has recently challenged the approach of Webster and others by pointing to a number of similar initiatives. Gorsky, 'Public Health', p. 182.

127. The decline of illegitimate institutional births is also noted by Nuttall for Edinburgh and by Gosling for Bristol, Nuttall, 'Maternal Charities', p. 377; Gosling, 'Charity and Change', p. 73.

128. MOH Leeds, *Annual Report*, 1928, p. 135.

129. Leeds Survey Report, TNA MH66/1072, Maternity Report, pp. 26–7.

130. Ibid., p. 26.

131. MOH Leeds, *Annual Report*, 1934, p. 14.

132. Ibid., p. 180.

133. Similar schemes existed in other cities with teaching hospitals, including Manchester and Edinburgh. Pickstone, *Medicine and Industrial Society*, pp. 243–7; Nuttall, 'Maternity Charities', p. 377. See ch. 7 for discussion of coordination of maternity services.

134. MOH Leeds, *Annual Report*, 1946, p. 9. For more detail see ch. 1.

135. Leeds Survey Report, TNA MH66/1072, Maternity Report, p. 4.

136. For example Reinarz, *Birmingham*, p. 198. For an alternative view, which emphasizes the small numbers involved in MMR deaths and the volatility of the figures, see Gorsky, 'Public Health', p. 182.

137. Leeds Survey Report, TNA MH66/1072, Maternity Report, p. 24. Most historians are of the opinion that hospitals made little difference to maternal mortality before sulphonamides. Hardy, *Health and Medicine*, p. 105; Pickstone, *Medicine and Industrial Society*, pp. 246–7.

138. LMH, *Annual Report*, 1935, pp. 5, 7, 12, 29; MOH Leeds, *Annual Report*, 1936, pp. 157–61.

139. MOH Leeds, *Annual Report*, 1935, p. 165.

140. See p. 106 for more discussion of this development in Sheffield.

141. Eason, *Hospital Survey: Yorkshire*, pp. 32–3. See also ch. 2.

142. MOH Sheffield, *Annual Report*, 1934, p. 112.

143. Sheffield Survey Report, TNA MH66/1076, p. 77.

144. See ch. 7.

145. MOH Sheffield, *Annual Report*, 1935, p. 97.

146. Ibid., p. 82.

147. Sheffield Survey Report, TNA MH66/1076, pp. 80–1. Recent work on the adjoining county of Derbyshire has found that doctors increased their share of births in the first two decades of the twentieth century but it would seem that this trend ceased from around 1925 as hospitals became the main competition for midwives. A. Reid, 'Mrs Killer and Dr Crook: Birth Attendants and Birth Outcomes in Early Twentieth-century Derbyshire', *Medical History*, 56:4 (2012), pp. 511–30.

148. Sheffield Survey Report, TNA MH66/1076, p. 82.

149. Appendices to Sheffield Survey Report, App Q; Minutes of subcommittee considering allocation of hospital beds, TNA MH66/873.

150. For further discussion of these issues see ch. 7.

151. *Sheffield Telegraph*, 2 June 1937; Jessop, *Annual Report*, 1937, pp. 11–2. For the Birmingham flying squad see Reinarz, *Birmingham*, p. 199.

152. Sheffield Survey Report, TNA MH66/1076, maternity section.

153. Parsons, *Hospital Survey: Sheffield*, pp. 19–20 makes no reference to integration of service between the two sectors.

5 Finance

1. Gorsky, Mohan and Powell, 'Financial Health'; Cherry, 'Regional Comparators', p. 61.
2. R. Titmuss, *Problems of Social Policy* (London: HMSO, 1950). This view is also promoted by Webster, *Health Services since the War*.
3. Cherry, 'Accountability, Entitlement and Control'; Cherry, 'Before the National Health Service', p. 307.
4. Gosling, 'Charity and Change'; Gosling, 'Open the Other Eye'.
5. Hayes, 'Our Hospitals'; Hayes and Doyle, 'Eggs, Rags and Whist Drives'.
6. J. Mohan, '"The Caprice of Charity". Geographical Variations in the Finances of British Voluntary Hospitals before the NHS', in Gorsky and Sheard (eds), *Financing Medicine*, pp. 77–92; Doyle, 'Labour and Hospitals'.
7. Gosling, 'Charity and Change'.
8. SRI, *Annual Report*, 1938 quoted in SHC, *Annual Report of the '1d in the £' Fund* (Sheffield: SHC, 1923–48) [hereafter SHC, *Annual Report*, followed by year], 1938, pp. 10–1.
9. Gorsky, Mohan and Powell, 'Financial Health', pp. 542–6. Abel-Smith, *The Hospitals*, p. 384; Webster, *Health Services since the War*, p. 4 suggest it was the voluntary hospitals desire to maintain their technical lead over the municipal sector that drove rising costs.
10. Pinker, *Hospital Statistics*, table 33, pp. 155–6.
11. Pickstone, *Medicine and Industrial Society*, p. 252; Gorsky, 'Bristol', figure 3; Doyle and Nixon, 'Voluntary Hospital Finance'; Doyle, *Hospitals in Middlesbrough*; Hayes and Doyle, 'Eggs, Rags and Whist Drives', table 1.
12. Gorsky, Mohan and Powell, 'Financial Health', pp. 542–6 especially figure 1; Sturdy and Cooter, 'Scientific Management', pp. 421–66. See chs 2 and 3, this volume.
13. LGI, *Annual Report*, 1919, p. 10.
14. Gorsky, 'Bristol', figure 3; *Annual Report of the Cottage Hospital, North Ormesby, Middlesbrough*, 1920 and 1938 (Middlesbrough, 1921, 1939).
15. Gorsky, Mohan and Powell, 'Financial Health', p. 544, figure 1.
16. Ibid., pp. 544–6; Webster, *Health Services since the War*, p. 4. See ch. 2 for attempts to attract nursing staff.
17. Jessop, *Annual Report*, 1937, supplement p. 6; LGI, *Annual Report*, 1936, p. 18.
18. Sturdy and Cooter, 'Scientific Management', pp. 16–26.
19. Cherry, 'Before the National Health Service'; Gorsky, Mohan and Willis, *Mutualism and Health Care*; Doyle, 'Power and Accountability'.
20. For a focus on other forms of payment see Gosling, 'Open the Other Eye'.
21. LHC, *Hospitals of Liverpool*, pp. 28–9; Gorsky, Mohan and Willis, *Mutualism and Health Care*, pp. 50–1.
22. Ibid., p. 44; Reinarz, *Birmingham*, pp. 184–5.
23. Doyle and Nixon, 'Voluntary Hospital Finance'.
24. Pickstone, *Medicine and Industrial Society*, p. 252, table 3.
25. Gosling, 'Charity and Change', p. 191; Gorsky, 'Bristol', sec. 3.3.
26. Hayes and Doyle, 'Eggs, Rags and Whist Drives', p. 718, table 1.
27. Cherry, 'Beyond National Health Insurance', Appendix 2.

28. This paragraph is based on the list of subscribers and donors and the annual accounts of the SRI, SRH and the Sheffield Hospitals Council published in the Annual Reports between 1920 and 1938. Endnotes will be reserved for specific information.
29. For example, SRH, *Annual Report* 1921, p. 15.
30. J. Roach, 'The Sheffield Community and Public Work, 1790–1914', *Yorkshire Archaeological Journal*, 77 (2005), pp. 225–40.
31. Hayes and Doyle, 'Eggs, Rags and Whist Drives', pp. 717–20.
32. Eleven Luptons and seven Kitsons also subscribed over £200 collectively. LGI, *Annual Report*, 1938, pp. 71–83.
33. S. Gunn, 'Class, Identity and the Urban: The Middle Class in England, 1800–1950', *Urban History*, 31:1 (2004), pp. 1–19. For a more optimistic interpretation see R. H. Trainor, 'The Middle Class', in Daunton (ed.), *The Cambridge Urban History of Britain*, pp. 673–713.
34. LGI, *Annual Report*, 1920, 1928, 1938.
35. For example LGI, *Annual Report* 1928, pp. 152–212 provides a list of all of the contributions from towns and villages along with the number of patients treated and the cost of treatment.
36. For difficulties extracting payment at a suitable rate from other schemes see Abel-Smith, *The Hospitals*, pp. 385–6; Gorsky, Mohan and Willis, *Mutualism and Health Care*, pp. 76–81.
37. LGI, *Annual Report*, for example 1920, p. 114; 1938, p. 88.
38. Hayes and Doyle, 'Eggs, Rags and Whist Drives', pp. 723–5.
39. LGI, *Annual Report*, 1920, pp. 111–20; 1928, pp. 46–123; 1938, pp. 84–95.
40. Cherry, 'Regional Comparators'.
41. SRI, *Annual Report*, 1924, p. 5.
42. Undated newscutting, Jessop Cuttings Book, SCA NHS17/1/9/1/6; SRH, *Annual Report*, 1919, p. 8.
43. SRI, *Annual Report*, 1938, p. 16.
44. LGI, *Annual Report*, 1919, p. 37, 1938, p. 51.
45. SRI, *Annual Report*, 1932, p. 19.
46. SRH, *Annual Report*, 1936, p. 16.
47. N. Hayes, 'Did We Really Want a National Health Service? Hospitals, Patients and Public Opinions before 1948', *English Historical Review*, 127 (2012), pp. 625–61. Leeds Voluntary Hospitals' Fund, Minutes, 1923–33, 8 July 1927, WYL 2295/25/3. [This body had various names including Leeds Employers' Contribution Fund, Leeds Voluntary Hospitals' Fund and Leeds Voluntary Hospitals' Committee but Leeds Voluntary Hospitals' Fund will be used throughout.]
48. SRI, *Annual Report*, 1935, p. 10.
49. SRI, *Annual Report*, 1921, p. 6.
50. SRI, *Annual Report*, 1922, p. 7; SRH, *Annual Report*, 1922, p. 7.
51. SRH, *Annual Report*, 1928, p. 12; SRI, *Annual Report*, 1929, p. 13; 1935, p. 10; SRH, *Annual Report*, 1937, p. 14. See also *Sheffield Independent*, 29 October 1929 for an article on the need to support the Rag.
52. LGI, *Annual Report*, 1926, p. 13–14.
53. C. Dyhouse, *Students: A Gendered History* (London: Routledge, 2005), pp. 191–6; Jessop, *Annual Report*, 1936, p. 7; 1926, p. 8 and SRI, *Annual Report*, 1940, p. 15.
54. *Sheffield Daily Telegraph*, 17 January 1935.
55. Reinarz, *Birmingham*, p. 186 for the collapse of subscriptions at the Ear Hospital.

56. Cherry, 'Regional Comparators', pp. 65–7; Doyle, 'Hospital Contributory Schemes', pp. 294–6, 299–301. See also chs 3, 6 and 7 in this volume.
57. The Joint Consultative and Advisory Hospitals Council, *General Statement of the Position of the Voluntary Hospitals of Sheffield, Prepared by the Collation Committee, for the Use of the Council* (Sheffield: Northend, 1920); Doyle, 'Labour and Hospitals'; SHC, *Sheffield 1d in the £ Scheme: 1919–1948*.
58. SHC, *Annual Report*, e.g. 1926, pp. 30–70.
59. See Gorsky, Mohan and Willis, *Mutualism and Health Care*, pp. 255–7 for additional benefits.
60. SHC, *Annual Report*, 1932, p. 32; 1933, p. 36. Sheffield and District Association of Hospital Contributors, Minutes of the Special Meeting of Delegates, 26 January, 1932. LHC, *Hospitals of Liverpool*, p. 30.
61. Doyle, 'Hospital Contributory Schemes', p. 294.
62. Leeds Workpeople's Hospital Fund, *Annual Report*, 1930 p. 16; 1931, pp. 13–14 [hereafter LWHF, *Annual Report*, followed by year]; *Leeds Hospital Magazine*, September 1931, p. 163.
63. Gorsky, Mohan and Willis, *Mutualism and Health Care*, pp. 73–6.
64. Abel-Smith, *The Hospitals*, p. 386.
65. *Yorkshire Post*, 27 September 1920. The scheme is mentioned favourably by Gorsky, Mohan and Willis, *Mutualism and Health Care*, p. 51.
66. LGI, *Annual Report*, for example 1919, pp. 17–18; 1920, p. 18; 1925, p. 11; 1928, p. 41. For the operation of this and subsequent committees see WYL 2295/25/2–3.
67. The system used for establishing the payments was similar to that developed in the Durham coalfield for funding workmen's compensation.
68. Gorsky, Mohan and Willis, *Mutualism and Health Care*, p. 51.
69. SHC, *Sheffield 1d in the £ Scheme*, p. 29.
70. LWHF, *Annual Report*, 1930, pp. 13–14; 1934, p. 16; 1938, p. 14; Doyle, 'Hospital Contributory Schemes', p. 300.
71. Leeds Voluntary Hospitals' Fund, Minutes 1933–49, 4 May 1933, 5 May 1937, 8 September 1937, WYL 2295/25/2; Leeds and District Employers' Hospitals Fund, *Annual Report*, 1934, p. 3.
72. Leeds and District Voluntary Hospital Fund, *Annual Report*, 1940, p. 10.
73. Leeds Voluntary Hospitals' Fund, Minutes 1933–49, 7 January 1942, WYL 2295/25/2.
74. LGI, *Annual Report*, 1945, p. 41.
75. Gorsky, Mohan and Willis point this out in *Mutualism and Health Care*, pp. 34–7. For the other schemes see Cherry, 'Beyond National Health Insurance', p. 467; LHC, *Hospitals of Liverpool*, p. 29; Reinarz, *Birmingham*, p. 195.
76. Willis, 'Health Care in Sheffield', p. 133.
77. Gorsky, Mohan and Willis, *Mutualism and Health Care*, pp. 51–2; Hayes and Doyle, 'Eggs, Rags and Whist Drives', p. 270.
78. Cherry, 'Before the National Health Service', p. 308.
79. See Doyle, 'Hospital Contributory Schemes' for further details.
80. Cherry, *Medical Services*, p. 73; Gorsky, Mohan and Powell, 'Financial Health' consider the importance of investments, especially at the end of the 1930s, pp. 540–2.
81. Cherry, 'Before the National Health Service', table 5; Gorsky, Mohan and Powell, 'Financial Health', table 5.
82. For the national picture see Cherry, 'Before the National Health Service', pp. 312–5, 321–2; Gorsky, Mohan and Powell, 'Financial Health', pp. 540–2.

83. LGI, *Annual Report*, 1934, p. 39; 1938, p. 49; SRI, *Annual Report*, 1934, p. 55; 1938, p. 57; SRH, *Annual Report*, 1934, p. 21; 1938, p. 29.

84. Webster, *Health Services since the War*, p. 4.

85. SRH, *Annual Report*, 1921, p. 6; SRI, *Annual Report*, 1922, p. 9.

86. See ch. 6.

87. LMH, *Annual Report*, 1928, p. 16; 1938, p. 14; 1947, p. 13.

88. Gorsky, 'Bristol', figure 6a.

89. LGI Weekly Board Minutes, 1919–29, 7 November 1924, 6 December 1924, WYL 2295/3/26. The document entitled 'General Infirmary at Leeds, September 1924' can be found loose in LGI Faculty Minutes, 1913–29, WYL 2295/5/3.

90. See LGI, *Annual Report*, for example 1928, for comments on OP almoner income p. 15. For almoners generally, see ch. 3.

91. LGI, *Annual Report*, 1930, p. 15.

92. LGI, *Annual Report*, 1931, p. 16.

93. LGI, *Annual Report*, 1935, p. 20; 1936, p. 23; 1937, p. 20.

94. LGI, *Annual Report*, 1933, p. 59; 1938, p. 51; 1939, p. 27.

95. In 1933 the LGI had refused to support an LWHF plan to take over all the out of city schemes, in all likelihood to prevent the Leeds scheme, with its inadequate contribution base, dominating the county.

96. Gosling, 'Charity and Change', ch. 5.

97. LHW, *Annual Report*, 1938, p. 16.

98. LGI, *Annual Report*, 1947, p. 45.

99. See ch. 7, p. 181 for details of services for VD and childhood orthopaedics.

100. SRH, *Annual Report*, 1935, p. 52.

101. LGI, *Annual Report*, 1927, pp. 17–18.

102. SRH, *Annual Report*, 1929, p. 14; SRI, *Annual Report*, 1929, p. 10; 1934, p. 18.

103. LGI, *Annual Report*, 1919, p. 121.

104. LGI, *Annual Report*, 1929.

105. Back page advert, SRI, *Annual Report*, 1935.

106. LGI, *Annual Report*, 1928, pp. 146–51.

107. Hayes, 'Our Hospitals', p. 101.

108. SHC, *Annual Report*, 1927, p. 12; 1934, p. 27; LGI, *Annual Report*, 1932, p. 19.

109. LGI, *Annual Report*, 1929, p. 156.

110. SRH, *Annual Report*, 1932, p. 11; 1933, p. 9.

111. Hayes and Doyle, 'Eggs, Rags and Whist Drives'.

112. Hayes, 'Our Hospitals'; Hayes and Doyle, 'Eggs, Rags and Whist Drives'; Reinarz, *Birmingham*, pp. 185, 200.

113. LGI, *Annual Report*, 1930, p. 29; 1938, p. 31.

114. SRI, *Annual Report*, 1930, p. 9; 1930, p. 9; 1938, p. 16.

115. SHC, *Annual Report*, 1924, p. 19; 1925, p. 8.

116. Doyle, *Hospitals in Middlesbrough*, pp. 38–9.

117. SRH, *Annual Report*, 1931, p. 16.

118. SRI, *Annual Report*, 1929, p. 15.

119. Gorsky, Mohan and Powell, 'Financial Health', pp. 536, 540; Cherry, 'Before the National Health Service', p. 309; The lack of uniform accounting methods makes a nationally based analysis impossible. Pinker, *Hospital Statistics*, p. 143.

120. LGI, *Annual Report*, 1935, p. 17. See also LGI, *Annual Report*, 1934, p. 29.

121. Hayes and Doyle, 'Eggs, Rags and Whist Drives', pp. 728–9; Reinarz, *Birmingham*, p. 206.
122. LGI, *Annual Report*, 1938, pp. 13–15.
123. SRH, *Annual Report,* 1921, p. 7.
124. Roach, 'Sheffield Community'.
125. *Sheffield Guardian*, 14 October 1926.
126. Gorsky, 'Bristol', sec. 3.1; Hayes, 'Our Hospitals', pp. 91, 100; Reinarz, *Birmingham*, pp. 82, 146, 201, 146.
127. Cherry, 'Before the National Health Service', pp. 321–2; Gorsky, Mohan and Powell, 'Financial Health', pp. 540–2.
128. *Sheffield Telegraph*, 28 December 1918.
129. *Sheffield Telegraph*, 4 January 1919; *Yorkshire Post*, 1 July 1924. For the role of leading donors elsewhere see Gorsky, 'Bristol', sec. 5.1; Reinarz, *Birmingham*, p. 213.
130. *Sheffield Telegraph*, 4 June 1932, p. 5.
131. SRH, *Annual Report*, 1932, pp. 17–18.
132. Sheffield Trades and Labour Council, Minutes of Executive Committee, 21 June 1932, SCA LD1645.
133. SRH, *Annual Report*, 1932, pp. 8–9, 18–21. The Graves Trust subsequently supported the building of the OP Department and the establishment of a Radium Institute in 1942.
134. LGI, *Annual Report*, 1933, pp. 14, 29.
135. LGI, *Annual Report*, 1935, p. 17. The largest contribution was the £15,000 voted by the Labour-led Leeds City Council.
136. LGI, *Annual Report*, 1935, pp. 39–43.
137. Sheffield United Hospitals Collection, Printed Brochure, 'Sheffield Voluntary Hospitals Million Pound Appeal', The City Hall, Tuesday, 19 July 1938, SCA NHS12/3/6/3.
138. Reinarz, *Birmingham*, p. 213.
139. Ellis to the Chief Medical Officer, 5 August 1938, TNA MH58/319.
140. Sheffield United Hospitals Collection, Eighth Annual Report, Sheffield Voluntary Hospitals Million Pound Appeal Fund, 1946, SCA NHS12/3/6/3.
141. Gorsky, Mohan and Willis, *Mutualism and Health Care*, pp. 92–123.
142. For example Reinarz, *Birmingham*, pp. 199, 202, 204, 206 for the joint appeal involving the Queens, General and Ear Hospitals around 1930.
143. Gorsky, Mohan and Powell, 'Financial Health', pp. 540–2 for a discussion of investments at the end of the 1930s.
144. For a discussion of this element of 'subscriber democracy' see the work of R. J. Morris, especially R. J. Morris, 'Structure, Culture and Society in British Towns', in Daunton (ed.), *The Cambridge Urban History of Britain*, pp. 395–426.
145. Martin Gorsky has, however, managed to unravel some aspects of this for the south-west, e.g. Gorsky, 'Local Government', pp. 396–9.
146. I am very grateful to Alysa Levene, John Stewart, Martin Powell and Becky Taylor for providing me with the spreadsheets for their calculations of annual per capita expenditure on health activities between 1922 and 1936 discussed in their book, Levene et al., *Cradle to Grave*, and especially in Levene, Powell and Stewart, 'Municipal Health Expenditure'.
147. Levene, Powell and Stewart, 'Municipal Hospital Care'. The following analysis is based on their data drawn from Levene, Powell and Stewart, 'Municipal Health Expenditure', which includes information on per capita spending across a range of public health headings in the eighty-three English and Welsh county boroughs between 1922 and 1936.

148. The top five spenders at this point were Salford, Manchester, West Bromwich, Liverpool and Rochdale.
149. For a discussion of the weakness of some of the sources and methods used by historians to estimate local authority health spending see Gorsky, 'Local Government', pp. 396–404.
150. For interwar municipal spending see Doyle, 'Changing Functions of Urban Government', pp. 293–5.
151. Gorsky, 'Local Government', pp. 409–10.
152. See ch. 6.
153. Sheffield Survey Report, TNA MH66/1076, p. 210, and ch. 3.
154. Leeds Survey Report, TNA MH66/1072, p. 69.
155. Gorsky, 'Local Government', table 1, p. 402.
156. Sheffield Survey Report, TNA MH66/1076, p. 210.
157. Contrast this with the enthusiastic use of almoners in Leeds. See ch. 6.
158. SHC, *Annual Report*, 1938, p. 29; 1946, p. 25.
159. Pickstone, *Medicine and Industrial Society*, pp. 256–64; Gorsky, 'Bristol', sec. 5.3.
160. TA CB/M/H 14, 'Matters Chatted about and Noted for Future Reference'. Special Reports of the Medical Officer of Health [1942] quoted in Doyle, 'Competition and Cooperation', p. 353.
161. Leeds Survey Report, TNA MH66/1072, report by Dame Janet Campbell on Infant and Child Welfare Services, p. 9.
162. Leeds Survey Report, TNA MH66/711, Appendix O.1, O.3.
163. Sheffield Survey Report, TNA MH66/1076, p. 209.
164. For similar criticisms see Gorsky, 'Local Government', pp. 404–5.
165. For example Bell and Millward, 'Public Health Expenditure and Mortality'.
166. Leeds Corporation Sanitary Committee, *Leeds City Hospitals: Seacroft and Killingbeck*.
167. Leeds Survey Report, TNA MH66/711, Appendix O.
168. The survey report references approval of a significant loan for improvements at St James's in 1931, Leeds Survey Report, TNA MH66/1072.
169. Mohan, *Planning*, pp. 40–1, 57; Levene, Powell and Stewart, 'Municipal Hospital Care', p. 10.
170. Leeds Survey Report, TNA MH66/1072, pp. 48–9.
171. Leeds Survey Report, TNA MH66/711, Appendix L.
172. Pickstone, *Medicine and Industrial Society*.
173. 'Sheffield Municipal and Voluntary Hospitals Joint Advisory Committee' Minutes, 18 July 1938, SCA NHS28/10/1; Sheffield Labour Party, *Labour Accomplishes*, pp. 5–6.
174. City of Leeds, *Opening of the New Extensions at St. James's Hospital*. See also ch. 2.
175. A minute from 1934 in the Leeds Survey file observed that there was little prospect of major work at St James's due in part to the slum clearance programme. The following year, the Labour Council was still expressing caution around major expenditure due to the economic situation. TNA MH66/711.
176. Hayes and Doyle, 'Eggs, Rags and Whist Drives'.
177. Hayes, 'Did We Really Want a National Health Service'.

6 The Politics of Hospital Provision

1. Brief surveys appear in Abel-Smith, *The Hospitals*; Cherry, *Medical Services*; Mohan, *Planning*.
2. This is what emerges from discussion of the debates around a national health service after 1938, for example in Webster, *Health Services Since the War*; Webster, 'Conflict

and Consensus'; Gorsky, Mohan and Willis, *Mutualism and Health Care*. But it is often simplified in general texts like R. Lowe, *The Welfare State in Britain since 1945*, 3rd edn (Basingstoke: Palgrave Macmilla, 2004) and Jones, *Health and Society*.

3. Pickstone, *Medicine and Industrial Society*; Welshman, *Municipal Medicine*; Mohan, *Planning*; Reinarz, *Birmingham*; Gorsky, 'Bristol'; Gorsky, 'Threshold of a New Era'; Rivett, *London Hospital System*; Levene et al., *Cradle to Grave*; Stewart, 'Healthy London', Willis, 'Health Care in Sheffield'.

4. Doyle, 'Labour and Hospitals'.

5. Levene, *Cradle to Grave*.

6. Gunn, 'Class, Identity and the Urban'; Morris, 'Structure, Culture and Society in British Towns'; Trainor, 'The Middle Class'; B. M. Doyle, 'The Structure of Elite Power in the Early Twentieth-Century City: Norwich, 1900–35', *Urban History*, 24:2 (1997), pp. 179–99.

7. For a discussion of similar questions in a municipal context see Levene et al., *Cradle to Grave* and, to a lesser extent, Pickstone, *Medicine and Industrial Society*.

8. These are most readily found in the older literature, including Abel-Smith, *The Hospitals*; Webster, *Health Services since the War*; and more recently Mohan, *Planning*.

9. Such distinctions are implicit in Pickstone, *Medicine and Industrial Society*, with the party clearly having some influence in much of Lancashire, though not in Tory Liverpool.

10. Levene et al., *Cradle to Grave*, chs 4, 7.

11. Gorsky, *Patterns of Philanthropy*, pp. 157–8; Waddington, *London Hospitals*, especially chs 5 and 6; Cherry, 'Accountability, Entitlement and Control'; Reinarz, *Birmingham*, in particular pp. 82–92 on the Hospital for Women.

12. Doyle, 'Power and Accountability'.

13. Ibid.

14. LGI, *Annual Report*, 1948, pp. 13–14.

15. Pickstone, *Medicine and Industrial Society*, pp. 253–4; N. Hayes, 'Counting Civil Society: Deconstructing Elite Participation in the Provincial English City, 1900–1950', *Urban History*, 40:2 (2013), pp. 287–314, on p. 297.

16. Trainor, 'The Middle Class', pp. 699–703; Gorsky, 'Bristol', sec. 5.1; Reinarz, *Birmingham*, p. 213; Hayes, 'Counting Civil Society', p. 297.

17. Anning, *General Infirmary: Vol. II*; Morris, 'Middle-Class Culture'.

18. For stability in the executive boards of Nottingham's medical charities see Hayes, 'Counting Civil Society'.

19. LPD, *Annual Report*, 1930–1, p. 3.

20. Some studies of nineteenth-century hospitals reveal the role of women, including Gorsky, *Patterns of Philanthropy*, pp. 162–77; Reinarz, *Birmingham*, pp. 82–92; Pickstone, *Medicine and Industrial Society*, pp. 114–16; Waddington, *London Hospitals*, pp. 146–8. However, these do tend to show women's influence rather than their power.

21. LHW, *Annual Report*, 1919, p. 2; 1931, p. 3.

22. Pickstone, *Medicine and Industrial Society*, pp. 114–18; LMH, *Annual Report*, 1913, p. 3.

23. Doyle, *Hospitals in Middlesbrough*, p. 26; Reinarz, *Birmingham*, p. 91; Hayes, 'Counting Civil Society', p. 304.

24. There is little discussion of the hospital administrator in the literature, but see Waddington, *London Hospitals*, pp. 139–41; Sturdy and Cooter, 'Scientific Management', p. 9 and M. J. Vogel, 'Managing Medicine: Creating a Profession of Hospital Administration in

the United States, 1895–1915', in Granshaw and Porter (eds), *The Hospital in History*, pp. 243–60. The development of the secretary mirrored developments in local government where administrators, especially town clerks, acquired considerable power. Doyle, 'Changing Functions of Urban Government', pp. 295–8.

25. SRI, *Annual Report*, 1932, p. 8; *Sheffield Daily Telegraph*, 23 December 1931. In Nottingham, the General Hospital's chairman in the early 1940, Sir Louis Pearson, claimed he spent 'two or three afternoons a week, at least' on hospital business. Hayes, 'Counting Civil Society', p. 297.

26. For Clayton Fryer's distrust of the contributory schemes, see S. Clayton Fryers, 'Voluntary Hospitals and Contributory Schemes', *Supplement to the British Medical Journal* (18 February 1939), pp. 73–6. For investments see Pickstone, *Medicine and Industrial Society*, p. 254; Hayes and Doyle, 'Eggs, Rags and Whist Drives', pp. 727–9 for the strength of investment income in Leicester and Nottingham where contributory schemes were weak.

27. For example Doyle, 'Power and Accountability'.

28. This was particularly the case in relation to the better-off members of the contributory schemes. For the prolonged standoff in Sheffield in 1938 around 'black-coated workers' see, for example, *Sheffield Independent*, 7 September 1938 and *Sheffield Telegraph*, 7 September 1938 and following weeks.

29. LHC, *Hospitals of Liverpool*, pp. 16–19 for a description of teams and Sturdy and Cooter, 'Scientific Management', pp. 5–6 for their consequences.

30. Doyle, 'Power and Accountability', pp. 219–23; Gorsky et al., *Mutualism and Health Care*, ch. 6.

31. For a discussion of the role of the MOH in one city see Welshman, *Municipal Medicine*.

32. Each year MOH Leeds, *Annual Report* published details of the membership of the Health Committee and its subcommittees, as did MOH Sheffield, *Annual Report*.

33. MOH Leeds, *Annual Report*, 1928, p. 5; 1930, p. 5; 1934, unpaginated front matter; 1938, p. vi–vii; MOH Sheffield, *Annual Report*, 1928, unpaginated front matter; 1932, unpaginated front matter; 1934, unpaginated front matter.

34. Digby, 'Politics of Gender'. There is a more positive literature which points to women's agency in both philanthropic and political fields in the second half of the nineteenth century, especially Gorsky, *Patterns of Philanthropy*, pp. 162–77; F. Prochaska, *Women and Philanthropy in Nineteenth Century England* (Oxford: Oxford University Press, 1980) and P. Hollis, *Ladies Elect: Women in English Local Government, 1865–1914* (Oxford: Oxford University Press, 1989).

35. MOH Leeds, *Annual Report*, 1935, unpaginated front matter.

36. MOH Sheffield, *Annual Report*, 1934, unpaginated front matter.

37. For comments on similar leading figures in Leicester see Welshman, *Municipal Medicine*, pp. 70–4.

38. J. Welshman, 'The Medical Officer of Health in England and Wales, 1900–74: Watchdog or Lapdog?', *Journal of Public Health Medicine*, 19:4 (1997), pp. 443–50.

39. For examples, Welshman, *Municipal Medicine*; Doyle, 'Pollution in Middlesbrough'; and B. M. Doyle, 'Mapping Slums in an Historic City: Representing Working Class Communities in Edwardian Norwich', *Planning Perspectives*, 16:1 (2001), pp. 47–65.

40. J. Lewis, *What Price Community Medicine? The Philosophy, Practice and Politics of Public Health since 1919* (Brighton: Wheatsheaf, 1986); Webster, 'Healthy or Hungry'; Welshman, *Municipal Medicine*; Pickstone, *Medicine and Industrial Society*; and Doyle, 'Competition and Cooperation' and 'Pollution in Middlesbrough'.

41. MOH Leeds, *Annual Report*, 1946, p. 2.
42. Sheffield Survey Report, TNA MH66/1076, pp. 24–30.
43. Leeds Survey Report, TNA MH66/1072, pp. 39–40.
44. Ibid., pp. 74–5.
45. Sheffield Survey Report, TNA MH66/1076, p. 29.
46. Ibid., p. 25; Leeds Survey Report, TNA MH66/1072, pp. 75, 40.
47. Ibid., p. 75.
48. Mohan, *Planning*, pp. 57–8; Pickstone, *Medicine and Industrial Society*, ch. 12; Gorsky, 'Bristol', sec. 5.3; Levene et al., *Cradle to Grave*, pp. 130–4; Doyle, 'Competition and Cooperation', pp. 352–3.
49. For its activities see SHC, *Annual Report*, various years from 1922.
50. Sheffield Voluntary Hospital Standing Committee, 1924–1942, evidence submitted to the Sankey Commission inserted in minutes, SCA NHS28/10/1.
51. Leeds Voluntary Hospital Committee Minutes and Rules 1934 and 1939. For the Maternity Hospital issue see ch. 7.
52. LJHAC, *Annual Reports*, 1936–9.
53. Sheffield Municipal and Voluntary Hospitals Joint Advisory Committee, minutes, SCA NHS28/10/1.
54. For further discussion of all these themes see ch. 7.
55. Sheffield Voluntary Hospital Standing Committee, 1924–1942, evidence submitted to the Sankey Commission inserted in minutes, SCA NHS28/10/1, p. 6.
56. Gorsky, Mohan and Willis, *Mutualism and Health Care*; Doyle, 'Power and Accountability'; Hayes, 'Our Hospitals'; Gorsky, 'Bristol'; Reinarz, *Birmingham*.
57. Doyle, 'Competition and Cooperation'.
58. SRI, *Annual Report*, 1939, p. 1.
59. SHC, *Annual Report*, 1923, p. 92; *Sheffield Daily Telegraph*, 7 September 1938.
60. Doyle, 'Labour and Hospitals'.
61. LGI Weekly Board Minutes, 1938–40, 15 July 1938, WYL 2295/3/28; Doyle, 'Labour and Hospitals'.
62. LGI Weekly Board, Minutes, 1919–29, 3 October 1924, WYL 2295/3/26; Leeds Voluntary Hospitals' Council Minutes [hereafter LVHC Minutes and date], 23 May 1935, WYL 2295/25/3.
63. For similar interrelatedness in Lancashire see Pickstone, *Medicine and Industrial Society*, pp. 253–5.
64. Leigh was on the Health Committee in the 1920s, a member of the LPD Committee and was appointed chair of the LWHF in 1936. His wife was also a Conservative councillor who served on the Health Committee.
65. Pickstone, *Medicine and Industrial Society*, p. 254; M. Savage, *The Dynamics of Working Class Politics: The Labour Movement in Preston, 1880–1940* (Cambridge: Cambridge University Press, 1987), pp. 168–9, 186–7; Welshman, *Municipal Medicine*, p. 73; Hayes, 'Counting Civil Society', p. 297.
66. Sheffield Survey Report, TNA MH66/1076, pp. 156–7; Parsons, *Hospital Survey: Sheffield*.
67. For the establishment of the scheme in 1928 see LGI Faculty Minutes, letter from Leeds Union, 4 January 1928, WYL 2295 5/3.
68. Leeds Survey Report, TNA MH66/1072, p. 44; Leeds Survey Report, TNA MH66/711, Appendix O1.A, part 4.

69. LVHC Minutes, 2 March 1935 and (inserted) Leeds Joint Hospitals Advisory Committee, 'Scheme for the Appointment of Consultant Staffs to Municipal and Voluntary Hospitals' operative from 1 June 1944, WYL 2295/25/3.
70. Pickstone, *Medicine and Industrial Society*, pp. 257, 285–93; Gorsky, 'Bristol', sec. 5.3.
71. Webster, *Health Services since the War*, p. 25.
72. Earwicker, 'Labour Movement'.
73. *Sheffield Daily Telegraph*, 6 May 1922.
74. Stewart, 'Healthy London'; Stewart, *Battle for Health*.
75. Doyle, 'Labour and Hospitals'; Earwicker, 'Labour Movement'.
76. H. R. S. Phillpott, *Where Labour Rules: A Tour through Towns and Counties* (London: Methuen, 1934); Davies and Morley, 'Voters in Yorkshire'; Cherry, 'Medical Care'; Eason, *Hospital Survey: Yorkshire*, pp. 62–5.
77. Levene et al., *Cradle to Grave*, pp. 127–35; Doyle, 'Competition and Cooperation', pp. 346–8.
78. LHC, *Hospitals of Liverpool*; Gorsky, 'Bristol', sec. 5.3 (includes reference to Birmingham); Willis, 'Bradford Municipal Hospital Experiment'; Pickstone, *Medicine and Industrial Society*, pp. 274–6; Levene et al., *Cradle to Grave*, pp. 175–80. For the view that Labour representation could make a difference see Powell, 'Did Politics Matter?'.
79. Willis, 'Health Care in Sheffield'; Doyle, 'Labour and Hospitals'.
80. *Sheffield Daily Telegraph*, 9 November 1921; 1 October 1921.
81. *Sheffield Daily Telegraph*, 22 June 1922.
82. See ch. 5.
83. *Sheffield Daily Telegraph*, 15 November 1921.
84. For examples of Fountain Pen's views see *Sheffield Daily Telegraph*, 26 September 1923; 6 February 1924; 12 February 1924.
85. Sheffield and District Association of Hospital Contributors, Minutes of 27 Quarterly Meeting, 5 September 1928; SRH, *Annual Report*, 1939, p. 1.
86. Doyle, 'Labour and Hospitals'.
87. Levene et al., *Cradle to Grave*, p. 132; S. Thompson, 'A Proletarian Public Sphere: Working-Class Provision of Medical Services and Care in South Wales, *c.* 1900–1948', in A. Borsay (ed.), *Medicine in Wales, c. 1800–2000: Public Service or Private Commodity?* (Cardiff: University of Wales Press, 2003), pp. 86–107; Doyle, 'Power and Accountability'.
88. *Sheffield Star*, 29 March 1933. For a similar remark the year before see *Sheffield Star*, 23 March 1932.
89. Gorsky, Mohan and Willis, *Mutualism and Health Care*, p. 102.
90. British Hospitals Contributory Schemes Association (BHCSA), *Report of Proceedings: Fifth Annual Conference Sheffield 19th to 22nd September 1935* (Sheffield: BHCSA, 1935), p. 24. See also Doyle, 'Labour and Hospitals'.
91. 'Sheffield Municipal and Voluntary Hospitals Joint Advisory Committee Minutes', 7 December 1937, SCA NHS28/10/1.
92. *Sheffield Independent*, 19 January 1931.
93. *Sheffield Telegraph and Independent*, 11 March 1939.
94. *Sheffield Daily Telegraph*, 30 July 1938.
95. *Leeds Weekly Citizen* [hereafter *Citizen*], 3 October 1924.
96. *Citizen*, 6 July 1928. See also Doyle 'Labour and Hospitals'.
97. Leeds Voluntary Hospital Committee Minutes, 8 July 1927, WYL 2295 25/3.
98. LPD, *Annual Report*, 1927–8, p. 16.

99. LWHF, *Annual Report*, 1928, p. 19.
100. LGI, *Annual Report*, 1928, p. 21.
101. *Citizen*, 22 September 1933.
102. *Citizen*, 7 May 1937.
103. *Citizen*, 10 October 1924.
104. *Citizen*, 6 March 1925.
105. *Citizen*, 28 October 1927.
106. *Citizen*, 24 September 1937, p. 10.
107. For further discussion of these themes see Doyle, 'Hospital Contributory Schemes'.
108. LWHF, *Annual Report*, 1925, p. 21.
109. LWHF, *Annual Report*, 1937, p. 20. Doyle, 'Hospital Contributory Schemes'.
110. LPD, *Annual Report*, 1918–19, p. 11.
111. LPD, *Annual Report*, 1921–2, p. 11.
112. LPD, *Annual Report*, 1924–5, pp. 15–16.
113. LPD, *Annual Report*, 1937, p. 12.
114. LPD, *Annual Report*, 1938, p. 11.
115. Hayes, 'Our Hospitals', p. 99.
116. Doyle, 'Labour and Hospitals'; Doyle, 'Hospital Contributory Schemes'.
117. LPD, *Annual Report*, 1925–6, p. 17.
118. *Sheffield Independent*, 10 October 1927.
119. *Sheffield Telegraph and Star*, 15 October 1927.
120. LPD, *Annual Report*, 1917–18, p. 13.
121. Hayes, 'Did We Really Want a National Health Service'; Hayes, 'Our Hospitals'.
122. *Sheffield Telegraph and Star*, 15 October 1927.
123. LPD, *Annual Report*, 1923–4, pp. 15–16.
124. *Sheffield Telegraph and Star*, 15 October 1927.
125. LPD, *Annual Report*, 1931–2, p. 12.
126. *Sheffield Telegraph*, 27 March 1929.
127. *Sheffield Telegraph*, 23 September 1935.
128. See for example Whittaker at the AGM of the Armley and Wortley Ward Committee in February 1931 when he stated 'If the infirmaries and hospitals got into Government hands it would be bad for the country'. *Leeds Hospital Magazine*, February 1931, p. 31.
129. LWHF, *Annual Report*, 1929, p. 20.
130. *Sheffield Telegraph and Star*, 5 October 1927.
131. *Sheffield Telegraph and Star*, 15 October 1927.
132. *Sheffield Telegraph*, 27 March 1929.
133. 'Current Topics', *Sheffield Telegraph*, 11 June 1919.
134. Hayes, 'Counting Civil Society', p. 297.
135. Gorsky, Mohan and Willis, *Mutualism and Health Care*; Doyle, 'Hospital Contributory Schemes'.
136. For the strength of voluntary income see Hayes and Doyle, 'Eggs, Rags and Whist Drives'.
137. This is equivalent to an increase of 7.5 per cent. *Sheffield Independent*, 10 October 1927.
138. *Sheffield Telegraph*, 10 June 1919.
139. 'Current Topics', *Sheffield Telegraph*, 11 June 1919.
140. *Sheffield Daily Telegraph*, 24 March 1932, 6 April 1938.
141. *Sheffield Telegraph*, 10 June 1919.
142. Leeds Voluntary Hospitals Fund, Minute Book, 6 November 1935, WYL 2295/25/3.
143. Leeds Voluntary Hospitals Fund, Minute Book, 13 October 1937, WYL 2295/25/3.

144. LPD, *Annual Report*, 1930–1, p. 14–15.

145. LWHF, *Annual Report*, 1937, p. 22.

146. LWHF, *Annual Report*, 1939, pp. 20–1.

147. Levene et al., *Cradle to Grave*, pp. 75–86; Levene, Powell and Stewart, 'Municipal Hospital Care', pp. 19–20.

148. For further discussion of the potential impact of party on health care spending see Powell, 'Did Politics Matter?'; Powell, 'An Expanding Service'.

149. *Sheffield Independent*, 6 October 1927.

150. *Sheffield Telegraph and Star*, 27 March 1929.

151. *Sheffield Independent*, 6 October 1927.

152. *Sheffield Telegraph and Star*, 15 October 1927.

153. *Citizen*, 27 January 1928, 28 September 1928.

154. Article by Councillor George Brett, *Citizen*, 22 November 1929.

155. For example views of Councillor O'Donnell cited in *Citizen*, 1 August 1930.

156. Gorsky, 'Bristol', sec. 4.3.

157. For the development of these services see chs 2 and 3.

158. These issues also underpinned opposition to appropriation elsewhere, Levene et al., *Cradle to Grave*, pp. 79–82.

159. Leeds Survey Report, TNA MH66/1072, p. 68, See ch. 5 for discussion of the recovery of contributions from patients.

160. Willis, 'Local Authority Health Care'.

161. Sheffield City Council Labour Group, *Six Years of Labour Rule*.

162. *Citizen*, 9 October 1931.

163. *Citizen*, 22 September 1933, 13 October 1933.

164. He and three other Conservatives abstained in the original 1931 vote to block appropriation. *Leeds Mercury*, 5 February 1931.

165. Leeds Survey Report, TNA MH66/1072, pp. 68–9.

166. *Citizen*, 4 May 1934; *Leeds Mercury*, 3 May 1934.

167. Sheffield City Council Labour Group, *Six Years of Labour Rule*, p. 18.

168. Sheffield Labour Party, *Labour Accomplishes*, pp. 4–5.

169. *Citizen*, 4 October 1935, 5 April 1935. Bold as in original.

170. *Citizen*, 21 October 1938.

171. See ch. 7.

172. LVHC Minutes, 6 January 1938, 14 July 1938, WYL 2295/25/1.

173. 'Second Annual Meeting of the Leeds Voluntary Hospitals' Fund Committee', LVHF Minutes, 28 March 1938, WYL 2295/25/2.

174. LVHC Minutes, 14 July 1938, WYL 2295/25/1.

175. 'Sheffield Municipal and Voluntary Hospitals Joint Advisory Committee' Minutes, 4 December 1936; 18 July 1938, SCA NHS28/10/1.

176. *Sheffield Telegraph and Independent*, 11 March 1939. Bold as in original.

7 Co-operation, Competition and the Development of Hospital Systems

1. Lowe, *The Welfare State*, p. 169.

2. Webster, *Health Services since the War*, p. 5.

3. Ibid., p. 20.

4. Abel-Smith, *The Hospitals*, p. 410.
5. For a particularly critical view of the latter case Mohan, *Planning*, ch. 3.
6. Doyle, *Hospitals in Middlesbrough*, p. 13; Levene et al., *Cradle to Grave*, pp. 131–4.
7. Gorsky, 'Bristol', sec. 5.3; Gosling, 'Charity and Change', pp. 149–56; Cherry, 'Beyond National Health Insurance'; Mohan, *Planning*, pp. 58–9.
8. Cherry, 'Beyond National Health Insurance'; M. Gorsky, 'The Gloucestershire Extension of Medical Services Scheme: An Experiment in the Integration of Health Services in Britain before the NHS', *Medical History*, 50:4 (2006), pp. 491–512; Topping to Sharpe, 'South West Division. Sankey Report. Grouping of Hospitals'. 27 July 1937 and subsequent discussion, TNA MH58/323.
9. Robinson-Hill, 19 May 1933, TNA MH55/4, quoted in Mohan, *Planning*, p. 57.
10. Gorsky, 'Bristol', sec. 5.3; Reinarz, *Birmingham*, pp. 213–14; Gorsky, Mohan and Willis, *Mutualism and Health Care*, pp. 82–4.
11. LHC, *Hospitals of Liverpool*, pp. 23–5; Powell, 'An Expanding Service', pp. 343–5.
12. British Hospitals Association (BHA), *Report of the Voluntary Hospitals Commission* (London: British Hospitals Association, 1937) [Sankey Commission].
13. See pp. 68–9; 119–22.
14. Most general and specialist studies make reference to the Dawson Report, Cave Committee and Onslow Commission which urged local organization in return for government grants. For example see Mohan, *Planning*, pp. 49–52.
15. Gorsky, 'Bristol', sec. 5.3; Reinarz, *Birmingham*, pp. 235–8; Pickstone, *Medicine and Industrial Society*, pp. 280–93.
16. 'Organisation of the Voluntary Hospital System and its Relationship to the Sheffield Appeal' [hereafter 'Voluntary Hospital System'] and 'Precis of Memorandum dated April 5th, 1938, prepared by the Honorary Staffs of the Voluntary Hospitals for presentation to the "Sheffield Municipal and Voluntary Advisory Committee"' [hereafter 'Precis']. Both are in 'Sheffield: Policy and Growth, 1938', TNA MH58/319.
17. BHA, *Voluntary Hospitals Commission*. See also news coverage of the positive impression of Sheffield presented in the report e.g. *Sheffield Telegraph*, 30 April 1937.
18. 'Precis', TNA MH58/319.
19. 'Voluntary Hospital System', TNA MH58/319, p. 6.
20. See for example Abel-Smith, *The Hospitals*, pp. 307–10; Mohan, *Planning*, p. 49.
21. Joint Consultative and Advisory Hospitals Council, *General Statement*. See also this volume, chs 3, 6.
22. A list of the membership was published annually in the SHC, *Annual Report*.
23. Doyle, 'Competition and Cooperation', p. 352. See also Gorsky, Mohan and Willis, *Mutualism and Health Care*, p. 82 for other examples.
24. SHC, *First Annual Report*, 1923, pp. 15–16.
25. SHC, *Annual Report*, 1924, p. 2.
26. LGI, *Annual Report*, 1920, p. 13.
27. Minutes of LGI Weekly Board, 1919–29 [hereafter LGI Board Minutes and date], 2 February 1923, WYL 2295/3/26. Sheffield stayed out as its hinterland covered Derbyshire, Nottinghamshire and even Lincolnshire.
28. Leeds and District Employers' Voluntary Hospital Fund, Minutes, WYL 2295/25/3.
29. Gorsky, 'Bristol', sec. 5.2; Gosling, 'Charity and Change', pp. 68–77 for changes by closure and removal amongst services for women and children.
30. Reinarz, *Birmingham*, p. 213.

31. LGI Sub-committees Minute Book, 'Co-ordination Scheme Sub-committee', 25 October 1929 and 31 January 1930 [hereafter 'Co-ordination Committee'] WYL 2295/7/1.
32. 'Co-ordination Committee', 12 February 1930, WYL 2295/7/1.
33. Ibid., 3 November, 27 November 1930, WYL 2295/7/1.
34. Ibid., 26 January 1933, WYL 2295/7/1.
35. *Rules of the Leeds Voluntary Hospitals Council* (Leeds, 1939) WYL 2295/315.
36. *Shape of Things*, TNA MH 58/319.
37. Extract from Jessop, *Annual Report* in SHC, *Annual Report*, 1937, p. 20.
38. Extract from Sheffield Children's Hospital, *Annual Report* in SHC, *Annual Report*, 1937, p. 22.
39. SHC, *Annual Report*, 1923, p. 20.
40. Extract from the SRI, *Annual Report* in SHC, *Annual Report*, 1935, p. 10.
41. SHC, *Annual Report*, 1936, pp. 10–1.
42. Extract from the SRI, *Annual Report* in SHC, *Annual Report*, 1937, p. 10.
43. Extract from SHC, *Annual Report*, 1937, p. 20.
44. For example fractures and rehabilitation and neuro-surgery as discussed in ch. 4.
45. *Rules of the Leeds Voluntary Hospitals Council*.
46. Extract from Edgar Allen Institute, *Annual Report* in SHC, *Annual Report*, 1937, p. 23.
47. SUH, *Annual Report*, 1947, p. 8.
48. Eason, *Hospital Survey: Yorkshire*, pp. 21, 32; Parsons, *Hospital Survey: Sheffield*, pp. 8, 13, 18.
49. See some of the comments noted by Mohan, *Planning*, p. 55.
50. See chs 2, 3.
51. MOH Sheffield, *Annual Report*, 1927, pp. 92, 80.
52. MOH Sheffield, *Annual Report*, 1930, p. 58.
53. Powell, 'An Expanding Service', p. 345 did highlight Nether Edge as one of the appropriated institutions which did not develop general services, but this was because it was part of a broader reallocation of activities across the city.
54. Survey Letter, 7 March 1935, Sheffield Survey Report, TNA MH66/1076.
55. Survey Letter to Leeds Corporation, 1933, Leeds Survey Report, TNA MH66/1072.
56. Leeds Survey Report, TNA MH66/1072, p. 65.
57. Jervis, *Utilization of Poor Law*, p. 3.
58. Leeds Survey Report, TNA MH66/1072, p. 65.
59. Jervis, *Utilization of Poor Law*, p. 8.
60. Ibid., Appendix.
61. Webster, *Health Services since the War*, p. 20; Abel-Smith, *The Hospitals*, pp. 407–10 and Mohan, *Planning*, p. 53 all mention Manchester, Oxford, Liverpool and Birmingham – largely because these either had published studies of their activities or were examined by the Ministry of Health, TNA MH58/323.
62. SHC, *Annual Report*, 1923, p. 22.
63. LGI Board Minutes, 2 November 1923, WYL 2295/3/26.
64. Welshman, *Municipal Medicine*, pp. 266–7.
65. Report by Medical Officer of Health to Board of LGI, LGI Board Minutes, 12 September 1924, WYL 2295/3/26.
66. LGI Board Minutes, 12 September 1924, WYL 2295/3/26.
67. LGI Board Minutes, 2 November 1923, WYL 2295/3/26.
68. LGI Board Minutes, 2 November 1923, WYL 2295/3/26.
69. LGI Board Minutes, 7 December 1923, 4 April 1924, WYL 2295/3/26.

70. LGI Board Minutes, 2 October 1924, WYL 2295/3/26.
71. LGI Faculty Minutes, 1913–29, 12 September 1924, WYL 2295/5/3.
72. Doyle, 'Hospital Contributory Schemes', p. 297.
73. *Leeds Hospital Magazine*, September 1931, p. 163; Doyle, 'Hospital Contributory Schemes', pp. 304–5.
74. Doyle, 'Competition and Cooperation', p. 350. See also Mohan, *Planning*, pp. 57–9 and Levene et al., *Cradle to Grave*, pp. 215–17 for the hostile relations in West Hartlepool.
75. SRH, *Annual Report*, 1930, p. 13.
76. Sheffield Survey Report, TNA MH66/1076, p. 181.
77. 'Co-ordination of Hospital Services'. This version of the meeting was clearly minuted by the MOH. There is a separate, broadly similar account, in 'Co-ordination Committee', 28 October 1936, WYL 2295/7/2.
78. LHC, *Hospitals of Liverpool*, p. 6; Powell, 'An Expanding Service'.
79. LJHAC, *First Annual Report*.
80. Report of Medical Superintendent, MOH Leeds, *Annual Report*, 1937, p. 98.
81. MOH Sheffield, *Annual Report*, 1934, p. 8.
82. Sheffield Survey Report, TNA MH66/1076; History of 'Sheffield Municipal and Voluntary Hospital Joint Advisory Committee' bound with 'Sheffield Municipal and Voluntary Hospitals Joint Advisory Committee' Minutes, SCA NHS/28/10/1.
83. Notes of joint meeting 'Co-ordination Committee', 28 October 1936, WYL 2295/7/2.
84. 'Co-ordination of Hospital Services', p. 3.
85. Pickstone, *Medicine and Industrial Society*, pp. 256–60; Doyle, 'Competition and Cooperation', pp. 352–3; Gorsky, 'Bristol', sec. 5.3.
86. Standing Committee for Sheffield Voluntary Hospitals, Minutes 1924–42. 'Commission of Enquiry with Reference to the Future of the Voluntary Hospitals of the Country: Summary of evidence to be submitted on behalf of The Sheffield Hospitals Council (Incorporated)', p. 4, SCA NHS/28/10/1.
87. LJHAC, *First Annual Report*, p. 5–6.
88. Leeds Survey Report, TNA MH66/1072, p. 62.
89. For the dumping ground fear see Doyle, 'Competition and Cooperation', p. 353; Parsons, *Hospital Survey: Sheffield*, p. 8.
90. LVHC Minutes, 11 October 1934, WYL 2295/25/3.
91. Leeds Survey Report, TNA MH66/1072, pp. 62–4.
92. 'Co-ordination of Hospital Services', p. 3.
93. The LGI minutes state only 'that it was not intended to refer only uninteresting cases to St James' and care would be taken to prevent any difficulties arising in this direction'. 'Co-ordination Committee', 14 January 1937, WYL 2295/7/2.
94. Pickstone, *Medicine and Industrial Society*, pp. 278–93; Gorsky, 'Bristol', sec. 5.3; Doyle, 'Competition and Cooperation', p. 353; Welshman, *Municipal Medicine*, pp. 267–71; Mohan, *Planning*, pp. 58–9. See also TNA MH58/323 for other examples.
95. LJHAC, *First Annual Report*.
96. 'Voluntary Hospital System', TNA MH58/319, pp. 4–5.
97. MOH Leeds, *Annual Report*, 1939, p. 104.
98. Pickstone, 'Contested Cumulations'; Murphy, 'History of Radiotherapy'; D. Cantor, 'Cancer', in W. F. Bynum and R. Porter (eds), *Companion Encyclopedia of the History of Medicine*, 2 vols (London: Routledge, 1993), vol. 1, pp. 536–60.

99. Pickstone, *Medicine and Industrial Society*, p. 201; T. W. Barnard, *Graves Institute of Radiotherapy Trust Fund: Memoir on the Origin and Progress of the Trust* (Sheffield: n.p., 1964), p. 4.

100. This was part of a flurry of activity at the end of the 1920s which saw radium departments established in Bradford and Burnley, Murphy, 'History of Radiotherapy', p. 5.69.

101. Murphy, 'History of Radiotherapy'.

102. Coombs, *History of Radiology*, pp. 46, 18.

103. *Independent*, 25 February 2006; 'Professor Frank Ellis FRCR in interview with Sir Christopher Paine, Oxford, 14 July 1997', Transcript of interview, Oxford Brookes University Library, 14 July 1997, MSVA 169. I am grateful to Don Marshall of Oxford Brookes University Library for helping me track this down.

104. LGI, *Annual Report*, 1939, pp. 25–6; *Independent*, 25 February 2006.

105. Gorsky, 'Bristol', sec 5.3; Murphy, 'History of Radiotherapy', p. 6.21.

106. MOH Sheffield, *Annual Report*, 1938, p. 15.

107. MOH Sheffield, *Annual Report*, 1929, p. 57.

108. Sheffield Survey Report, TNA MH66/1076, p. 162. For more detail see ch. 3.

109. MOH Leeds, *Annual Report*, 1937, p. 104; Pickstone, *Medicine and Industrial Society*, p. 273.

110. LJHAC, *First Annual Report*, p. 7.

111. Sheffield Survey Report, TNA MH66/1076, p. 162.

112. See ch. 4 and *Sheffield Telegraph*, 2 and 3 October 1936 for criticism of the council's services.

113. LGI Faculty Minutes, 1913–29, 30 October 1925, WYL 2295/5/3.

114. Document entitled 'Medical Teaching', LGI Board Minutes, 6 December 1924, WYL 2295/3/26.

115. Board of Faculty of Medicine, Minutes, 1910–30, 28 January 1930, University of Leeds Archives, School of Medicine, Box 12.1.

116. 'Precis', TNA MH58/319, p. 5.

117. 'Hospital Resources, 1939', 15 September 1939, Medical Faculty (General) 1931–57, University of Sheffield Archives, VC/2/M//17; Parsons, *Hospital Survey: Sheffield*, p. 19.

118. MOH Leeds, *Annual Report*, 1945, p. 64.

119. Mohan, 'Voluntarism, Municipalism and Welfare', p. 59.

120. Parsons, *Hospital Survey: Sheffield*, p. 7.

121. 'Co-ordination Committee', 25 October 1929, WYL 2295/7/1.

122. 'Sheffield Municipal and Voluntary Hospitals Joint Advisory Committee' Minutes, 1 June 1937; 7 December 1937; 18 July 1938, SCA NHS/28/10/1.

123. Ibid., 1 June 1937; 7 December 1937, SCA NHS/28/10/1.

124. LGI Faculty minutes 1913–29, 12 September 1924, WYL 2295/5/3.

125. Doyle, 'Competition and Cooperation', p. 353.

126. Eason, *Hospital Survey: Yorkshire*, p. 33.

127. 'Precis', TNA MH58/319, pp. 4–5.

128. Ibid., p. 3.

129. 'Voluntary Hospital System', TNA MH58/319 and this volume, ch. 3.

130. See ch. 4, p. 91.

131. 'Precis', TNA MH58/319, p. 5.

132. For example Middlesbrough in 1928, Doyle, *History of Hospitals in Middlesbrough*, p. 72.

133. Note of Interview with Mr P. Austyn Barran by J. H. Turnbull, 15 June 1934. Survey File following Survey Appendices, TNA MH66/711.
134. Dr Turnbull to Dr Macewen 15 June 1934 and T S McIntosh to Dr Turnbull, 5 July 1934, Leeds Survey File following Survey Appendices, TNA MH66/711.
135. LVHC Minutes, 12 April 1934, WYL 2295/25/3.
136. LVHC Minutes, 10 January 1935, WYL 2295/25/3.
137. LVHC Minutes, April 1935, WYL 2295/25/3.
138. 'Maternity Service of the City of Leeds', in LVHC Minutes, 23 May 1935, WYL 2295/25/3.
139. LVHC Minutes, 23 May 1935, WYL 2295/25/3.
140. LVHC Minutes, 10 October 1935, WYL 2295/25/3.
141. Austyn Barran to Knigsley Wood, 17 January 1936, and Kingsley Wood to Barran, 4 February 1936, Leeds Survey File following Survey Appendices, TNA MH66/711.
142. LJHAC, *First Annual Report*, p. 8. Though see also Barran's thoughts on 'misleading comments', LVHC Section 13 Committee meeting, 6 January 1938, WYL 2295/25/3.
143. Eason, *Hospital Survey: Yorkshire*, p. 32.
144. *Sheffield Telegraph and Independent*, 11 March 1939.
145. 'Sheffield Municipal and Voluntary Hospitals Joint Advisory Committee' Minutes, 4 December 1936, SCA NHS/28/10/1.
146. Memorandum on the history of the committee, 'Sheffield Municipal and Voluntary Hospitals Joint Advisory Committee' Minutes, SCA NHS/28/10/1.
147. See ch. 5.
148. See ch. 3 and Gorsky, Mohan and Willis, *Mutualism and Health Care*, pp. 80–2.
149. Summary of evidence submitted to Sankey Commission, SCA NHS/28/10/1.
150. Ibid. and discussion in Gosling, 'Charity and Change', pp. 149–56.
151. LGI, *Annual Report*, 1945, p. 26; Eason, *Hospital Survey: Yorkshire*, p. 35; SHC, *Annual Report*, 1945, pp. 25, 27–8.
152. Extract from the SRH, *Annual Report* in SHC, *Annual Report*, 1936, pp. 16–17.
153. See ch. 4.
154. 'Proposed Radium Institute', in LGI Board Sub-committees, 1934–41, 'Radium', 4 January 1938, WYL 2295/7/2. SRI, *Annual Report*, 1938.
155. 'Radium Department: Memo: On Need for Radium Institute or Radio-Therapeutic Block', in LGI Board Sub-committees, 1934–41, 'Radium', 15 November 1937, WYL 2295/7/2.
156. *Shape of Things*, p. 4.
157. 'On Need for Radium Institute', WYL 2295/7/2.
158. Parsons, *Hospital Survey: Sheffield*, p. 13.
159. 'Voluntary Hospital System', TNA MH58/319.
160. For Labour opposition in Sheffield see ch. 6 and 'Sheffield Municipal and Voluntary Hospitals Joint Advisory Committee' Minutes, 18 July 1938, SCA NHS/28/10/1.
161. See LVHC Minutes, various dates 1939–45, WYL 2295/25/2.
162. Eason, *Hospital Survey: Yorkshire*, pp. 21–2.
163. Ibid., p. 32.
164. Parsons, *Hospital Survey: Sheffield*, p. 18.
165. Ibid., p. 19. See also ch. 4.
166. Ibid., p. 23.
167. In particular, see favourable comments in Eason, *Hospital Survey: Yorkshire*, p. 32.

168. Contrast the criticisms of Parsons, *Hospital Survey: Sheffield*, pp. 18–19 with evidence from SUH, *Annual Report*, 1945, pp. 5–10; 1946, p. 8; 1947, pp. 11–2.
169. Powell, 'An Expanding Service', pp. 345–9; Levene et al., *Cradle to Grave*, pp. 76–8.

Conclusion

1. Gorsky, Mohan and Powell, 'British Voluntary Hospitals'; Levene et al., *Cradle to Grave*.
2. Granshaw, 'Fame and Fortune'; Sturdy and Cooter, 'Scientific Management'.
3. Cherry, 'Before the National Health Service'; Gorsky, Mohan and Powell, 'Financial Health'.
4. Powell, 'Did Politics Matter?'; Stewart, *Battle for Health*; Doyle, 'Labour and Hospitals'.
5. Gorsky, 'Bristol'; Pickstone, *Medicine and Industrial Society*; Mohan, *Planning*.
6. Pickstone, *Medicine and Industrial Society*, p. 267.
7. Sturdy and Cooter, 'Scientific Management'.
8. Hayes and Doyle, 'Eggs, Rags and Whist Drives'.
9. Pickstone, *Medicine and Industrial Society*, pp. 286–8; Sheffield Survey Report, TNA MH66/1076, p. 78.
10. Gorsky, Mohan and Willis, *Mutualism and Health Care*, pp. 44–6.
11. Pickstone, *Medicine and Industrial Society*, p. 252; Gosling, 'Charity and Change'; Hayes and Doyle, 'Eggs, Rags and Whist Drives', p. 718.
12. Sturdy and Cooter, 'Scientific Management'.
13. Reinarz, *Birmingham*, pp. 227–30; Cooter, *ODNB*.
14. Gorsky, Mohan and Willis, *Mutualism and Health Care*, pp. 80–7 and ch. 6.
15. See also Cherry, 'Regional Comparators', pp. 69–71 for some discussion of the networks around Sheffield.
16. Doyle, 'Power and Accountability', pp. 222–3.
17. Levene et al., *Cradle to Grave*, p. 132; Pickstone, *Medicine and Industrial Society*, p. 254; Doyle, 'Competition and Cooperation', p. 352.
18. Abel-Smith, *The Hospitals*, pp. 409–10; Webster, *Health Services since the War*, p. 20; while Mohan, *Planning*, provides the most vigorous recent assertion of the failure of cooperation.
19. Reinarz, *Birmingham*.
20. There was a joint faculty in Bristol by 1939 and a joint board for the four teaching hospitals instituted in Liverpool. Gorsky, 'Bristol', sec. 5.3; TNA MH58/323.
21. Mohan, 'Voluntarism, Municipalism and Welfare'.
22. Gosling, 'Charity and Change', pp. 149–55.
23. As suggested by Anuerin Bevan in a letter to Sheffield Hospital Contributors' Association in 1946 quoted above, p. 1. Sheffield Hospitals Contributors Association, 'Annual Report of the Executive Committee for the Year Ended 31st December, 1946', in *Annual Report*, 1946, p. 27.
24. Webster, *Health Services since the War*, p. 14.
25. Cherry, 'Regional Comparators'.
26. Mohan, *Planning*, p. 59.
27. Reinarz, *Birmingham*, which is concerned largely with the development of the medical school; Gorsky, 'Bristol', sec. 5.3; LHC, *Hospitals of Liverpool*, pp. 23–4.
28. Levene, Powell and Stewart, 'Municipal Hospital Care'.

29. One survey of a rural area using political science methodologies is J. Neville, 'Explaining Local Authority Choices on Public Hospital Provision in the 1930s: A Public Policy Hypothesis', *Medical History*, 56:1 (2012), pp. 48–71.

WORKS CITED

Primary Sources

Unpublished

Leeds Local Studies Department, Minutes of 'Members of the Health Committee Meeting with Representatives of the Voluntary Hospitals Committee to Discuss Co-ordination of Hospital Services', 19 October 1936.

The National Archives [TNA], 'Leeds', in *Survey Reports, County Boroughs: Hastings to Leicester*, Ministry of Health [MH]66/1072. Survey Appendices, MH66/711.

The National Archives [TNA], Minutes of subcommittee considering allocation of hospital beds, TNA MH66/873.

The National Archives [TNA], 'Sheffield', in *Survey Reports, County Boroughs: Rotherham to Southampton*, Ministry of Health [MH] 66/1076. Survey Appendices O–Z, MH66/873.

The National Archives [TNA], 'Sheffield: Policy and Growth, 1938', TNA MH58/319.

Oxford Brookes University Library, 'Professor Frank Ellis FRCR in interview with Sir Christopher Paine, Oxford, 14 July 1997', Transcript of interview, 14 July 1997, MSVA 169.

Sheffield City Archives [SCA], 'Jessop Hospital for Women Newscuttings Book vol. 6, 1938–48', SCA NHS12/1/7/1/6.

Sheffield City Archives [SCA], 'Sheffield Municipal and Voluntary Hospitals Joint Advisory Committee' Minutes, SCA NHS28/10/1.

Sheffield City Archives [SCA], Sheffield Royal Infirmary Collection, SCA NHS17.

Sheffield City Archives [SCA], Sheffield Trades and Labour Council, Minutes of Executive Committee, SCA LD1645.

Sheffield City Archives [SCA], Sheffield United Hospitals Collection, 'Sheffield Voluntary Hospitals Million Pound Appeal', SCA NHS12/3/6/3.

University of Leeds Archives, Board of Faculty of Medicine, Minutes, 1910–30, School of Medicine, box 12.1.

University of Sheffield Archives, Medical Faculty (General) 1931–57, VC/2/M//17.

West Yorkshire Archives Leeds [WYL], LGI Board Sub-committees, 1934–41, 'Radium', WYL 2295/7/2.

West Yorkshire Archives Leeds [WYL], LGI Faculty Minutes, 1913–29, WYL 2295/5/3.

West Yorkshire Archives Leeds [WYL], LGI Sub-committees Minute Book, 'Co-ordination Scheme Sub-committee', WYL 2295/7/1.

West Yorkshire Archives Leeds [WYL], LGI Weekly Board Minutes, 1919–29, WYL 2295/3/26; 1938–40, WYL 2295/3/28.

West Yorkshire Archives Leeds [WYL], LVHC Minutes, 1923–33, WYL 2295/25/3.

West Yorkshire Archives Leeds [WYL], LVHF Minutes, 1923–33, WYL 2295/25/3; 1933–49, WYL 2295/25/2.

West Yorkshire Archives Leeds [WYL], Leeds and District Employers' Voluntary Hospital Fund, Minutes 1923–33, WYL 2295/25/3.

West Yorkshire Archives Leeds [WYL], *Rules of the Leeds Voluntary Hospitals Council* (Leeds, 1939) WYL 2295/315.

Published

Abercrombie, R. G., 'The Pathology of Adolescent Scoliosis', *BMJ* (27 January 1938), pp. 215–17.

Asbury, W., 'Presidential Address on "Smoke Abatement"', *Journal of the Royal Sanitary Institute*, 50 (1929–30), pp. 389–93.

British Hospitals Association [BHA], *Report of the Voluntary Hospitals Commission* (London: British Hospitals Association, 1937).

British Hospitals Contributory Schemes Association [BHCSA], *Report of Proceedings: Fifth Annual Conference Sheffield 19th to 22nd September 1935* (Sheffield: BHCSA, 1935).

City of Leeds, *Opening of the New Wards for Women at Killingbeck Sanatorium by the Minister of Health ... July 9th 1936* (Leeds: Leeds Corporation, 1936).

—, *Opening of the New Extensions at St. James's Hospital by the Minister of Health ... September 30th 1940* (Leeds: Leeds Corporation, 1940).

Cottage Hospital, North Ormesby, Middlesbrough, *Annual Report*, 1920, 1938.

Eason, H., R. Veitch Clark and W. H. Harper, *Hospital Survey: The Hospital Services of the Yorkshire Area* (London: HMSO, 1945).

Edgar Allan Institute, *Annual Report*, 1933–4, 1936–7.

Final Report of the Inter-departmental Committee on the Rehabilitation of Persons Injured by Accidents (London: HMSO, 1939).

General Infirmary at Leeds, *Annual Report*, 1917–47.

Jervis, J. J., *Scheme for the Utilization of Poor Law Institutions under the Local Government Act, 1929* (Leeds: Leeds Corporation, 1934).

—, *The Health Services of the City after the War* (Leeds: City of Leeds, 1945).

—, 'Foreword: A Review of the Public Health Services of the City during the Thirty-One Years 1916–1948', in MOH Leeds, *Annual Report*, 1946, pp. 1–19.

Jessop Hospital for Women, Sheffield, *Annual Report*, 1922–38.

Joint Consultative and Advisory Hospitals Council, *General Statement of the Position of the Voluntary Hospitals of Sheffield, Prepared by the Collation Committee, for the Use of the Council* (Sheffield: Northend, 1920).

Leeds and District Employers' Hospitals Fund, *Annual Report* (Leeds, 1934).

Leeds and District Voluntary Hospital Fund, *Annual Report*, 1940.

Leeds Board of Guardians, *Yearbook, 1925–26* (Leeds, 1926).

Leeds Board of Guardians, *Yearbook, 1929–30* (Leeds, 1930).

Leeds Corporation Sanitary Committee, *Leeds City Hospitals: Seacroft and Killingbeck. Opened by the Right Nonourable, the Lord Mayor and Lady Mayoress, September 29th 1904* (Leeds: Leeds Corporation, 1904).

Leeds (Group A) Hospital Management Committee, *Report for the Period, 5th July 1948 to 31st December 1949* (Leeds: Leeds HMC, 1950).

Leeds (Group B) Hospital Management Committee No. 22, *First Annual Report for the Period Ended 31st March 1949 with Statistical Tables for the Year Ended 31st December 1948* (Leeds: Leeds HMC, 1949).

Leeds Hospital for Women and Children, *Annual Report*, 1917–44.

Leeds Hospital Management Committee B Group, *50th Anniversary of the Opening of Seacroft and Killingbeck Hospitals* (Leeds: Leeds HMC, 1954).

Leeds Joint Hospitals Advisory Committee, *Annual Report*, 1936–8.

Leeds Maternity Hospital, *Annual Report*, various years 1908–47.

Leeds Public Dispensary, *Annual Report*, 1915–44.

Leeds Voluntary Hospital Committee Minutes and Rules 1934, 1939.

Leeds Workpeople's Hospital Fund, *Annual Report*, 1918–40.

Liverpool Hospitals Commission, *Report on the Voluntary Hospitals of Liverpool* (Liverpool: Liverpool University Press, 1935).

Medical Officer of Health, *Annual Report on the Health of the City of Sheffield*, 1927–35, 1938–47.

Medical Officer of Health City of Leeds, *Report on the Health and Sanitary Administration of the City*, 1917–48.

North Riding Infirmary, *Annual Report For the Year Ending 31st December 1933* (Middlesbrough: Appleyard, 1934).

'Obituary: J. B. Ferguson Wilson, M.S. F.R.C.S.', *BMJ* (24 October 1959), p. 829.

'Obituary: R. G. Abercrombie', *BMJ* (10 June 1961), p. 1690.

'Obituary Notices: Sir Frank Holdsworth, M.A., M.Chir, F.R.C.S.', *BMJ* (27 December 1969), p. 812.

Parsons, L. G., S. Clayton Fryers and G. E. Godber, *Hospital Survey: The Hospital Services of the Sheffield and East Midlands Area* (London: HMSO, 1945).

'Rehabilitation of Injured Miners', *BMJ* (24 June 1944), p. 851.

Royal Sheffield Infirmary and Hospital, *Annual Report*, 1944–8.

The Shape of Things to Come: The Sheffield Voluntary Hospitals' Million Pound Appeal (Sheffield: Appeal Committee, 1938).

Sheffield and District Association of Hospital Contributors, Published Minutes of Quarterly Meetings, 1928, 1932.

Sheffield Children's Hospital, *Annual Report*, 1932–3.

Sheffield City Council Labour Group, *Six Years of Labour Rule in Sheffield, 1926–32* (Sheffield: E. G. Rowlinson, 1932).

Sheffield Hospital Contributors Association, 'Annual Report of the Executive Committee for the Year Ended 31st December, 1946', in Sheffield Hospital Council, *Annual Report, 1946*, pp.25–32.

Sheffield Hospitals Council, *Annual Report of the '1d in the £' Fund*, 1924–48.

Sheffield Hospitals Council Incorporated, *Sheffield 1d in the £ Scheme: 1919–1948* (Sheffield: Sheffield Hospitals Council, 1949).

Sheffield Joint Hospitals' Council, *A Record of 1923* (Sheffield: Sheffield Hospitals Council, 1923).

Sheffield Labour Party, *Labour Accomplishes: What Has Been Done – What Will Be Done* (Sheffield: n.p., 1945).

Sheffield Royal Hospital, *Rules of Sheffield Royal Hospital* (Sheffield: n.p., 1911).

—, *Annual Report*, 1911–43.

Sheffield Royal Infirmary, *Annual Report*, 1912–43.

The United Leeds Hospitals, *First Report Covering the Period 5th July 1948 to 31st March 1950* (Leeds: Kelly & Barratt, 1950).

Newspapers

Independent, 2006.

Leeds Hospital Magazine, 1900–39.

Leeds Mercury, 1931, 1934.

Leeds Weekly Citizen, 1924–5, 1927–31, 1933–5, 1937–8.

Sheffield Daily Telegraph, 1921–4, 1931, 1935, 1938.

Sheffield Guardian, 1926.

Sheffield Independent, 1927, 1931–2, 1935, 1938.

Sheffield Star, 1926, 1932–3.

Sheffield Telegraph, 1918–19, 1929, 1932, 1935–8.

Sheffield Telegraph and Star, 1927, 1929.

Sheffield Telegraph and Independent, 1939.

Yorkshire Post, 1920, 1924.

Websites

Disability and Industrial Society: A Comparative Cultural History of British Coalfields, 1780–1948, at http://www.dis-ind-soc.org.uk/en/index.htm [accessed 12 December 2013].

Oxford Dictionary of National Biography, Oxford University Press, 2004, at http://www.oxforddnb.com [accessed 21 August 2013].

Plarr's Lives of the Fellows Online, at http://livesonline.rcseng.ac.uk [accessed 20 November 2013].

A Vision of Britain through Time, at http://www.visionofbritain.org.uk [accessed 26 September 2013].

The Voluntary Hospitals Database Project, at http://www.hospitalsdatabase.lshtm.ac.uk/the-voluntary-hospitals-database-project.php [accessed 9 September 2010].

Broadcasts

'Health before the NHS: A Medical Revolution' (BBC4 *Timeshift* programme, 1 October 2012).

Secondary Sources

Abel-Smith, B., *The Hospitals, 1800–1948: A Study in Social Administration in England and Wales* (London: Heinemann, 1964).

Adams, T., 'Labour and the First World War: Economy, Politics and the Erosion of Local Peculiarity?', *Journal of Regional and Local Studies*, 10 (1990), pp. 23–47.

Airth A. D., and D. J. Newell, *The Demand for Hospital Beds: Results of an Enquiry on Tees-side* (Newcastle: King's College, Newcastle, 1962).

Anning, S. T., *The General Infirmary at Leeds: The First Hundred Years, 1767–1869* (Edinburgh: Livingstone, 1963).

—, *The General Infirmary at Leeds: Volume II the Second Hundred Years, 1869–1965* (Edinburgh: Livinstone, 1966).

—, 'The History of Medicine in Leeds', *Proceedings of the Leeds Philosophical and Literary Society: Literary and Historical Section*, 16 (1978), pp. 207–46.

Anning, S. T., and W. K. J. Walls, *A History of the Leeds School of Medicine: One and a Half Centuries, 1831–1981* (Leeds: Leeds University Press, 1981).

Atkinson, P., 'Cultural Causes of the Nineteenth-Century Fertility Decline: A Study of Three Yorkshire Towns' (PhD thesis, University of Leeds, 2010).

Barber, B. J., 'Aspects of Municipal Government, 1835–1914', in Fraser (ed.), *A History of Modern Leeds*, pp. 301–26.

Barnard, T. W., *Graves Institute of Radiotherapy Trust Fund: Memoir on the Origin and Progress of the Trust* (Sheffield: n.p., 1964).

Bell, F., *At the Works: A Study of a Manufacturing Town with a New Introduction by Jim Turner* (1907; Middlesbrough: University of Teesside, repub. 1997).

Bell F., and R. Millward, 'Public Health Expenditure and Mortality in England and Wales, 1870–1914', *Continuity and Change*, 13:2 (1998), pp. 221–49.

Benson, J., *The Rise of Consumer Society in Britain, 1880–1980* (London: Longman, 1994).

Beresford, M. W., 'Prosperity Street and Others: An Essay in Visible Urban History', in M. W. Beresford and G. R. J. Jones (eds), *Leeds and its Region* (Leeds: For the British Association for the Advancement of Science, 1967), pp. 186–99.

Berridge, V., 'Health and Medicine', in F. M. L. Thompson (ed.), *The Cambridge Social History of Britain, 1750–1950: Volume 3 Social Agencies and Institutions* (Cambridge: Cambridge University Press, 1990), pp. 171–242.

Binfield, C., R. Childs, R. Harper, D. Hey, D. Martin and G. Tweedale (eds), *The History of the City of Sheffield 1843–1993*, 3 vols (Sheffield: Sheffield Academic Press, 1993).

Binfield, C., and D. Hey (eds), *Mesters to Masters: A History of the Company of Cutlers in Hallamshire* (Oxford: Oxford University Press, 1997).

Borowy, I., 'Road Traffic Injuries: Social Change and Development', *Medical History*, 57:1 (2013), pp. 108–38.

Borsay, A., '"Fit to Work": Representing Rehabilitation on the South Wales Coalfield during the Second World War', in A. Borsay (ed.), *Medicine in Wales c. 1800–2000: Public Service or Private Commodity?* (Cardiff: University of Wales Press, 2003), pp. 128–53.

—, 'Disciplining Disabled Bodies: The Development of Orthopaedic Medicine in Britain, c. 1800–1939', in D. M. Turner and K. Stagg (eds), *Social Histories of Disability and Deformity: Bodies, Images and Experiences* (London: Routledge, 2006), pp. 97–116.

Brown, V., 'Public Health Issues and General Practice in the Area of Middlesbrough, 1880–1980' (PhD thesis, University of Durham, 2012).

Brumby, A., 'From "Pauper Lunatics" to "Rate-Aided Patients": Dismantling the Poor Law of Lunacy in Mental Health Care: 1888–1930' (PhD in progress, University of Huddersfield).

Buckman, J., 'Later Phases of Industrialisation, to 1918', in Beresford and Jones (eds), *Leeds and its Region*, pp. 156–66.

Bufton, M. W., and J. Melling, 'Coming Up for Air: Experts, Employers and Workers in Campaigns to Compensate Silicosis Sufferers in Britain, 1918–1939', *Social History of Medicine*, 18:1 (2005), pp. 63–86.

Cantor, D., 'Cancer', in W. F. Bynum and R. Porter (eds), *Companion Encyclopedia of the History of Medicine*, 2 vols (London: Routledge, 1993), vol. 1, pp. 536–60.

Chartres, J., 'John Waddington PLC, 1890s to 1990s: A Strategy of Quality and Innovation', in Chartres and Honeyman (eds), *Leeds City Business*, pp. 145–85.

—, 'Joshua Tetley and Son, 1890s to 1990s: A Century in the Tied Trade', in Chartres and Honeyman (eds), *Leeds City Business*, pp. 112–44.

Chartres, J. and K. Honeyman (eds), *Leeds City Business, 1893–1993: Essays Marking the Centenary of the Incorporation* (Leeds: Leeds University Press, 1993).

Cherry, S., 'Beyond National Health Insurance: The Voluntary Hospitals and Hospital Contributory Schemes: A Regional Study', *Social History of Medicine*, 5:3 (1992), pp. 455–82.

—, 'Accountability, Entitlement and Control Issues and Voluntary Hospital Funding, *c.* 1860–1939', *Social History of Medicine*, 9:2 (1996), pp. 215–33.

—, *Medical Services and the Hospitals in Britain, 1860–1939* (Cambridge: Cambridge University Press, 1996).

—, 'Before the National Health Service: Financing the Voluntary Hospitals, 1900–1939', *Economic History Review*, 50 (1997), pp. 309–27.

—, 'Hospital Saturday, Workplace Collections and Issues in Late Nineteenth-Century Hospital Funding', *Medical History*, 44:4 (2000), pp. 461–88.

—, 'Medical Care since 1750', in C. Rawcliffe and R. Wilson (eds), *Norwich since 1550* (London: Hambledon and London, 2004), pp. 271–94.

—, 'Regional Comparators in the Funding and Organisation of the Voluntary Hospital System, *c.* 1860–1939', in M. Gorsky and S. Sheard (eds), *Financing Medicine* (London; New York: Routledge, 2006), pp. 59–76.

Claye, A. M., *A Short History of the Hospital for Women at Leeds, 1853–1953* (Leeds: Walter Gardham Ltd., 1953).

Clayton Fryers, S., 'Voluntary Hospitals and Contributory Schemes', *Supplement to the British Medical Journal* (18 February 1939), pp. 73–6.

—, 'The General Infirmary at Leeds: A Short History', *University of Leeds Review*, 3 (1952–3), pp. 341–9.

Coleman, D., and J. Salt, *The British Population: Patterns, Trends and Processes* (Oxford: Oxford University Press, 1992).

Collins, M., 'The History of Leeds Permanent Building Society, 1893–1993', in Chartres and Honeyman (eds), *Leeds City Business*, pp. 57–79.

Connell, E. J., and M. Ward, 'Industrial Development, 1780–1914', in Fraser (ed.), *A History of Modern Leeds*, pp. 142–76.

Coombs, W. H. J., *The History of Radiology and Radiography in the United Sheffield Hospitals* (Sheffield: Privately printed, 1981).

Cooter, R., 'The Meaning of Fractures: Orthopaedics and the Reform of British Hospitals in the Inter-War Period', *Medical History*, 31:3 (1987), pp. 306–32.

—, *Surgery and Society in Peace and War: Orthopaedics and the Organization of Modern Medicine, 1880–1948* (Basingstoke: Macmillan in Association with the Centre for the History of Science, Technology and Medicine, University of Manchester, 1993).

Craven, A. M., 'Housing before the First World War', in Binfield et al. (eds), *The History of the City of Sheffield*, vol. 2, pp. 65–75.

Crook, A. D. H., 'Needs, Standards and Affordability: Housing Policy after 1914', in Binfield et al. (eds), *The History of the City of Sheffield*, vol. 2, pp. 76–99.

—, 'Appendix: Population and Boundary Changes, 1801–1981', in Binfield et al. (eds), *The History of the City of Sheffield*, vol. 2, pp. 482–5.

Daunton, M., 'Payment and Participation: Welfare and State-Formation in Britain 1900–1951', *Past and Present*, 150:1 (1996), pp. 169–216.

— (ed.), *The Cambridge Urban History of Britain: Volume 3, 1830–1950* (Cambridge: Cambridge University Press, 2001).

Davies, S., and B. Morley, 'The Reactions of Municipal Voters in Yorkshire to the Second Labour Government, 1929–32', in M. Worley (ed.), *Labour's Grass Roots: Essays on the Activities of Local Labour Parties and Members, 1918–45* (Aldershot: Ashgate, 2005), pp. 124–46.

Digby, A., *Making a Medical Living: Doctors and Patients in the English Market for Medicine, 1720–1911* (Cambridge: Cambridge University Press, 1994).

—, 'Poverty, Health, and the Politics of Gender in Britain 1870–1948', in A. Digby and J. Stewart (eds), *Gender, Health and Welfare* (London: Routledge, 1996), pp. 67–90.

—, *The Evolution of British General Practice, 1850–1948* (Oxford: Oxford University Press, 1999).

Digby, A., and J. Stewart, 'Welfare in Context', in Digby and Stewart (eds), *Gender, Health and Welfare*, pp. 1–30.

Dingwall, R., A. M. Rafferty and C. Webster, *An Introduction to the Social History of Nursing* (London: Routledge, 1988).

Doyle, B. M., 'The Structure of Elite Power in the Early Twentieth-Century City: Norwich, 1900–35', *Urban History*, 24:2 (1997), pp. 179–99.

—, 'Mapping Slums in an Historic City: Representing Working Class Communities in Edwardian Norwich', *Planning Perspectives*, 16:1 (2001), pp. 47–65.

—, 'The Changing Functions of Urban Government: Councillors, Officials and Pressure Groups', in Daunton (ed.), *The Cambridge Urban History of Britain*, pp. 287–313.

—, *A History of Hospitals in Middlesbrough* (Middlesbrough: South Tees Hospitals NHS Trust, 2002).

—, 'Competition and Cooperation in Hospital Provision in Middlesbrough, 1918–48', *Medical History*, 51:3 (2007), pp. 337–56.

—, 'Power and Accountability in the Voluntary Hospitals of Middlesbrough, 1900–1948', in A. Borsay and P. Shapley (eds), *Medicine, Charity and Mutual Aid: The Consumption of Health and Welfare, c. 1550–1950* (Aldershot: Ashgate, 2007), pp. 207–24.

—, 'Labour and Hospitals in Three Yorkshire Towns: Middlesbrough, Leeds, Sheffield, 1919–1938', *Social History of Medicine*, 23:2 (2010), pp. pp. 374–92.

—, 'Managing and Contesting Industrial Pollution in Middlesbrough, 1880–1940', *Northern History*, 47:1 (2010), pp. 135–54.

—, 'The Economics, Culture and Politics of Hospital Contributory Schemes: The Case of Inter War Leeds', *Labour History Review*, 77:3 (2012), pp. 289–315.

Doyle, B. M., and R. Nixon, 'Voluntary Hospital Finance in North-East England: The Case of North Ormesby Hospital, Middlesbrough, 1900–1947', *Cleveland History*, 80 (2001), pp. 5–19.

Dyhouse, C., *Students: A Gendered History* (London: Routledge, 2005).

Earwicker, R., 'The Labour Movement and the Creation of the National Health Service 1906–1948' (PhD thesis, University of Birmingham, 1982).

Elliott, B. J., 'The Last Five Years of the Sheffield Guardians', *Transactions of the Hunter Archaeological Society* (1977), pp. 132–7.

Ellis, R., 'The Asylum, the Poor Law and the Growth of County Asylums in Nineteenth-Century Yorkshire', *Northern History*, 45:2 (2008), pp. 279–93.

Flett, J., *The Story of the Workhouse and the Hospital at Nether Edge* (Sheffield: n.p., [1984]).

Fowler, F. J., 'Urban Renewal, 1918–1966', in Beresford and Jones (eds), *Leeds and its Region*, pp. 175–85.

Fraser, D., *Urban Politics in Victorian England: The Structure of Politics in Victorian Cities* (Leicester: Leicester University Press, 1976).

— (ed.), *A History of Modern Leeds* (Manchester: Manchester University Press, 1980).

Gorsky, M., *Patterns of Philanthropy: Charity and Society in Nineteenth-Century Bristol* (Woodbridge: Boydell and Brewer, 1999).

—, '"For the Treatment of Sick Persons of All Classes": The Transformation of Bristol's Hospital Service, 1918–39', in P. Wardley (ed.), *Bristol Historical Resource CD-ROM* (Bristol: University of the West of England, 2000).

—, '"Threshold of a New Era": The Development of an Integrated Hospital System in North-East Scotland, 1900–39', *Social History of Medicine*, 17:2 (2004), pp. 247–67.

—, 'The Gloucestershire Extension of Medical Services Scheme: An Experiment in the Integration of Health Services in Britain before the NHS', *Medical History*, 50:4 (2006), pp. 491–512.

—, 'Public Health in Interwar England and Wales: Did It Fail?', *Dynamis*, 28 (2008), pp. 175–98.

—, 'Local Government Health Services in Interwar England: Problems of Quantification and Interpretation', *Bulletin of the History of Medicine*, 85:3 (2011), pp. 384–412.

Gorsky, M., J. Mohan and M. Powell, 'British Voluntary Hospitals, 1871–1938: The Geography of Provision and Utilization', *Journal of Historical Geography*, 25 (1999), pp. 463–82.

—, 'British Voluntary Hospitals and the Public Sphere: Contribution and Participation before the National Health Service', in S. Sturdy (ed.), *Medicine, Health and the Public Sphere in Britain, 1600–2000* (Abingdon and New York: Routledge, 2002), pp. 123–44.

—, 'The Financial Health of Voluntary Hospitals in Interwar Britain', *Economic History Review*, 55:3 (2002), pp. 533–57.

Gorsky, M., J. Mohan and T. Willis, 'Hospital Contributory Schemes and the NHS Debate 1937–1946: The Rejection of Social Insurance in the British Welfare State?', *Twentieth Century British History*, 16 (2005), pp. 170–92.

—, *Mutualism and Health Care: British Hospital Contributory Schemes in the Twentieth Century* (Manchester: Manchester University Press, 2006).

Gorsky, M., and S. Sheard (eds), *Financing Medicine: The British Experience since 1750* (London: Routledge, 2006).

Gosling, G. C., '"Open the Other Eye": Payment, Civic Duty and Hospital Contributory Schemes in Bristol, *c.* 1927–1948', *Medical History*, 54:4 (2010), pp. 475–94.

—, 'Charity and Change in the Mixed Economy of Healthcare in Bristol, 1918–1948' (PhD thesis, Oxford Brookes University, 2012).

Grady, K., 'Commercial, Marketing and Retailing Amenities, 1700–1914', in Fraser (ed.), *A History of Modern Leeds*, pp. 177–99.

Granshaw, L., 'Introduction', in L. Granshaw and R. Porter (eds), *The Hospital in History* (London: Routledge, 1989).

—, '"Fame and Fortune by Means of Bricks and Mortar": The Medical Profession and Specialist Hospitals in Britain, 1800–1948', in L. Granshaw and R. Porter (eds), *The Hospital in History*, pp. 199–220.

—, 'The Hospital', in W. F. Bynum and R. Porter (eds), *Companion Encyclopedia of the History of Medicine*, 2 vols (London: Routledge, 1993), vol. 2, pp. 1180–203.

Gray, J., *Edinburgh City Hospital* (East Linton: Tuckwell, 1999).

Gunn, S., *The Public Culture of the Victorian Middle Class: Ritual and Authority in the English Industrial City 1840–1914* (Manchester: Manchester University Press, 2000).

—, 'Class, Identity and the Urban: The Middle Class in England, 1800–1950', *Urban History*, 31:1 (2004), pp. 1–19.

Hall, L. A., 'Venereal Diseases and Society in Britain from the Contagious Diseases Act to the National Health Service', in R. Davidson and L. A. Hall (eds), *Sex, Sin and Suffering: Venereal Disease and European Society since 1870* (London: Routledge, 2001), pp. 120–36.

Hardy, A., *Health and Medicine in Britain since 1860* (Basingstoke: Palgrave, 2001).

Harrison, M., *The Medical War: British Military Medicine in the First World War* (Oxford: Oxford University Press, 2010).

Harvey, P., *Up the Hill to Western Bank: A History of the Children's Hospital, Sheffield, 1876–1976* (Sheffield: The Centenary Committee, Children's Hospital, 1976).

Hayes, N., 'Did We Really Want a National Health Service? Hospitals, Patients and Public Opinions before 1948', *English Historical Review*, 127 (2012), pp. 625–61.

—, '"Our Hospitals"? Voluntary Provision, Community and Civic Consciousness in Nottingham before the NHS', *Midland History*, 37 (2012), pp. 84–105.

—, 'Counting Civil Society: Deconstructing Elite Participation in the Provincial English City, 1900–1950', *Urban History*, 40:2 (2013), pp. 287–314.

Hayes, N., and B. M. Doyle, 'Eggs, Rags and Whist Drives: Popular Munificence and the Development of Provincial Medical Voluntarism between the Wars', *Historical Research*, 86:234 (November 2013), pp. 712–40.

Heaman, E. A., *St Mary's: The History of a London Teaching Hospital* (Montreal and Liverpool: McGill-Queen's University Press, 2003).

Hey, D., 'Continuities and Perceptions', in Binfield et al. (eds), *The History of the City of Sheffield*, vol. 2, pp. 7–16.

Hodgkinson, R. G., *The Origins of the National Health Service: The Medical Services of the New Poor Law, 1834–1871* (London: Wellcome History Medical Library, 1967).

Hollis, P., *Ladies Elect: Women in English Local Government, 1865–1914* (Oxford: Oxford University Press, 1989).

Honeyman, K., 'Montague Burton Ltd.: The Creators of Well-dressed Men', in J. Chartres and K. Honeyman (eds), *Leeds City Business*, pp. 186–216.

—, '"Soapy Joes": The History of Joseph Watson and Sons Ltd., 1893–1993', in Chartres and Honeyman (eds), *Leeds City Business*, pp. 217–43.

—, *Well Suited: A History of the Leeds Clothing Industry, 1850–1990* (Oxford and New York: Pasold Research Fund: Oxford University Press, 2000).

Jamieson, A., 'More Than Meets the Eye: Revealing the Therapeutic Potential of "Light", 1896–1910', *Social History of Medicine*, 26:4 (2013), pp. 715–37.

Jones, H., *Health and Society in Twentieth Century Britain* (Harlow: Longman, 1994).

Kershen, A. J., *Uniting the Tailors: Trade Unionism Amongst the Tailors of London and Leeds, 1870–1939* (Ilford: Frank Cass, 1995).

Law, M. J., 'Speed and Blood on the Bypass: The New Automobilities of Inter-War London', *Urban History*, 39:3 (2012), pp. 490–509.

Laybourn, K., *Britain on the Breadline: A Social and Political History of Britain, 1918–1939* (Stroud: Sutton, 1998).

Levene, A., 'Between Less Eligibility and the NHS: The Changing Place of Poor Law Hospitals in England and Wales, 1929–1939', *Twentieth Century British History*, 20:3 (2009), pp. 322–45.

Levene, A., M. Powell and J. Stewart, 'Patterns of Municipal Health Expenditure in Interwar England and Wales', *Bulletin of the History of Medicine*, 78 (2004), pp. 635–69.

—, 'The Development of Municipal Hospital Care in English County Boroughs in the 1930s', *Medical History*, 50:1 (2006), pp. 3–28.

Levene, A., M. Powell, J. Stewart and B. Taylor, *Cradle to Grave: Municipal Medicine in Interwar England and Wales* (Bern: Peter Lang, 2011).

Lewis, J., *What Price Community Medicine? The Philosophy, Practice and Politics of Public Health since 1919* (Brighton: Wheatsheaf, 1986).

Lewis, R., R. Nixon and B. Doyle, 'Health Services in Middlesbrough: North Ormesby Hospital 1900–1948' (Unpublished AHRC Final Report, Middlesbrough, 1999).

Lloyd-Jones, R., and M. J. Lewis, 'Business Structure and Political Economy in Sheffield: The Metal Trades, 1880–1920', in Binfield et al. (eds), *The History of the City of Sheffield*, vol. 2, pp. 211–33.

Lomax, E., 'Small and Special: The Development of Hospitals for Children in Victorian Britain', *Medical History Supplement*, 16 (1996), pp. 50–2.

Lowe, R., *The Welfare State in Britain since 1945*, 3rd edn (Basingstoke: Palgrave Macmillan, 2004).

Luckin, B., 'Accidents, Disasters and Cities', *Urban History*, 20:2 (1993), pp. 177–90.

—, 'War on the Roads: Traffic, Accidents and Social Tension in Britain, 1939–45', in Luckin and Cooter (eds), *Accidents*, pp. 234–54.

Luckin, B., and R. Cooter (eds), *Accidents in History: Injuries, Fatalities and Social Relations* (Amsterdam: Rodopi, 1997).

Luckin, B., and D. Sheen, 'Defining Early Modern Automobility: The Road Traffic Accident Crisis in Manchester, 1939–45', *Cultural and Social History*, 6:2 (2009), pp. 211–30.

McIntosh, T., '"A Price Must be Paid for Motherhood": The Experience of Maternity in Sheffield, 1879–1939' (PhD thesis, University of Sheffield, 1997).

—, '"An Abortionist City": Maternal Mortality, Abortion and Birth Control in Sheffield, 1920–1940', *Medical History*, 44:1 (2000), pp. 75–96.

McIvor, A., 'Germs at Work: Establishing Tuberculosis as an Occupational Disease in Britain, c. 1900–1951', *Social History of Medicine*, 25:4 (2012), pp. 812–29.

McIvor, A., and R. Johnson, *Miners' Lung: A History of Dust Disease in British Coal Mining* (Aldershot: Ashgate, 2007).

Marland, H., *Medicine and Society in Wakefield and Huddersfield, 1780–1870* (Cambridge: Cambridge University Press, 1987).

Marshall, R. J., 'Town Planning in Sheffield', in Binfield et al. (eds), *The History of the City of Sheffield*, vol. 2, pp. 17–32.

Mathers, H. E., 'Sheffield Municipal Politics, 1893–1926: Parties, Personalities and the Rise of Labour' (PhD thesis, University of Sheffield, 1979).

Mathers, H., 'The City of Sheffield, 1893–1926', in Binfield et al. (eds), *The History of the City of Sheffield*, vol. 1, pp. 53–84.

Meadowcroft, M., 'The Years of Political Transition', in Fraser (ed.), *A History of Modern Leeds*, pp. 410–36.

Melling, J., and P. Dale, 'Britain's Medical Officers of Health, Gender and the Provision of Cancer Services by Local and National Government, c. 1900–1940', *Medical History*, 53:4 (2009), pp. 537–60.

Meyer, W. R., 'Charles Henry Wilson: The Man Who was Leeds', *Publications of the Thoresby Society*, second series, 8 (1998), pp. 78–96.

Mitchell, M., 'The Effects of Unemployment on the Social Condition of Women and Children in the 1930s', *History Workshop Journal*, 19 (1985), pp. 105–27.

Mohan, J., *Planning, Markets and Hospitals* (London: Routledge, 2002).

—, 'Voluntarism, Municipalism and Welfare: The Geography of Hospital Utilization in England in 1938', *Transactions of the Institute of British Geographers*, new series, 28 (2003), pp. 56–74.

—, '"The Caprice of Charity". Geographical Variations in the Finances of British Voluntary Hospitals before the NHS', in M. Gorsky and S. Sheard (eds), *Financing Medicine*, pp. 77–92.

Moran, J., 'Crossing the Road in Britain', *Historical Journal*, 49:2 (2006), pp. 477–96.

Morgan, C. J., 'Demographic Change, 1771–1911', in Fraser (ed.), *A History of Modern Leeds*, pp. 46–71.

Morris, R. J., 'Middle-Class Culture, 1700–1914', in Fraser (ed.), *A History of Modern Leeds*, pp. 200–22.

—, *Class, Sect and Party: The Making of the British Middle Class, Leeds 1820–1850* (Manchester: Manchester University Press, 1990).

—, 'Structure, Culture and Society in British Towns', in Daunton (ed.), *The Cambridge Urban History of Britain*, pp. 395–426.

—, *Men, Women and Property in England, 1780–1870* (Cambridge: Cambridge University Press, 2005).

Mosley, S., *The Chimney of the World: A History of Smoke Pollution in Victorian and Edwardian Manchester* (London: White Horse, pb edn, 2008).

Murphy, C., 'A History of Radiotherapy to 1950: Cancer and Radiotherapy in Britain, 1850–1950' (PhD thesis, University of Manchester, 1986).

—, 'From Friedenheim to Hospice: A Century of Cancer Hospitals', in Granshaw and Porter (eds), *The Hospital in History*, pp. 221–41.

Neville, J., 'Explaining Local Authority Choices on Public Hospital Provision in the 1930s: A Public Policy Hypothesis', *Medical History*, 56:1 (2012), pp. 48–71.

Nuttall, A., 'Maternity Charities, the Edinburgh Maternity Scheme and the Medicalisation of Childbirth, 1900–1925', *Social History of Medicine*, 24:2 (2011), pp. 370–88.

O'Connell, S., *The Car and British Society: Class, Gender and Motoring, 1896–1939* (Manchester: Manchester University Press, 1998).

Pennock, P. M., 'The Evolution of St James's, 1845–94: Leeds Moral and Industrial Training School, Leeds Union Workhouse and Leeds Union Infirmary', *Publications of the Thoresby Society*, 59 (1984), pp. 129–76.

Phillpott, H. R. S., *Where Labour Rules: A Tour through Towns and Counties* (London: Methuen, 1934).

Pickstone, J. V., *Medicine and Industrial Society: A History of Hospital Development in Manchester and its Region* (Manchester: Manchester University Press, 1985).

—, 'Contested Cumulations: Configurations of Cancer Treatments through the Twentieth Century', *Bulletin of the History of Medicine*, 81:1 (2007), pp. 164–96.

Pinker, R., *English Hospital Statistics, 1861–1938* (London: Heinemann, 1966).

Pollard, S., 'Labour', in Binfield et al. (eds), *The History of the City of Sheffield*, vol. 2, pp. 260–78.

Pooley, C., and J. Turnbull, 'Commuting, Transport and Urban Form: Manchester and Glasgow in the Mid-Twentieth Century', *Urban History*, 27:3 (2000), pp. 360–83.

Porter, W. S., *The Royal Infirmary, Sheffield: An Epitome* (Oldham: Allan Hanson, 1921).

Powell, M., 'Hospital Provision before the NHS: A Geographic Study of the 1945 Hospital Survey', *Social History of Medicine*, 5:3 (1992), pp. 483–504.

—, 'Hospital Provision before the NHS: Territorial Justice or Inverse Care Law', *Journal of Social Policy*, 21:2 (1992), pp. 145–63.

—, 'Did Politics Matter? Municipal Public Health Expenditure in the 1930s', *Urban History*, 22:3 (1995), pp. 360–79.

—, 'An Expanding Service: Municipal Acute Medicine in the 1930s', *Twentieth Century British History*, 8 (1997), pp. 334–57.

Prochaska, F., *Women and Philanthropy in Nineteenth Century England* (Oxford: Oxford University Press, 1980).

Proctor, P., 'St. James's Hospital Leeds: 1900 to 1970, A Study of its Development, from Poor Law Infirmary to the Largest General Hospital in this Country' (Unpublished typescript, Leeds, 1970).

Rainnie, G. F., and R. K. Williamson, 'The Economic Structure', in Beresford and Jones (eds), *Leeds and its Region*, pp. 215–39.

Ravetz, A., *Model Estate: Planned Housing at Quarry Hill* (London: Croom Helm in association with Joseph Rowntree Memorial Trust, 1974).

Reid, A., 'Mrs Killer and Dr Crook: Birth Attendants and Birth Outcomes in Early Twentieth-century Derbyshire', *Medical History*, 56:4 (2012), pp. 511–30.

Reinarz, J., *Healthcare in Birmingham: A History of the Birmingham Teaching Hospitals, 1779–1939* (Woodbridge: Boydell and Brewer, 2009).

Reynolds, J., and K. Laybourn, *Labour Heartland* (Bradford: Bradford University Press, 1986).

Rivett, G., *The Development of the London Hospital System, 1823–1982* (London: King Edward's Hospital Fund, 1986).

Roach, J., 'The Sheffield Community and Public Work, 1790–1914', *Yorkshire Archaeological Journal*, 77 (2005), pp. 225–40.

Rosen, G., *Specialization in Medicine* (New York: Froben Press, 1944).

Savage, M., *The Dynamics of Working Class Politics: The Labour Movement in Preston, 1880–1940* (Cambridge: Cambridge University Press, 1987).

Shaw, C., 'Aspects of Public Health', in Binfield et al. (eds), *The History of the City of Sheffield*, vol. 2, pp. 110–17.

Shepherd, J., J. Davis and C. Wrigley (eds), *The Second Labour Government: A Reappraisal* (Manchester: Manchester University Press, 2011).

Skinner, E. F., *A Short History of the Sheffield Royal Hospital: 1832–1932* (Sheffield: Printed by Greenup & Thompson, Limited, 1932).

Speck, P., et al., *The Institution and Hospital at Fir Vale, Sheffield: A Centenary History of the Northern General Hospital* (Sheffield: Northern General Hospital, 1978).

Spencer, E. M., 'Notes on the History of Dental Dispensaries', *Medical History*, 26:1 (1982) pp. 47–66.

Stevens, C., 'The Conservative Club Movement in the Industrial West Riding, 1880–1914', *Northern History*, 38:1 (2001), pp. 121–43.

Stevens, R., *Medical Practice in Modern England: The Impact of Specialization and State Medicine* (New Haven, CT: Yale University Press, 1966).

Stewart, J., '"For a Healthy London": The Socialist Medical Association and the London County Council in the 1930s', *Medical History*, 41:4 (1997), pp. 417–36.

—, *'The Battle for Health': A Political History of the Socialist Medical Association, 1930–51* (Aldershot: Ashgate, 1999).

—, '"The Finest Municipal Hospital Service in the World"? Contemporary Perceptions of the London County Council's Hospital Provision, 1929–1939', *Urban History*, 32:2 (2005), pp. 327–44.

Sturdy, S., 'The Political Economy of Scientific Medicine: Science, Education and the Transformation of Medical Practice in Sheffield, 1890–1922', *Medical History*, 36:2 (1992), pp. 125–59.

—, 'Looking for Trouble: Medical Science and Clinical Practice in the Historiography of Modern Medicine', *Social History of Medicine*, 24:3 (2011), pp. 739–57.

Sturdy, S., and R. Cooter, 'Science, Scientific Management, and the Transformation of Medicine in Britain, *c.* 1870–1950', *History of Science*, 36 (1998), pp. 1–47.

Swan, H., 'Medical Education', in Binfield et al. (eds), *The History of the City of Sheffield*, vol. 2, pp. 130–41.

Taylor, B., J. Stewart and M. Powell, 'The Development of Central-Local Relations in the 1930s', *English Historical Review*, 122:496 (2007), pp. 397–426.

Taylor, J., *The Rebirth of the Norfolk and Norwich Hospital, 1874–1883: An Architectural Exploration* (Norwich: Wellcome Unit for the History of Medicine, 2000).

Taylor, S., 'The Industrial Structure of the Sheffield Cutlery Trades, 1870–1914', in Binfield et al. (eds), *The History of the City of Sheffield*, vol. 2, pp. 194–210.

Thompson, S., 'A Proletarian Public Sphere: Working-Class Provision of Medical Services and Care in South Wales, c. 1900–1948', in A. Borsay (ed.), *Medicine in Wales, c. 1800–2000: Public Service or Private Commodity?* (Cardiff: University of Wales Press, 2003), pp. 86–107.

Thorpe, A., 'The Consolidation of a Labour Stronghold 1926–1951', in Binfield et al. (eds), *The History of the City of Sheffield*, vol. 1, pp. 85–118.

Timmins, N., *The Five Giants: A Biography of the Welfare State* (London: Fontana, 1995).

Titmuss, R., *Problems of Social Policy* (London: HMSO, 1950).

Trainor, R. H., 'The Middle Class', in Daunton (ed.), *The Cambridge Urban History of Britain*, pp. 673–713.

Tweedale, G., 'The Business and Technology of Sheffield Steelmaking', in Binfield et al. (eds), *The History of the City of Sheffield*, vol. 2, pp. 142–93.

—, *Steel City: Entrepreneurship, Strategy, and Technology in Sheffield 1743–1993* (Oxford: Clarendon, 1995).

—, 'Steelmakers as Masters Cutler: A Look at a Sheffield Industrial Elite', in C. Binfield and D. Hey (eds), *Mesters to Masters*, pp. 63–84.

Vogel, M. J., 'Managing Medicine: Creating a Profession of Hospital Administration in the United States, 1895–1915', in Granshaw and Porter (eds), *The Hospital in History*, pp. 243–60.

Waddington, K., *Charity and the London Hospitals, 1850–1898* (Woodbridge: Boydell and Brewer, 2000).

Wainwright, P., 'Chas. F. Thackray Ltd.: Suppliers to the Surgeons', in Chartres and Honeyman (eds), *Leeds City Business*, pp. 244–69.

Ward, A. J., and T. Ashton (eds), *Cookridge Hospital, 1867–1972* (Leeds: Cookridge Hospital, 1997).

Webster, C., 'Healthy or Hungry Thirties?', *History Workshop*, 13 (1982), pp. 110–29.

—, *The Health Services since the War: Problems of Health Care. The National Health Service before 1957* (London: HMSO, 1988).

—, 'Conflict and Consensus: Explaining the British Health Service', *Twentieth Century British History*, 1:2 (1990), pp. 115–51.

— (ed.), *Caring for Health: History and Diversity*, 2nd edn (Buckingham: Open University Press, 1993).

—, *The National Health Service: A Political History*, 2nd edn (Oxford: Oxford University Press, 2002).

Welshman, J., 'The Medical Officer of Health in England and Wales, 1900–1974: Watchdog or Lapdog?', *Journal of Public Health Medicine*, 19:4 (1997), pp. 443–50.

—, 'Dental Health as a Neglected Issue in Medical History: the School Dental Service in England and Wales, 1900–40', *Medical History*, 42:3 (1998), pp. 306–27.

—, *Municipal Medicine: Public Health in Twentieth-Century Britain* (Oxford and New York: Peter Lang, 2000).

Willis, T., 'Politics, Ideology and the Governance of Health Care in Sheffield before the NHS', in R. J. Morris and R. H. Trainor (eds), *Urban Governance: Britain and Beyond since 1750* (Aldershot: Ashgate, 2000), pp. 218–49.

—, 'The Bradford Municipal Hospital Experiment of 1920: The Emergence of the Mixed Economy in Hospital Provision in Inter-War Britain', in M. Gorsky and S. Sheard (eds), *Financing Medicine: The British Experience since 1750* (London: Routledge, 2006), pp. 130–41.

—, 'The Politics and Ideology of Local Authority Health Care in Sheffield, 1918–1948' (PhD thesis, Sheffield Hallam University, 2009).

Winter, J., 'Unemployment, Nutrition and Infant Mortality in Britain, 1920–1950', in J. M. Winter (ed.), *The Working Class in Modern British History* (Cambridge: Cambridge University Press, 1983), pp. 232–56.

Woodhouse, T., 'The Working Class', in Fraser (ed.), *A History of Modern Leeds*, pp. 327–52.

—, *Nourishing the Liberty Tree: Liberals and Labour in Leeds, 1880–1914* (Keele: Keele University Press, 1996).

INDEX

Milton Keynes UK
Ingram Content Group UK Ltd.
UKHW031144141024
449569UK00024B/1093